Optic Nerve Disorders

Ophthalmology Monographs

A series published by Oxford University Press in cooperation with the American Academy of Ophthalmology

Series Editor: Richard K. Parrish, II, Bascom Palmer Eye Institute

American Academy of Ophthalmology Clinical Education Secretariat:
Thomas J. Liesegang, Mayo Clinic
Gregory L. Skuta, Dean A. McGee Eye Institute

2. *Electrophysiologic Testing in Disorders of the Retina, Optic Nerve, and Visual Pathway*, second edition
   Gerald Allen Fishman, David G. Birch, Graham E. Holder, and Mitchell G. Brigell

3. *Visual Fields: Examination and Interpretation*, second edition
   Thomas J. Walsh

4. *Glaucoma Surgery: Principles and Techniques*, second edition
   Edited by Robert N. Weinreb and Richard P. Mills

5. *Fluorescein and Indocyanine Green Angiography: Technique and Interpretation*, second edition
   Joseph W. Berkow, Robert W. Flower, David H. Orth, and James S. Kelley

7. *Cataract Surgery and Intraocular Lenses: A 21st-Century Perspective*, second edition
   Edited by Jerry G. Ford and Carol L. Karp

8. *Surgery of the Eyelid, Orbit and Lacrimal System*, volumes 1, 2, and 3.
   Edited by William B. Stewart

9. *Surgical Anatomy of the Ocular Adnexa: A Clinical Approach*
   David R. Jordan and Richard L. Anderson

10. *Optic Nerve Disorders*, second edition
    Edited by Lanning B. Kline and Rod Foroozan

11. *Laser Photocoagulation of the Retina and Choroid* (includes slide set)
    James C. Folk and José S. Pulido

12. *Low Vision Rehabilitation: Caring for the Whole Person*
    Edited by Donald C. Fletcher

13. *Glaucoma Medical Therapy: Principles and Management*
    Edited by Peter A. Netland and Robert C. Allen

14. *Diabetes and Ocular Disease: Past, Present, and Future Therapies*
    Edited by Harry W. Flynn and William E. Smiddy

15. *HIV/AIDS and the Eye: A Global Perspective*
    Emmett T. Cunningham and Rubens Belfort

16. *Corneal Dystrophies and Degenerations*
    Edited by Ming X. Wang

17. *Strabismus Surgery: Basic and Advanced Techniques*
    Edited by David A. Plager; written by Edward G. Buckley, David A. Plager, Michael X. Repka, and M. Edward Wilson; contributions by Marshall M. Parks and Gunter K. von Noorden
    www.oup.com/us/aao/plager/strabismus

18. *A Compendium of Inherited Disorders and the Eye*
    Elias I. Traboulsi
    www.oup.com/us/aao/traboulsi/genetic

OPTIC NERVE DISORDERS,
Second Edition

Edited by

LANNING B. KLINE AND ROD FOROOZAN

Published by Oxford University Press
In cooperation with
The American Academy of Ophthalmology

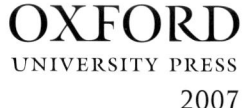

OXFORD
UNIVERSITY PRESS
2007

OXFORD

UNIVERSITY PRESS

Oxford University Press, Inc., publishes works that further
Oxford University's objective of excellence
in research, scholarship, and education.

Oxford   New York
Auckland   Cape Town   Dar es Salaam   Hong Kong   Karachi
Kuala Lumpur   Madrid   Melbourne   Mexico City   Nairobi
New Delhi   Shanghai   Taipei   Toronto

With offices in

Argentina   Austria   Brazil   Chile   Czech Republic   France   Greece
Guatemala   Hungary   Italy   Japan   Poland   Portugal   Singapore
South Korea   Switzerland   Thailand   Turkey   Ukraine   Vietnam

Published by Oxford University Press, Inc.
198 Madison Avenue, New York, New York 10016

www.oup.com

Oxford is a registered trademark of Oxford University Press

Library of Congress Cataloging-in-Publication Data
Optic nerve disorders / edited by Lanning B. Kline and Rod Foroozan.—2nd ed.
p. cm. — (Ophthalmology monographs ; 10)
ISBN-13: 978-0-19-531281-2
ISBN-10: 0-19-531281-3
1. Optic nerve—Diseases.   I. Kline, Lanning B.   II. Foroozan, Rod.   III. Series.
RE727.O65 2006
617.7'32—dc22   2006006735

9 8 7 6 5 4 3 2 1

Printed in China
on acid-free paper

To William Fletcher Hoyt

. . . a scholar, and a ripe and good one;

Exceeding wise, fair-spoken, and persuading:

Lofty and sour to them that lov'd him not;

But to those men that sought him sweet as summer.

—Shakespeare, *King Henry VIII*

Preface

Just as neuro-ophthalmology links ophthalmology with other medical specialties, so too the optic nerve links the eye with the central nervous system. Thus, the ophthalmologist must be familiar with a wide variety of optic nerve diseases, which may occur in isolation or may form part of a generalized neurologic or systemic disorder.

While this monograph was initially published over a decade ago, with publication of a second edition the basic organization remains unchanged. Chapter 1 reviews the major anatomic aspects of the optic nerve at both a macroscopic and a microscopic level. The introductory chapter also discusses the critical role of axonal transport in optic nerve physiology. Chapter 2 takes the reader "back to basics," emphasizing the importance of obtaining a detailed patient history and performing a careful ophthalmologic examination. Electrophysiologic and imaging studies play complementary roles in the assessment of optic nerve function. Chapters 3 through 9 cover the major clinical disorders affecting the optic nerve: papilledema, optic neuritis, ischemic optic neuropathy, compression of the anterior visual pathways, developmental and hereditary optic nerve disorders, toxic and nutritional optic neuropathy, and traumatic optic neuropathy. The last chapter of the monograph, Chapter 10, summarizes those optic neuropathies that cannot easily be categorized but that frequently confront the general ophthalmologist in clinical practice.

The educational objectives of this publication are to

- Provide a succinct yet comprehensive review of optic nerve disorders commonly encountered in clinical practice
- Review briefly the anatomy and physiology of the optic nerve

- Outline those techniques of particular importance during clinical testing of optic nerve function
- Afford the clinician a handy reference to assist in both diagnosis and management of a wide variety of optic nerve disorders
- Publish an up-to-date guide to the relevant literature on clinical diseases of the optic nerve

Our gratitude is extended to the contributors of this monograph, all experts in their fields, whose enthusiasm and skill have helped make this publication possible. Our editor, Catharine Carlin, facilitated revisions of the text and kept production on schedule. Our assistant, Dawn Self, did a superb job assisting in compilation of new and previously published material. Finally, we are grateful to the American Academy of Ophthalmology for supporting and publication of an updated version of *Optic Nerve Disorders*.

Contents

Contributors, xv

Legal Notice, xvii

1. Anatomy and Physiology of the Optic Nerve, 3
   John C. Morrison

   1-1 Anatomy of the Optic Nerve, 3
      1-1-1 Intraocular Optic Nerve, 4
         1-1-1-1 Nerve Fiber Layer, 4
         1-1-1-2 Lamina Choroidalis, 6
         1-1-1-3 Lamina Cribrosa, 7
      1-1-2 Intraorbital Optic Nerve, 8
      1-1-3 Intracanalicular Optic Nerve, 10
      1-1-4 Intracranial Optic Nerve, 10
   1-2 Topographic Organization of the Optic Nerve, 11
   1-3 Blood Supply of the Optic Nerve, 12
      1-3-1 Intraocular Optic Nerve, 12
      1-3-2 Intraorbital Optic Nerve, 15
      1-3-3 Intracanalicular Optic Nerve, 15
      1-3-4 Intracranial Optic Nerve, 16
   1-4 Axonal Physiology of the Optic Nerve, 16

2. Clinical Testing of Optic Nerve Function, 25
   Lawrence M. Buono

   2-1 Evaluation of the Patient, 25
      2-1-1 History Taking, 25
      2-1-2 Visual Acuity, 26

2-1-3 Visual Field, 26
2-1-4 Color Vision, 27
2-1-5 Brightness Comparison, 27
2-1-6 Pupillary Testing, 28
2-1-7 Photostress Recovery Test, 28
2-1-8 Contrast Sensitivity, 28
2-1-9 Ophthalmoscopy, 29
2-1-10 Electrophysiology, 30
2-1-11 Imaging Studies, 31
2-2 Assessment of the Findings, 31
2-2-1 Clinical Examples, 33
2-2-1-1 Optic Disc Drusen, 33
2-2-1-2 Optociliary Shunt Vessels, 34
2-2-1-3 Optic Atrophy, 34
2-2-1-4 Functional Visual Loss, 34
2-2-1-5 Optic Neuritis, 35
2-2-1-6 Craniopharyngioma, 36

3. Papilledema, 41
Rod Foroozan and Lanning B. Kline

3-1 Pathogenesis of Papilledema, 41
3-1-1 Ophthalmoscopic Findings, 42
3-2 Classification of Papilledema, 43
3-2-1 Early Papilledema, 43
3-2-2 Fully Developed Papilledema, 43
3-2-3 Chronic Papilledema, 46
3-2-4 Postpapilledema Optic Atrophy, 46
3-3 Associated Clinical Features, 47
3-3-1 Visual Symptoms, 47
3-3-2 Visual Acuity, 48
3-3-3 Visual Field Defects, 48
3-3-4 Pupillary Function, 49
3-3-5 Diplopia, 49
3-4 Visual Prognosis, 49
3-5 Foster Kennedy Syndrome, 50
3-6 Neurologic Symptoms, 52
3-7 Causes of Papilledema, 53
3-8. Patient Evaluation, 54
3-9 Idiopathic Intracranial Hypertension, 57
3-10 Management of Papilledema, 60

4. Optic Neuritis, 65
Michael S. Vaphiades and Lanning B. Kline

4-1 Clinical Features, 65
4-1-1 Visual Symptoms, 65
4-1-2 Color Vision, 66

    4-1-3 *Pupillary Function, 66*
    4-1-4 *Visual Field Defects, 67*
    4-1-5 *Optic Disc Abnormalities, 67*
    4-1-6 *Uhthoff's Symptom, 67*
    4-1-7 *Visual Evoked Response, 67*
    4-1-8 *Neuroimaging Abnormalities, 69*
  4-2 Optic Neuritis and Multiple Sclerosis, 70
  4-3 Optic Neuritis Treatment Trial, 71
  4-4 The CHAMPS Trial, 73
  4-5 Optic Neuritis in Children, 73
  4-6 Neuromyelitis Optica, 74
  4-7 Chiasmal and Optic Tract Neuritis, 75
  4-8 Differential Diagnosis, 76
    4-8-1 *Demyelinating Disorders, 76*
    4-8-2 *Infectious Agents, 76*
    4-8-3 *Intraocular Inflammation, 78*
    4-8-4 *Systemic Diseases, 78*
  4-9 Mimickers of Optic Neuritis, 81
  4-10 Conclusion, 81

5. Ischemic Optic Neuropathy, 85
   Lawrence M. Buono

  5-1 Nonarteritic Anterior Ischemic Optic Neuropathy, 85
    5-1-1 *Idiopathic NAION, 86*
      5-1-1-1 *Risk Factors, 86*
      5-1-1-2 *Clinical Characteristics, 87*
      5-1-1-3 *Progressive Disease, 89*
      5-1-1-4 *Recurrent and Sequential Disease, 89*
      5-1-1-5 *Visual Acuity Outcome, 89*
      5-1-1-6 *Treatment, 89*
      5-1-1-7 *Atypical Features, 90*
      5-1-1-8 *Differential Diagnosis, 90*
    5-1-2 *Nonarteritic Anterior Ischemic Optic Neuropathy Attributable to a Specific Condition, 91*
      5-1-2-1 *Postcataract Extraction, 91*
      5-1-2-2 *Amiodarone Toxicity, 91*
      5-1-2-3 *Sildenafil Toxicity, 92*
      5-1-2-4 *Embolic Occlusion, 92*
      5-1-2-5 *Hypotension, 92*
      5-1-2-6 *Uremia, 93*
      5-1-2-7 *Diabetic Papillopathy, 93*
      5-1-2-8 *Migraine, 93*
  5-2 Arteritic Anterior Ischemic Optic Neuropathy, 93
    5-2-1 *Giant Cell Arteritis, 93*
      5-2-1-1 *Clinical Features, 94*
      5-2-1-2 *Serologic Markers, 94*

5-2-1-3 Treatment, 94

5-2-1-4 Temporal Artery Biopsy, 95

5-3 Posterior Ischemic Optic Neuropathy, 95

6. Compression of the Anterior Visual Pathways, 101
Rod Foroozan and Lisa Hinckley

6-1 Causes of Compressive Optic Neuropathy, 101

6-2 Symptoms of Compressive Optic Neuropathy, 101

6-3 Signs of Compressive Optic Neuropathy, 105

6-3-1 Optic Disc Findings, 106

6-4 Patient Evaluation, 111

6-5 Glioma, 111

6-5-1 Optic Nerve Glioma, 112

6-5-1-1 Clinical Features, 112

6-5-1-2 Histopathology, 113

6-5-1-3 Natural History, 113

6-5-1-4 Management Options, 113

6-5-2 Chiasmal Glioma, 113

6-5-2-1 Clinical Features, 113

6-5-2-2 Natural History, 114

6-5-2-3 Management Options, 114

6-6 Craniopharyngioma, 116

6-6-1 Clinical Features, 116

6-6-2 Histopathology, 116

6-6-3 Management Options, 117

6-7 Pituitary Adenoma, 118

6-7-1 Clinical Features, 118

6-7-1-1 Visual Signs, 119

6-7-1-2 Endocrine Signs, 120

6-7-2 Neuroimaging, 121

6-7-3 Management Options, 121

6-7-3-1 Therapy of Prolactinoma, 121

6-7-3-2 Therapy of Other Secreting Tumors, 122

6-7-3-3 Therapy of Nonsecreting Tumors, 122

6-7-3-4 Adverse Outcomes, 122

6-8 Meningioma, 122

6-8-1 Suprasellar Meningioma, 122

6-8-1-1 Clinical Features, 123

6-8-1-2 Neuroimaging, 125

6-8-1-3 Management Options, 126

6-8-2 Optic Nerve Sheath Meningioma, 127

6-8-2-1 Clinical Features, 127

6-8-2-2 Neuroimaging, 128

6-8-2-3 Management Options, 128

6-9 Intracranial Aneurysm, 129

6-9-1 Clinical Features, 131

6-9-2 *Neuroimaging, 133*
6-9-3 *Management Options, 135*
6-10 Optic Neuropathy from Thyroid-Associated Orbitopathy, 136
6-10-1 *Clinical Features, 136*
6-10-2 *Management Options, 137*

7. Developmental and Hereditary Optic Nerve Disorders, 151
Lanning B. Kline, Eugene H. Eng, and R. Michael Siatkowski

7-1 Developmental Optic Nerve Disorders, 151
7-1-1 *Anomalous Elevation of the Optic Nerve, or Pseudopapilledema, 151*
7-1-2 *Optic Nerve Hypoplasia, 156*
7-1-3 *Superior Segmental Optic Hypoplasia, 159*
7-1-4 *Hemioptic Hypoplasia, 159*
7-1-5 *Coloboma, 160*
7-1-6 *Optic Pit, 160*
7-1-7 *Tilted Disc, 161*
7-1-8 *Morning-Glory Syndrome, 161*
7-1-9 *Astrocytic Hamartoma, 163*
7-1-10 *Melanocytoma, 164*
7-2 Hereditary Optic Neuropathies, 165
7-2-1 *Dominant Optic Atrophy, 165*
7-2-2 *Recessive Optic Atrophy, 166*
7-2-3 *Leber's Hereditary Optic Neuropathy, 167*
7-2-4 *Neurologic Syndromes, 169*
7-2-5 *Metabolic Disease, 170*

8. Toxic and Nutritional Optic Neuropathy, 177
John B. Kerrison

8-1 Optic Neuropathies Caused by Toxins and Adverse Drug Reactions, 178
8-1-1 *Clinical Presentations, 178*
8-1-2 *Optic Neuropathies Caused by Toxins, 178*
8-1-2-1 *Methanol, 178*
8-1-2-2 *Ethylene Glycol, 180*
8-1-2-3 *Solvents (Toluene, Styrene, Others), 180*
8-1-2-4 *Carbon Monoxide, 180*
8-1-3 *Medication-Induced Toxic Optic Neuropathies, 180*
8-1-3-1 *Antibiotics, 180*
8-1-3-2 *Immunosuppressants and Immunomodulators, 181*
8-1-3-3 *Chemotherapeutic Agents, 182*
8-1-3-4 *Miscellaneous, 182*
8-1-3-5 *Tobacco and Alcohol, 182*
8-1-4 *Medication-Induced Optic Neuropathies Caused by a Nontoxic Mechanism, 183*
8-1-5 *Amiodarone-Associated Optic Neuropathy, 183*
8-2 Differential Diagnosis, Workup, Treatment, 184
8-3 Optic Neuropathies Caused by Nutritional Deficiency, 185

8-3-1 Clinical Presentation, 185
8-3-2 Differential Diagnosis and Workup, 187
8-3-3 Pathology, Etiology, and Treatment, 187

9. Traumatic Optic Neuropathy, 191
   Lanning B. Kline

   9-1 Optic Nerve Evulsion, 191
   9-2 Direct Optic Nerve Injury, 193
   9-3 Indirect Optic Nerve Injury, 195
       9-3-1 Anatomic Considerations, 195
       9-3-2 Types of Indirect Injuries, 196
           9-3-2-1 Anterior Indirect Injury, 196
           9-3-2-2 Posterior Indirect Injury, 197
       9-3-3 Clinical Features, 197
       9-3-4 Pathophysiology, 198
       9-3-5 Management Options, 200
       9-3-6 Visual Prognosis, 203

10. Miscellaneous Optic Neuropathies, 209
    Lanning B. Kline

    10-1 Radiation Optic Neuropathy, 209
    10-2 Neuroretinitis, 211
    10-3 Carcinomatous Optic Neuropathy, 213
    10-4 Diabetic Papillopathy, 216
    10-5 Papillophlebitis, 218
    10-6 Optic Perineuritis, 219
    10-7 Autoimmune-Related Retinopathy and Optic Neuropathy Syndrome
         (ARRON), 221
    10-8 Nonglaucomatous Optic Disc Cupping, 222

Index, 229

Contributors

Lawrence M. Buono, MD
Duke University Eye Center
Durham, North Carolina

Eugene H. Eng, MD
Dean McGee Eye Institute
University of Oklahoma
Oklahoma City, Oklahoma

Rod Foroozan, MD
Baylor College of Medicine
Houston, Texas

Lisa Hinckley, MD
Weill Cornell Medical College
Houston, Texas

John B. Kerrison, MD
Charleston Neuroscience Institute
Division of Retina and
    Neuro-ophthalmology
Charleston, South Carolina

Lanning B. Kline, MD
UAB Department of Ophthalmology
Callahan Eye Foundation Hospital
Birmingham, Alabama

John C. Morrison, MD
Casey Eye Institute
Oregon Health and Science University
Portland, Oregon

R. Michael Siatkowski, MD
Dean McGee Institute
University of Oklahoma
Oklahoma City, Oklahoma

Michael S. Vaphiades, DO
UAB Department of Ophthalmology
Callahan Eye Foundation Hospital
Birmingham, Alabama

Legal Notice

The American Academy of Ophthalmology provides the opportunity for a material to be presented for educational purposes only. The material represents the approach, ideas, statement or opinion of the author, not necessarily the only or best method or procedure in every case, nor the position of the Academy. Unless specifically stated otherwise, the opinions expressed and statements made by various authors in this monograph reflect the author's observations and do not imply endorsement by the Academy. The material is not intended to replace a physician's own judgment or give specific advice for case management. The Academy does not endorse any of the products or companies, if any, mentioned in this monograph.

Some material on recent developments may include information on drug or device applications that are not considered community standard, that reflect indications not included in approved FDA labeling, or that are approved for use only in restricted research settings. This information is provided as education only so physicians may be aware of alternative methods of the practice of medicine, and should not be considered endorsement, promotion, or in any way encouragement to use such applications. The FDA has stated that it is the responsibility of the physician to determine the FDA status of each drug or device he or she wishes to use in clinical practice, and to use these products with appropriate patient consent and in compliance with applicable law.

The Academy and Oxford University Press (OUP) do not make any warranties, as to the accuracy, adequacy or completeness of any material presented here, which is provided on an "as is" basis. The Academy and OUP are not liable to anyone for any errors, inaccuracies, omissions obtained here. The Academy specifically disclaims any and all liability for injury or other damages of any kind for any and all claims that may arise out of the use of any practice, technique, or drug described in any material by any author, whether such claims are asserted by a physician or any other person.

Optic Nerve Disorders

Anatomy and Physiology
of the Optic Nerve

JOHN C. MORRISON

The optic nerve is unique. It contains approximately 1.2 million axons, each originating from a single retinal ganglion cell, and experiences several "environmental" changes in its course from the eye to the brain. For example, optic nerve fibers are initially unmyelinated, satisfying the optical needs of the retina, but they become myelinated behind the globe, so as to provide rapid and efficient propagation of visual impulses to the lateral geniculate nucleus.

In order to accommodate these diverse needs as well as to withstand mechanical stresses such as changes in intraocular pressure (IOP) and eye movement, a variety of special structural features are required.[1] These include the lamina cribrosa and associated astrocytes within the prelaminar and laminar optic nerve head, which provide structural and metabolic support for potentially vulnerable axons. Similar considerations probably underlie the multiple sources of blood supply to the optic nerve head, ensuring steady and reliable perfusion of this anatomically complex region.

This chapter reviews the anatomy and physiology of the optic nerve, with emphasis on those characteristics that maintain homeostasis and lead to recognizable findings in various disease states.

1-1 ANATOMY OF THE OPTIC NERVE

Traditionally, the optic nerve is divided into four segments: (1) intraocular, (2) intraorbital, (3) intracanalicular, and (4) intracranial. Embryologically and anatomically, the optic nerve resembles a tract of the brain more than it does a typical cranial nerve. Basically, it is a myelinated white matter pathway with little if any regenerative capacity. It is invested by dural, arachnoidal, and pial membranes from the external scleral surface to the cranial cavity. Like nerve fibers in the brain and spinal cord, optic nerve fibers have no sheaths or Schwann cells. Instead, oligodendrocytes provide the myelin for optic nerve fibers from the posterior edge of the lamina cribrosa (where myelination begins), while supporting astrocytes are present throughout the course of the optic nerve.

1-1-1 *Intraocular Optic Nerve.* The axons of the optic nerve experience rapid and dramatic changes at the level of the optic disc, where they exit the posterior sclera. As unmyelinated fibers, the axons traverse the multiple layers of the optic nerve head, withstanding an abrupt pressure drop from the eye (IOP) to the central nervous system (subarachnoid pressure). The axons within the optic disc also receive their blood supply from several sources, including the central retinal artery, the posterior ciliary arteries, and the ophthalmic artery, and ultimately become myelinated at the origin of the retrobulbar optic nerve.

The optic nerve head is composed of three main regions: the (1) nerve fiber layer, (2) lamina choroidalis, and (3) lamina cribrosa, or lamina scleralis (Figs. 1–1 and 1–2).[2–4]

1-1-1-1 *Nerve Fiber Layer.* Occupying the innermost layer of the retina, the nerve fiber layer is composed of astrocytes and retinal ganglion cell axons. These unmyelinated axons allow maximal light transmission to the photoreceptors and gradually coalesce into bundles separated by glial cell columns as they enter the optic nerve head. As the nerve fibers approach the optic nerve head, the thickness of the nerve fiber layer increases to a maximum of 200 μm. This increase in thickness

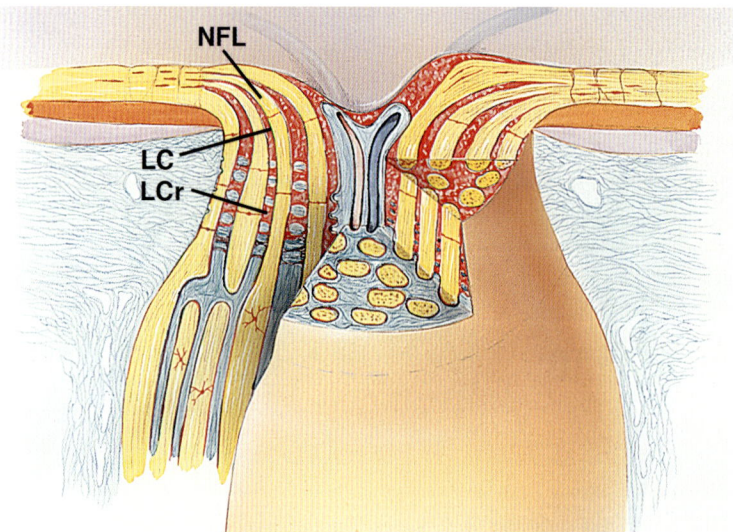

Figure 1–1. Three major portions of optic disc. NFL, nerve fiber layer; LC, lamina choroidalis; LCr, lamina cribrosa. Modified from Anderson DR: Ultrastructure of human and monkey lamina cribrosa and optic nerve head. Arch Ophthalmol 1969;82:800–814.

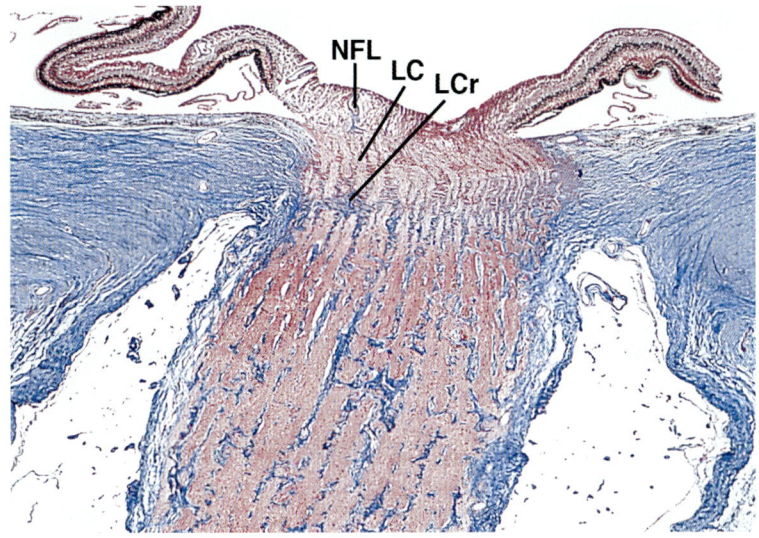

Figure 1–2. Longitudinal section of human optic nerve, stained to differentiate collagenous connective tissue (blue) from glial cells (red). NFL, nerve fiber layer; LC, lamina choroidalis; LCr, lamina cribrosa. (Masson trichrome, original magnification 10X.)

occurs in an arcuate pattern along the major vascular arcades, where the nerve fiber layer is most easily seen clinically with the red-free light of the ophthalmoscope.[5,6]

The topographic organization of the nerve fiber layer is best categorized into three zones (Fig. 1–3). Papillomacular fibers course directly from the fovea and nasal macula into the temporal side of the optic disc. Fibers from the nasal peripheral retina enter the nasal disc. Ganglion cells located above and below the horizontal midline in the temporal macula send fibers to the superior and inferior poles of the optic disc. These fibers arch above and below the papillomacular fibers; they are

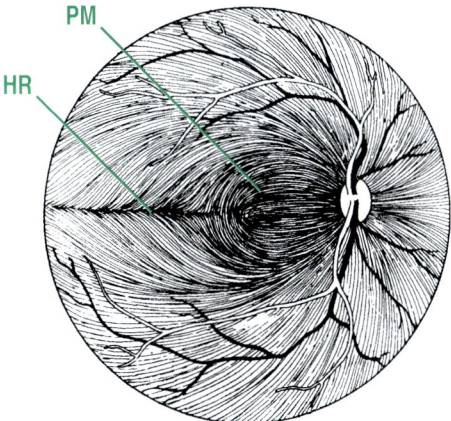

Figure 1–3. Pattern of nerve fiber layer of axons from ganglion cells to optic disc. Superior, inferior, and nasal fibers take a fairly straight course. Temporal axons originate above and below horizontal raphe (HR) and take an arching course to the disc. Axons arising from ganglion cells in nasal macula project directly to the disc as the papillomacular bundle (PM).

called arcuate bundles and are the thickest parts of the nerve fiber layer. They do not cross the horizontal raphe, a fact that produces the arcuate and nasal "step" visual field defects characteristic of glaucoma and other diseases of the optic nerve head.

The organization of nerve fibers with respect to their distance of origin from the optic nerve head is only partly understood. Most work suggests that peripherally originating axons are located in the inner superficial zones of the nerve fiber layer.[7] Ultimately, these fibers occupy the peripheral portion of the optic nerve; those of more proximal origin lie centrally.[8] Thus, the nerve fibers are reorganized at the edge of the optic nerve head.[9–11]

1-1-1-2 *Lamina Choroidalis.* Overlying the scleral canal, nerve fibers enter the optic nerve head and turn to exit the globe. This occurs at the level of the choroid; the support tissue at this level is termed the *lamina choroidalis.* The lamina choroidalis consists primarily of glial cells with intertwining cell processes. When viewed in profile, the glial cells appear stellate, their processes extending toward each other and forming a basket-like arrangement.

Longitudinal sections of the lamina choroidalis demonstrate that the glial cells, or astrocytes, are arranged in columns extending anteriorly from the lamina cribrosa. Astrocytes surround and support the nerve fiber bundles as they turn into the nerve head. The astrocytes send processes into the bundles to make intimate contact with axons (Fig. 1–4). These contacts suggest that astrocytes, which are interconnected by gap junctions to form a syncytium, provide important physiologic support for unmyelinated axons, as by storing glycogen and absorbing excess potassium ions released during axonal depolarization. Astrocytes may also aid in the transport of nutrients from capillaries lying within the glial columns.

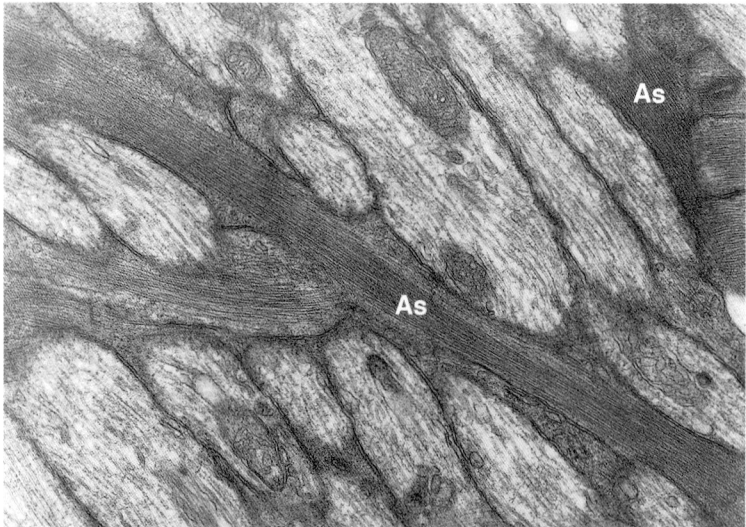

Figure 1–4. Transmission electron micrograph of optic nerve axons (lighter cells) of lamina choroidalis. Axons make intimate contact with astrocyte processes (As), dark cells that are filled with intermediate filaments and interconnect with each other. (Original magnification 13,000X.)

1-1-1-3 *Lamina Cribrosa*. At the level of the sclera, the main support for nerve fibers appears to be the lamina cribrosa (also known as the *lamina scleralis*), comprising 6 to 10 connective tissue plates that span the scleral opening at the back of the eye (see Figs. 1–1 and 1–2). Each plate contains perforations, or pores, which are aligned with those of adjacent plates to allow passage of nerve fiber bundles through the sclera into the intraorbital optic nerve.

Histologic cross sections and scanning electron microscopic analysis of trypsin-digested optic nerves from normal human eyes reveal that the laminar pores of the superior and inferior optic nerve head are larger than those located nasally and temporally.[12,13] The laminar beams of these regions, which contain the arcuate nerve fiber bundles, are fewer in number and generally thinner than in the horizontal regions. Because nerve fibers in these regions appear to be damaged first in glaucoma,[14] this anatomic association strongly supports the argument that the optic nerve head, and specifically the lamina cribrosa, is the site of initial injury in glaucoma. Some investigators have proposed that the thinner laminar beams in the superior and inferior optic nerve head are more easily distorted by IOP and more likely to compress and injure nerve fibers in these regions (the mechanical hypothesis).[12,15] Others point out that capillaries are contained within the laminar beams, leading to a relative decrease in the axonal blood supply; thus they theorize that axons are damaged by an ischemic mechanism (the vascular hypothesis).[16] To date, there has been little compelling evidence to absolutely prove or disprove either theory.

Immunohistochemical studies of the primate optic nerve head have greatly enhanced our understanding of the biochemical composition of the lamina cribrosa. Such studies confirm the presence of fibrillar collagens. These include collagens I (the major collagen of tendon), III, V, and VI.[17–22] Although collagen I contributes to laminar strength, collagen III is more distensible and may lend resiliency to the lamina cribrosa.

Another component that provides resiliency is elastin. Demonstrated initially by conventional histochemical stains and transmission electron microscopy, elastin fibrils are abundant within the laminar beams. This finding has been confirmed by both light and electron microscopic immunolocalization studies (Fig. 1–5).[23,24] The structural and resilient properties of the lamina cribrosa may protect ganglion cell axons from the stress of repeated changes in IOP due to ocular movement, eye rubbing, and diurnal fluctuation.

Numerous other constituents have been described in the lamina cribrosa, many of them components of basement membranes. These include laminin, collagen type IV, fibronectin, and the heparan sulfate-containing proteoglycan.[17–25] Lining the margins of the laminar beams, these basement membranes may be deposited by glial cells common to other regions of the central nervous system, wherever they come into contact with connective tissue. This distribution has been confirmed by transmission electron microscopy, along with the presence of basement-membrane materials within the beams themselves. This finding suggests that, rather than existing as several distinct plates of connective tissue, the laminar beams may interconnect. Interconnections between beams also exist in the form of astrocytic processes whose basement membranes are interposed between successive plates.[21]

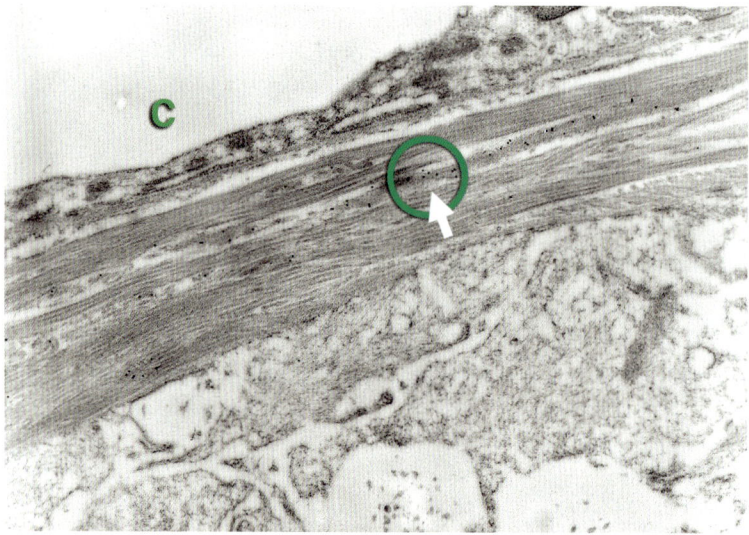

Figure 1–5. Transmission electron microscopic immunolocalization of elastin in monkey optic nerve head. Colloidal gold particles (arrow) are restricted to amorphous portions of laminar beam, within bundles of cross-banded collagen fibers. C,= capillary contained within laminar beam. (Original magnification 15,000X.)

Although the possibility of independent movement of laminar beams in response to elevated IOP has been proposed as a cause of mechanical compression and damage to optic nerve fibers, the presence of these two types of interconnections may limit the actual extent of such interlamellar movement.

The laminar beams also contain capillaries that supply this region of the optic nerve head (see Fig. 1–5). Derived mostly from the choroidal circulation, these capillaries consist primarily of vascular endothelium, their basement membranes, and pericytes. Details of the vascular anatomy and physiology of this region of the optic nerve head are discussed later in the chapter.

Figure 1–6 is an electron micrograph of axon bundles adjacent to a laminar beam. Astrocytes lining these beams send numerous processes into the bundles, with secondary projections that intimately contact the nerves. This arrangement allows the laminar beams to provide metabolic as well as anatomic support to the optic nerve fibers.

1-1-2 *Intraorbital Optic Nerve.* The posterior border of the lamina cribrosa marks the posterior sclera and presumably the posterior extent of the transition from intraocular to extraocular pressure. This border also marks the beginning of optic nerve myelination.

The intraorbital portion of the optic nerve extends from the sclera to the anterior end of the optic canal. It lies in the shape of an elongated "S" and measures 20 to 30 mm, which is longer than the distance from the eye to the optic canal. This slight redundancy of the nerve allows freedom of rotation of the globe without placing tension along the nerve. The axons are invested in myelin, while the nerve itself is surrounded by pia, arachnoid, and dura mater. The dura is the outermost

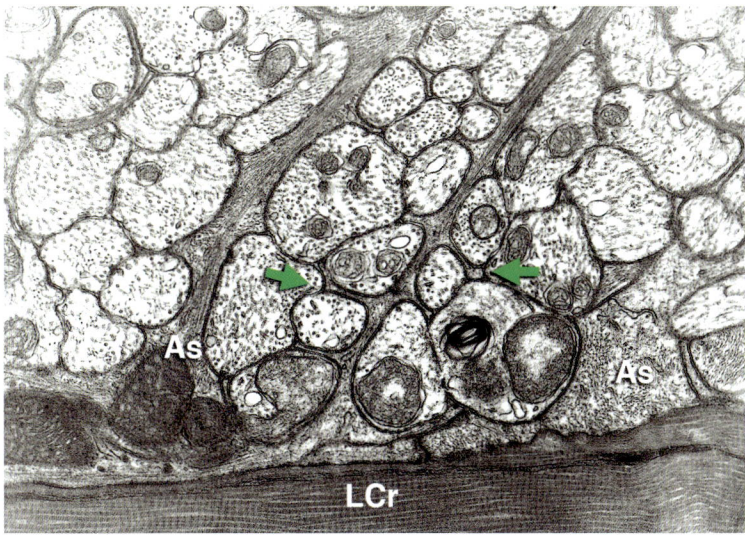

Figure 1–6. Transmission electron micrograph of lamina cribrosa beam (LCr), showing its adjacent astrocytes (As). Note numerous projections (arrows) of astrocytes between axons, filling nearly all interaxonal spaces. (Original magnification 13,000X.)

dense collagenous sheath that is continuous anteriorly with the sclera. At the apex of the orbit, the dura fuses with the periosteum of the sphenoid bone and with the annulus of Zinn. Lying within the dura, the arachnoid is a more cellular and less vascular tissue. Fine arachnoid trabeculae connect this membrane with the dura and the pia mater. The pia is the most vascular of the sheaths covering the optic nerve. It contains the capillaries that enter the substance of the nerve along fibrous septa and provide its major vascular supply. At the orbital apex, the optic nerve is surrounded by the four rectus muscles arising from the annulus of Zinn. This proximity of the muscles to the optic nerve leads to pain with eye movement during an episode of optic neuritis.[26]

The microanatomy of the intraorbital, intracanalicular, and intracranial portions of the optic nerves is virtually the same. At the origin of the intraorbital optic nerve, immediately behind the lamina cribrosa, optic nerve septa originate, blending gradually with the posterior lamina cribrosa. Oriented longitudinally within the optic nerve, the optic nerve septa consist of fibrillar collagen, elastin, and proteoglycans, usually less compactly arranged than in the laminar beams. The septa are lined with glial cells, which deposit basement membranes similar to those lining the laminar beams. Other basement-membrane materials are seen within the septa, associated with capillaries derived from the short posterior ciliary arteries and the pial system. This septal system divides the nerve fibers into a series of fasciculi that carry blood vessels throughout the optic nerve.

Within the intraorbital, intracanalicular, and intracranial segments of the optic nerve, oligodendroglia form myelin sheaths around the axons.[27] Processes from glial cells lining the septa and from glial cells lying within the myelinated nerve fiber bundles intimately contact the nerve fibers. The exact function of astrocytes in this region of the optic nerve is not known, although, as with peripheral nerves, they may serve to maintain the extracellular environment, particularly at the nodes of Ranvier.[28,29]

1-1-3 Intracanalicular Optic Nerve. The optic canal lies within the lesser wing of the sphenoid bone and contains the optic nerve, the ophthalmic artery, and portions of the carotid sympathetic plexus (Fig. 1–7). Each canal runs posteriorly and medially and from orbit to cranium, ascending at approximately 45 degrees. The distance between the two orbital openings averages 28 mm; and between the two cranial openings, 14.7 mm. The orbital plate of the frontal bone separates the frontal lobe of the brain from the optic canal. In some people, the frontal sinus may extend into the roof of the canal. Medially, the sphenoid sinus and posterior ethmoid air cells border on the canal. In some individuals, there is no medial bony wall to the canal and only the meningeal sheaths and sinus mucosa separate the optic nerve from the sphenoid sinus.

The intracanalicular nerve is firmly fixed within the canal and is 6 to 10 mm long. The dura of the intraorbital optic nerve fuses with the periosteum at the optic foramen. These anatomic relationships render this portion of the nerve most susceptible to trauma and to the compressive effects of even small lesions arising within the optic canal.

1-1-4 Intracranial Optic Nerve. The optic nerves emerge from the optic canals to converge toward each other at the optic chiasm (Fig. 1–8). The length of each intracranial optic nerve is variable, from 3 to 16 mm, depending on the relationship of the chiasm to the sella turcica. In 79% of individuals, the chiasm is centered over the posterior two-thirds of the sella. In 17%, the chiasm is prefixed, with its center lying over the chiasmatic sulcus or the anterior one-third of the sella. In such cases, the optic nerves are relatively short. In 4%, the chiasm is postfixed, lying on or

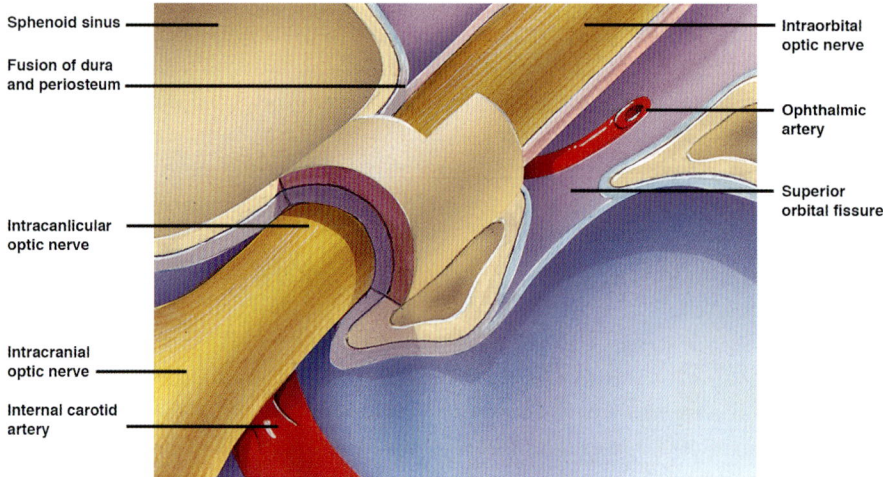

Figure 1–7. Intracanalicular portion of optic nerve traversing optic canal with ophthalmic artery. Orbital periosteum and dura of orbital optic nerve fuse at orbital apex.

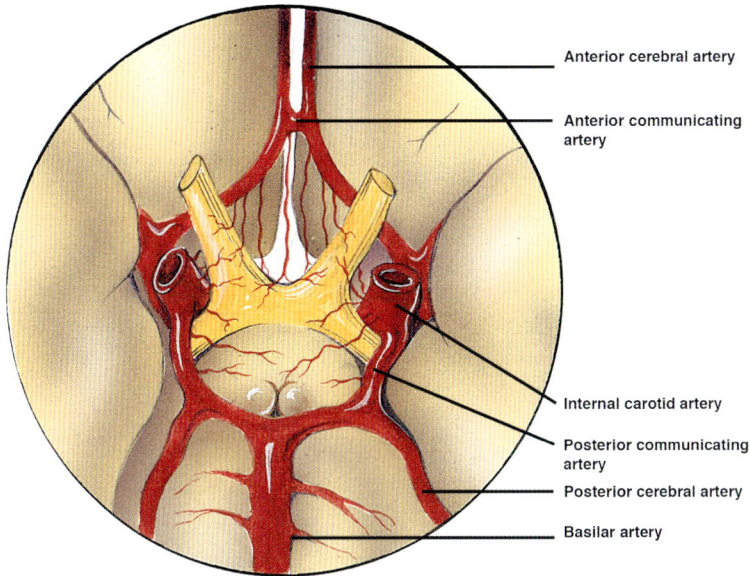

Figure 1–8. Intracranial segments of optic nerves and their blood supply.

behind the dorsum sellae. The intracranial segments of each optic nerve are relatively long. The variable anatomic relationship of the chiasm to the sella affects the types of visual field defects seen with compressive lesions.

The olfactory nerves and frontal lobes of the brain lie above each intracranial optic nerve; between these structures lie the anterior cerebral and anterior communicating arteries. On the lateral side of each intracranial optic nerve lies the internal carotid artery as it emerges from the cavernous sinus. The ophthalmic artery arises from the internal carotid artery just lateral and below the intracranial optic nerve and travels within the dural sheath as the nerve enters the optic canal. The planum sphenoidale lies above and anteriorly and the pituitary gland below and medial to each intracranial optic nerve.

1-2 TOPOGRAPHIC ORGANIZATION OF THE OPTIC NERVE

Ganglion cell axons traveling within the optic nerve follow a highly organized, precise course. Classic experiments mapping axonal degeneration in monkeys after lesions of specific fundus locations with laser photocoagulation have provided an understanding of these pathways.[30–33]

Macular fibers occupy one-third of the temporal portion of the anterior optic nerve. By the middle third of the intraorbital optic nerve, these fibers lie more centrally within the nerve. Within the chiasm, macular fibers originating nasal to the vertical meridian of the fundus begin crossing almost immediately in the anterosuperior chiasm. Crossing of macular fibers occupies nearly the entire chiasm, and crossed fibers are distributed in nearly two-thirds of the optic tract, primarily centrally and dorsolaterally.

Peripheral and paracentral fibers travel in more discrete bundles throughout the optic nerve and chiasm. Superior and inferior nasal fibers occupy the superior and inferior nasal sectors of the optic nerve up to the chiasm (Fig. 1–9A,B). Here, superior and inferior fibers decussate in the dorsal and ventral chiasm, respectively; this is the most dense crossing occurring posteriorly. The course of the inferonasal fiber projection deserves emphasis. Prior to decussating within the chiasm, this fiber bundle projects anteriorly into the contralateral optic nerve for approximately 4 mm (Fig. 1–9B). This portion of the inferior projection, often referred to as *Wilbrand's knee*, is important in understanding the basis for the junctional scotoma of chiasmal disease. Although the presence of Wilbrand's knee has been challenged,[34] it still appears to have clinical relevance.[35]

Within the optic tract, the crossed fibers immediately occupy discrete locations: the superior fibers within the medial tract and the inferior fibers ventrolaterally. Paracentral arcuate optic nerve fiber bundles contain axons originating both nasally and temporally to the fovea. Immediately posterior to the globe, fibers arising from ganglion cells located superior to the horizontal midline occupy a discrete wedge of the optic nerve superior to the temporally located macular fibers (Fig. 1–9C). Axons from the inferior ganglion cells are located inferior to the macular fibers (Fig. 1–9D). These wedges gradually widen as they approach the chiasm. Once again, fibers originating nasal to the fovea begin crossing in the anterior chiasm, arching slightly into the opposite optic nerve (Wilbrand's knee). Decussating superior and inferior fibers maintain their altitudinal position throughout their course to the chiasm. Nondecussating fibers originate temporal to the fovea and accompany their corresponding decussating fibers within the superior and inferior wedges of the optic nerve. Once in the chiasm, these fibers remain ipsilateral and mix with the decussating fibers of the contralateral optic nerve.

Although superior and inferior arcuate nerve fibers maintain their superior and inferior positions throughout the optic chiasm, all nondecussating fibers occupy the ipsilateral optic tract along with corresponding nasal decussating fibers. Superior arcuate nerve fibers lie nasally within the optic tract and inferior fibers lie laterally.

In summary, there are three basic anatomic "rules" of the optic chiasm:

1. The nasal retinal fibers (including the nasal half of the macula) of each eye cross in the chiasm to the contralateral optic tract. Temporal fibers remain uncrossed.
2. Lower retinal fibers project through the optic nerve and chiasm to lie laterally in the tract; upper retinal fibers lie medially. Thus, there is a 90-degree rotation of visual fibers from the optic nerve and chiasm into the optic tracts.
3. Inferonasal retinal fibers cross in the chiasm but course anteriorly in the contralateral optic nerve (Wilbrand's knee) before turning back to join the uncrossed inferotemporal fibers of the other eye in the optic tract.

1-3 BLOOD SUPPLY OF THE OPTIC NERVE

1-3-1 *Intraocular Optic Nerve.* The blood supply of the optic nerve is derived from the ophthalmic artery (Fig. 1–10). Although most studies agree that the bulk of the

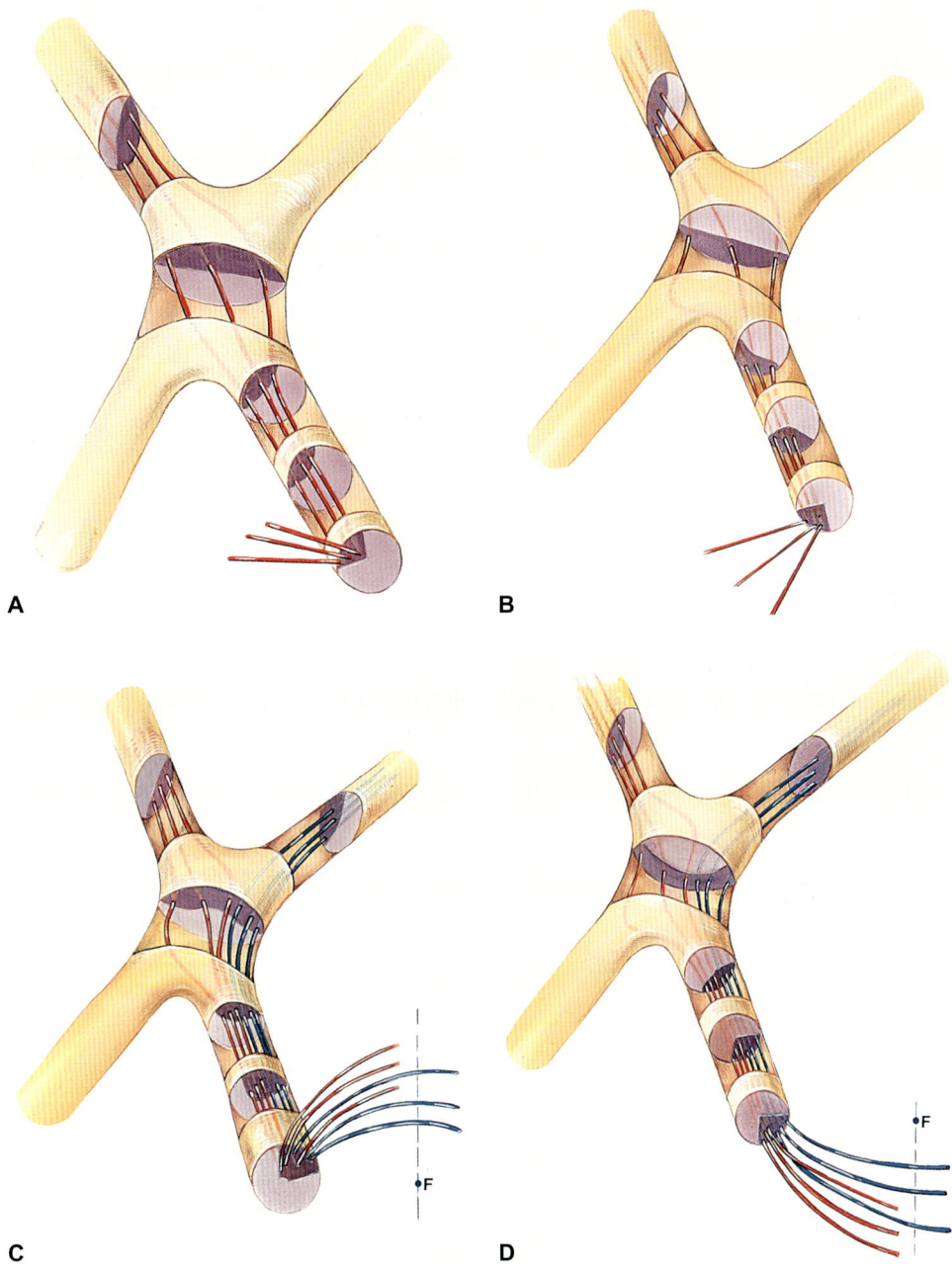

A

B

C

D

Figure 1–9. Nerve fiber bundles traversing optic nerves and chiasm into optic tracts for fibers originating nasal (A superior, B inferior) and temporal to disc (C superior, D inferior). Those arising temporally (arcuate bundles) may or may not decussate, depending on their relationship to vertical midline (hatched line) passing through fovea (F).

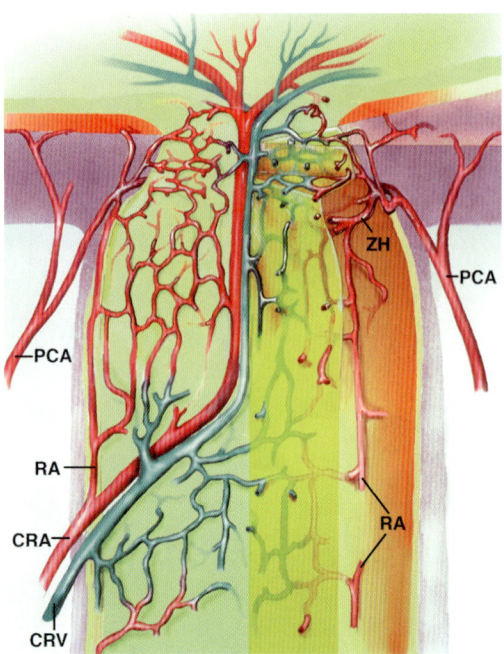

Figure 1–10. Partial cutaway view of vasculature of optic nerve head. Short posterior ciliary arteries (PCA) supply centripetal capillary beds of anterior optic nerve head. Central retinal artery (CRA) contribution is restricted to nerve fiber layer capillaries and those of anterior intraorbital optic nerve. Capillary beds at all levels drain into central retinal vein (CRV). ZH, intrascleral circle of Zinn-Haller; RA, recurrent posterior ciliary artery to pial plexus.

blood supply to the optic nerve head is from the short posterior ciliary arteries, the contribution of the central retinal artery remains controversial.[36,37]

The blood supply to the nerve fiber layer is derived entirely from branches of the central retinal artery. Cilioretinal arteries, when present, also supply precapillary branches to the superficial nerve fiber layer. The superficial capillary bed of the optic nerve head also receives scattered branches from the peripapillary capillaries and communicates freely with capillaries of the lamina choroidalis. Most of the venous drainage from the nerve fiber layer is into the central retinal vein.

The lamina choroidalis is perfused by a capillary bed that is continuous with that of the nerve fiber layer anteriorly and the lamina cribrosa posteriorly. Arterial supply in these capillaries is derived entirely from the short posterior ciliary arteries, either by intrascleral branches from the circle of Zinn-Haller or by choroidal vessels that supply the choriocapillaris. There are also sparse vessels that bridge the intermediate tissue of Kundt, an accumulation of astrocytes that separates the retina and choroid from the optic nerve.

As in the prelaminar region, the capillary bed of the lamina cribrosa receives its centripetal blood supply from intrascleral arterioles derived from the short posterior ciliary arteries. These capillaries, encased by laminar beams, are arranged in several layers and encircle the axon bundles. As with other regions of the optic nerve head, this capillary bed is continuous with the capillaries both anterior and posterior to it and drains into the central retinal vein.

The capillaries of the optic nerve head, whether derived from the central retinal artery or from the posterior ciliary arteries, are apparently capable of autoregulation.[33–43] In autoregulation, vessels respond to local stimuli to maintain constant perfusion in the face of changing physiologic conditions, such as hypertension (constriction), elevated IOP (dilation), and elevated carbon dioxide level (dilation). In addition, capillaries of the optic nerve head are surrounded by pericytes and possess nonfenestrated endothelium. Although this endothelium effectively creates a blood–brain barrier, blood-borne molecules can still enter the extravascular tissues of the optic nerve head by escaping the fenestrated peripapillary choriocapillaris and diffusing into the nerve head and lamina cribrosa.[47–49] Pericytes have the ability to contract and alter capillary bed perfusion,[50,51] and adenosine appears to relax pericytes and improve blood flow when metabolic demand is high.[52] Additional mechanisms for controlling vascular tone include nitric oxide, which can increase capillary perfusion,[53] and endothelins. Chronic administration of endothelin 1 in animal models has been shown to induce vasoconstriction and loss of retinal ganglion cells.[54,55]

1-3-2 Intraorbital Optic Nerve Myelinated nerve fibers of the intraorbital optic nerve are supplied by capillaries lying entirely within collagenous septa (Fig. 1–11). Anteriorly, these capillaries arise partly from the central retinal artery after it enters the optic nerve, usually 10 to 15 mm posterior to the globe, and partly from the pial plexus, which is supplied by recurrent branches of the short posterior ciliary arteries as well as branches of the ophthalmic artery. Capillaries in the remainder of the intraorbital optic nerve are supplied by the pial plexus; they are derived principally from the ophthalmic artery. However, there is often extensive collateral circulation to the intraorbital optic nerve through the external carotid system. Anastomotic branches frequently arise from the middle meningeal, superficial temporal, and transverse facial arteries.

1-3-3 Intracanalicular Optic Nerve. The intracanalicular optic nerve receives its blood supply from the pial plexus, which arises from the internal carotid artery and, in

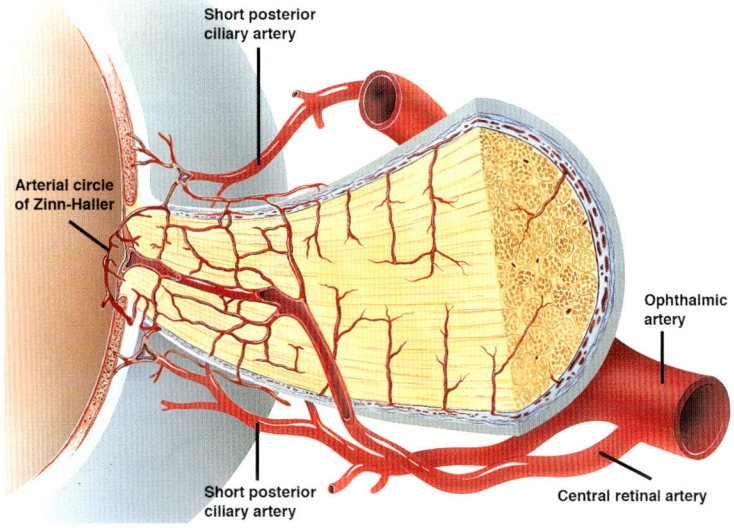

Figure 1–11. Intraorbital optic nerve and its peripheral and periaxial vascular network.

some individuals, from collateral branches of the ophthalmic artery. As in the intraorbital optic nerve, the capillary networks travel within fibrous septa of this portion of the optic nerve.

1-3-4 *Intracranial Optic Nerve*. The intracranial optic nerve also receives blood from the pial plexus of capillary branches traversing collagenous septa. The pial plexus for this portion of the nerve arises from various sources, including the internal carotid artery, the first (A1) segment of the anterior cerebral artery, and the anterior communicating artery (see Fig. 1–8). Two factors determine the relative contributions of these sources: (1) the embryologic development in a particular individual, and (2) the length of the intracranial portion of the optic nerve.

1-4 AXONAL PHYSIOLOGY OF THE OPTIC NERVE

The anterior visual system appears to provide visual information through two pathways.[56] One, most sensitive to low light levels and motion, relies on larger ganglion cells and axons that synapse in the magnocellular layer of the lateral geniculate body. This is called the *luminance*, or *M* (magnocellular) *pathway*. The other contains the majority of retinal ganglion cells, which are generally smaller and whose axons synapse in the parvocellular layer of the lateral geniculate. This *P* (parvocellular) *pathway* appears to be responsible for color vision and fine discrimination.

There is evidence that the energy demands of the optic nerve at the level of the optic nerve head are unique. This includes observations of high concentrations of mitrochondria, possibly contained in focal dilations of axons at the level of the lamina cribrosa.[57,58]

Like all neurons, ganglion cells rely on axoplasmic transport for intracellular communication.[59–61] Axonal transport is a complex, energy-dependent process that moves molecules and subcellular organelles away from (anterograde or orthograde) and toward (retrograde) the cell body. In this way, the cell body can remain "informed" of conditions along the axon and at the synapse while at the same time maintaining the size and functional properties of the axon.

Anterograde axonal transport occurs at slow, intermediate, and fast speeds. Although little is known of the intermediate phase, slow and fast transport rely on the axonal cytoskeleton, which is composed of microtubules, neurofilaments, and microfilaments (Figs. 1–12 and 1–13).[62] This cytoskeleton comprises the majority of the axonal volume. Microtubules and neurofilaments measure about 10 to 100 micrometers in length and are oriented parallel to the long axis of the axon (Fig. 1–13). Most of these three components are located centrally in the axon. Here, lying within the neurofilaments, microtubules form bundles with interspersed microfilaments and a surrounding dense matrix of globular proteins, many of which appear to be attached directly to the surface of the microfilaments. These attachments are thought to organize the matrix of the microtubular bundles, or domains, lying within the neurofilaments. Many proteins, including enzymes of intermediary metabolism, have been associated with the microfilaments. Microtubules, composed of alpha and beta tubulin, are highly polarized with a stable, or minus, end located at the

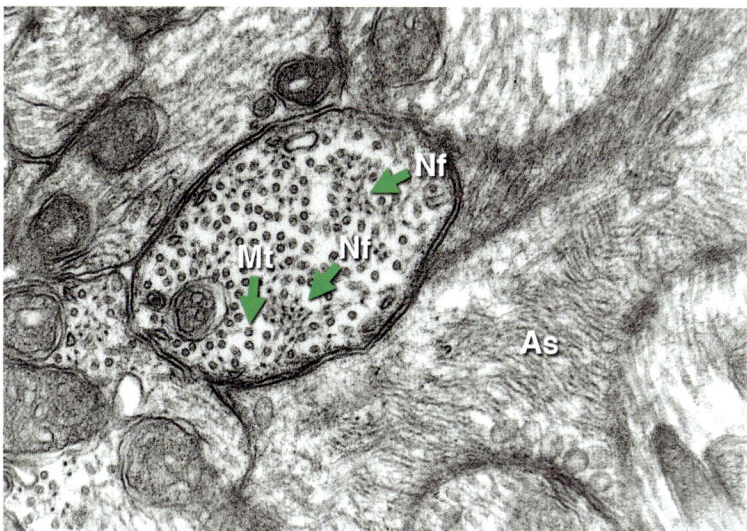

Figure 1–12. Transmission electron micrograph of optic nerve axon within lamina choroidalis. Microtubules (Mt) (arrow), interspersed bundles of neurofilaments (Nf) (arrows), and closely associated astrocytes (As). (Original magnification 25,000X.)

cell body and an unstable, or positive, end near the end of the axon. Microtubules possess side arms composed of microtubule-associated proteins, which may help to link the microtubules to neighboring microfilaments and neurofilaments.

Outside of the microtubular bundles, regions containing predominantly neurofilaments appear less dense owing to their relative lack of microfilaments. Like microtubules, neurofilaments also have side arms projecting from their surface; these allow interaction with neighboring neurofilaments and microtubules. These side arms may participate in the translocation of polymers down the axon for both microtubules and neurofilaments, producing slow axonal transport.

Depending on the nerve and the species, slow axonal transport often segregates into two components of different velocities: SCa = slow component, type a (1 mm/day), and SCb = slow component, type b (2.7 mm/day).[63] SCa appears to consist primarily of neurofilament proteins and the microtubular protein tubulin, along with other proteins that associate with neurofilaments and microtubules, such as spectrin. In contrast, SCb contains many more proteins, including actin (associated with microfilaments) and tubulin. The actual mechanism of slow axonal transport is not completely understood. However, it is likely that proteins transported in this fashion move as part of the cytoskeleton of the axons, although their movement may be intermittent.[64]

Fast axonal transport (from 20 to 400 mm/day), both anterograde and retrograde, is fundamentally distinct from slow transport.[59] Fast anterograde transport conveys membrane-bound vesicles, such as synaptic vesicles and plasma membrane components, as well as mitochondria and enzymes involved in neurotransmitter metabolism to the distal axon.[65] Retrograde transport moves lysosomes containing membrane receptors and neurotrophins, pinocytic vesicles, and degraded multivesiculate bodies in addition to mitochondria, which can apparently move bidirectionally.

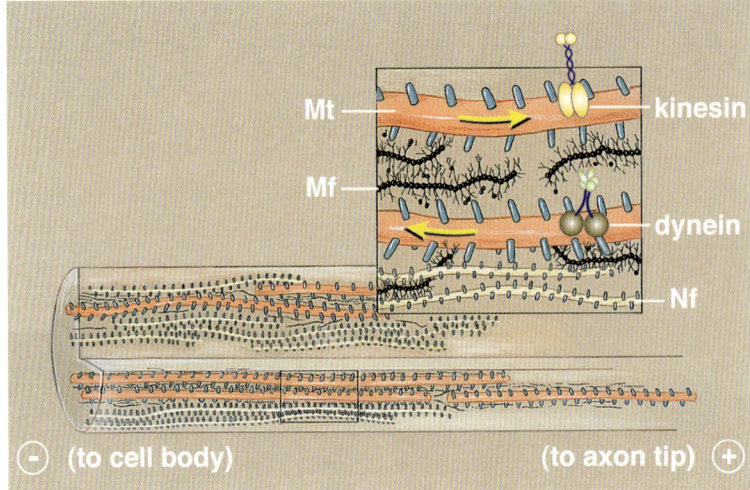

Figure 1–13. Representation of axonal cytoskeleton with bundles of microtubules and inter-spersed neurofilaments. Inset shows relationship of microtubules (Mt) and neurofilaments (Nf) with side arms and of microfilaments (Mf) with associated globular proteins. Motor proteins kinesin and dynein are important in anterograde and retrograde axonal transport, respectively.

In fast axonal transport, the movement of organelles in close association with microtubules appears to require adenosine triphosphate (ATP) and can proceed in either direction along a single microtubule.[66] This finding indicates that distinct "motor proteins" are responsible for anterograde and retrograde axonal transport. (Fig. 1–13). One such protein, kinesin, has been associated with anterograde axonal transport.[67,68] In fact, several kinesin motor proteins are now thought to exist,[69] which, along with axonal myosins,[70] may regulate different rates of transport for different cargos. Another motor protein, dynein, or microtubule-associated pro-tein 1C (MAP 1C), appears to catalyze vesicular movement in a direction opposite to that of kinesin and is thought to associate with specific organelles throughout their journey along the axon.[71,72] Dynein, synthesized in the cell body, travels by anterograde transport to the tip of the axon, where it becomes activated to begin transport to the cell body.[73–75]

In recent years, it has been recognized that protein synthesis may also occur within the axon itself, rather than requiring slow transport of proteins synthesized in the cell body and transported along the length of the axon.[76] This is supported by the finding of ribosomal plaques along axons.[77]

Axoplasmic transport in the optic nerve has been extensively studied in many optic nerve disorders, including glaucoma. Both anterograde and retrograde trans-port are affected by acutely elevated IOP.[78–82] Chronic elevation of IOP in mon-keys [83–85] and glaucoma in humans[86] have also been shown to disrupt axoplasmic flow, leading to a visible buildup of mitochondria and organelles primarily at the level of the lamina cribrosa.

Although not a proven factor in glaucomatous optic nerve damage, disruption of axoplasmic transport may lead to axonal and ganglionic cell death. This result could be due to the interruption of the supply of materials necessary to maintain the distal axon and synapse (anterograde transport) as well as loss of feedback or trophic factors (retrograde transport) needed to inform the cell body of changing environmental conditions. In fact, experimental models of chronic IOP elevation have demonstrated reduced delivery of brain-derived neurotrophic factor (BDNF) to the retinal ganglion cells[87,88] and trkB, its receptor. In addition, supplementation of BDNF using adeno-associated viral transfer has been linked to reduced loss of retinal ganglion cells.[89]

Obstruction of axoplasmic flow has been demonstrated in experimental papilledema and appears to be a primary cause of optic disc swelling in this condition.[90] Because many factors impede axoplasmic transport—including ischemia, mechanical compression, and toxins—this disturbance may well represent a final common pathway for many diseases affecting the optic nerve.

References

1. Morrison JC, Pollack IH. Glaucoma: Science and Practice. New York: Thieme, 2003.
2. Anderson DR. Ultrastructure of human and monkey lamina cribrosa and optic nerve head. Arch Ophthalmol 1969;82:800–14.
3. Anderson DR. Ultrastructure of the optic nerve head. Arch Ophthalmol 1970;83:63–73.
4. Anderson DR, Hoyt WF, Hogan MJ. The fine structure of the astroglia in the human optic nerve and optic nerve head. Trans Am Ophthalmol Soc 1967;65:275–305.
5. Quigley HA, Sommer A. How to use nerve fiber layer examination in the management of glaucoma. Trans Am Ophthalmol Soc 1987;85:254–72.
6. Quigley HA. Examination of the retinal nerve fiber layer in the recognition of early glaucoma damage. Trans Am Ophthalmol Soc 1986;84:920–66.
7. Ogden TE. Nerve fiber layer of the macaque retina: retinotopic organization. Invest Ophthalmol Vis Sci 1983;24:85–98.
8. Naito J. Retinogeniculate projection fibers in the monkey optic nerve: a demonstration of the fiber pathways by retrograde axonal transport of WGA-HRP. J Comp Neurol 1989;284:174–86.
9. FitzGibbon T. The human fetal retinal nerve fiber layer and optic nerve head: a DiI and DiA tracing study. Vis Neurosci 1997;14:433–47.
10. Fitzgibbon T, Taylor SF. Retinotopy of the human retinal nerve fibre layer and optic nerve head. J Comp Neurol 1996;375:238–51.
11. Morgan JE, Jeffery G, Foss AJ. Axon deviation in the human lamina cribrosa. Br J Ophthalmol 1998;82:680–3.
12. Quigley HA, Addicks EM. Regional differences in the structure of the lamina cribrosa and their relation to glaucomatous optic nerve damage. Arch Ophthalmol 1981;99:137–43.
13. Radius RL. Regional specificity in anatomy at the lamina cribrosa. Arch Ophthalmol 1981;99:478–80.
14. Quigley HA, Green WR. The histology of human glaucoma cupping and optic nerve damage: clinicopathologic correlation in 21 eyes. Ophthalmology 1979;86:1803–30.
15. Maumenee A. Visual field loss in glaucoma. In: Cairns JE, New Orleans Academy of Ophthalmology, eds. Symposium on Glaucoma : transactions of the New Orleans Academy of Ophthalmology. St. Louis: Mosby, 1981.

16. Flammer J, Orgul S. Optic nerve blood-flow abnormalities in glaucoma. Prog Retin Eye Res 1998;17:267–89.

17. Hernandez MR, Igoe F, Neufeld AH. Extracellular matrix of the human optic nerve head. Am J Ophthalmol 1986;102:139–48.

18. Hernandez MR, Luo XX, Igoe F, Neufeld AH. Extracellular matrix of the human lamina cribrosa. Am J Ophthalmol 1987;104:567–76.

19. Hernandez MR, Luo XX, Andrzejewska W, Neufeld AH. Age-related changes in the extracellular matrix of the human optic nerve head. Am J Ophthalmol 1989;107:476–84.

20. Morrison JC, Jerdan JA, L'Hernault NL, Quigley HA. The extracellular matrix composition of the monkey optic nerve head. Invest Ophthalmol Vis Sci 1988;29:1141–50.

21. Morrison JC, L'Hernault NL, Jerdan JA, Quigley HA. Ultrastructural location of extracellular matrix components in the optic nerve head. Arch Ophthalmol 1989;107:123–9.

22. Morrison JC, Dorman-Pease ME, Dunkelberger GR, Quigley HA. Optic nerve head extracellular matrix in primary optic atrophy and experimental glaucoma. Arch Ophthalmol 1990;108:1020–4.

23. Morrison JC, Jerdan JA, Dorman ME, Quigley HA. Structural proteins of the neonatal and adult lamina cribrosa. Arch Ophthalmol 1989;107:1220–4.

24. Hernandez MR. Ultrastructural immunocytochemical analysis of elastin in the human lamina cribrosa. Changes in elastic fibers in primary open-angle glaucoma. Invest Ophthalmol Vis Sci 1992;33:2891–903.

25. Morrison JC, Rask P, Johnson EC, Deppmeier L. Chondroitin sulfate proteoglycan distribution in the primate optic nerve head. Invest Ophthalmol Vis Sci 1994;35:838–45.

26. Lepore FE. The origin of pain in optic neuritis. Determinants of pain in 101 eyes with optic neuritis. Arch Neurol 1991;48:748–9.

27. Anderson DR, Hoyt WF. Ultrastructure of intraorbital portion of human and monkey optic nerve. Arch Ophthalmol 1969;82:506–30.

28. Butt AM, Ransom BR. Visualization of oligodendrocytes and astrocytes in the intact rat optic nerve by intracellular injection of lucifer yellow and horseradish peroxidase. Glia 1989;2:470–5.

29. Butt AM, Colquhoun K, Berry M. Confocal imaging of glial cells in the intact rat optic nerve. Glia 1994;10:315–22.

30. Hoyt WF, Luis O. Visual fiber anatomy in the infrageniculate pathway of the primate. Arch Ophthalmol 1962;68:94–106.

31. Hoyt WF. Anatomic considerations of arcuate scotomas associated with lesions of the optic nerve and chiasm. A Nauta axon degeneration study in the monkey. Bull Johns Hopkins Hosp 1962;111:57–71.

32. Hoyt WF, Luis O. The primate chiasm. Details of visual fiber organization studied by silver impregnation techniques. Arch Ophthalmol 1963;70:69–85.

33. Hoyt WF, Tudor RC. The course of parapapillary temporal retinal axons through the anterior optic nerve. A Nauta degeneration study in the primate. Arch Ophthalmol 1963;69:503–7.

34. Horton JC. Wilbrand's knee of the primate chiasm is an artifact of monocular enucleation. Trans Am Ophthalmol Soc. 1997; 95: 579–609.

35. Karanjia N, Jacobson DM. Compression of the prechiasmatic optic nerve produces a junctional scotoma. Am J Ophthalmol. 1999;128:256–258.

36. Hayreh SS. The 1994 Von Sallman Lecture. The optic nerve head circulation in health and disease. Exp Eye Res 1995;61:259–72.

37. Onda E, Cioffi GA, Bacon DR, Van Buskirk EM. Microvasculature of the human optic nerve. Am J Ophthalmol 1995;120:92–102.

38. Geijer C, Bill A. Effects of raised intraocular pressure on retinal, prelaminar, laminar, and retrolaminar optic nerve blood flow in monkeys. Invest Ophthalmol Vis Sci 1979;18: 1030–42.
39. Alm A, Bill A. Ocular and optic nerve blood flow at normal and increased intraocular pressures in monkeys (*Macaca irus*): a study with radioactively labelled microspheres including flow determinations in brain and some other tissues. Exp Eye Res 1973;15:15–29.
40. Alm A, Bill A. The oxygen supply to the retina. II. Effects of high intraocular pressure and of increased arterial carbon dioxide tension on uveal and retinal blood flow in cats. A study with radioactively labelled microspheres including flow determinations in brain and some other tissues. Acta Physiol Scand 1972;84:306–19.
41. Pillunat LE, Stodtmeister R, Wilmanns I, Christ T. Autoregulation of ocular blood flow during changes in intraocular pressure. Preliminary results. Graefes Arch Clin Exp Ophthalmol 1985;223:219–23.
42. Weinstein JM, Funsch D, Page RB, Brennan RW. Optic nerve blood flow and its regulation. Invest Ophthalmol Vis Sci 1982;23:640–5.
43. Weinstein JM, Duckrow RB, Beard D, Brennan RW. Regional optic nerve blood flow and its autoregulation. Invest Ophthalmol Vis Sci 1983;24:1559–65.
44. Quigley HA. The possibility of measuring blood flow in the optic nerve head in the live eye. Ophthalmology 1987;94:87–9.
45. Quigley HA, Hohman RM, Sanchez R, Addicks EM. Optic nerve head blood flow in chronic experimental glaucoma. Arch Ophthalmol 1985;103:956–62.
46. Pillunat LE, Anderson DR, Knighton RW, et al. Autoregulation of human optic nerve head circulation in response to increased intraocular pressure. Exp Eye Res 1997;64:737–44.
47. Grayson MC, Laties AM. Ocular localization of sodium fluorescein. Effects of administration in rabbit and monkey. Arch Ophthalmol 1971;85:600–3 passim.
48. Olsson Y, Kristensson K. Permeability of blood vessels and connective tissue sheaths in retina and optic nerve. Acta Neuropathol (Berl) 1973;26:147–56.
49. Tso MO, Shih CY, McLean IW. Is there a blood-brain barrier at the optic nerve head? Arch Ophthalmol 1975;93:815–25.
50. Anderson DR. Glaucoma, capillaries and pericytes. 1. Blood flow regulation. Ophthalmologica 1996;210:257–62.
51. Anderson DR, Davis EB. Glaucoma, capillaries and pericytes. 5. Preliminary evidence that carbon dioxide relaxes pericyte contractile tone. Ophthalmologica 1996;210:280–4.
52. Matsugi T, Chen Q, Anderson DR. Adenosine-induced relaxation of cultured bovine retinal pericytes. Invest Ophthalmol Vis Sci 1997; 38: 2695–701.
53. Schmetterer L, Polak K. Role of nitric oxide in the control of ocular blood flow. Prog Retin Eye Res 2001;20:823–47.
54. Cioffi GA, Orgul S, Onda E, et al. An in vivo model of chronic optic nerve ischemia: the dose-dependent effects of endothelin-1 on the optic nerve microvasculature. Curr Eye Res 1995;14:1147–53.
55. Chauhan BC, LeVatte TL, Jollimore CA, et al. Model of endothelin-1-induced chronic optic neuropathy in rat. Invest Ophthalmol Vis Sci 2004;45:144–52.
56. Shapley R. Visual sensitivity and parallel retinocortical channels. Annu Rev Psychol 1990;41:635–58.
57. Barron MJ, Griffiths P, Turnbull DM, et al. The distributions of mitochondria and sodium channels reflect the specific energy requirements and conduction properties of the human optic nerve head. Br J Ophthalmol 2004;88:286–90.

58. Andrews RM, Griffiths PG, Johnson MA, Turnbull DM. Histochemical localisation of mitochondrial enzyme activity in human optic nerve and retina. Br J Ophthalmol 1999; 83:231–5.

59. Grafstein B, Forman DS. Intracellular transport in neurons. Physiol Rev 1980;60:1167–283.

60. Schwartz JH. Axonal transport: components, mechanisms, and specificity. Annu Rev Neurosci 1979;2:467–504.

61. Vallee RB, Bloom GS. Mechanisms of fast and slow axonal transport. Annu Rev Neurosci 1991;14:59–92.

62. McQuarrie IG, Brady ST, Lasek RJ. Diversity in the axonal transport of structural proteins: major differences between optic and spinal axons in the rat. J Neurosci 1968;6: 1593–605.

63. Hoffman PN, Lasek RJ. The slow component of axonal transport. Identification of major structural polypeptides of the axon and their generality among mammalian neurons. J Cell Biol 1975;66:351–66.

64. Wang L, Ho CL, Sun D, et al. Rapid movement of axonal neurofilaments interrupted by prolonged pauses. Nat Cell Biol 2000;2:137–41.

65. Morgan JE. Circulation and axonal transport in the optic nerve. Eye 2004;18:1089–95.

66. Allen RD, Weiss DG, Hayden JH, et al. Gliding movement of and bidirectional transport along single native microtubules from squid axoplasm: evidence for an active role of microtubules in cytoplasmic transport. J Cell Biol 1985;100:1736–52.

67. Hirokawa N, Takemura R. Molecular motors and mechanisms of directional transport in neurons. Nat Rev Neurosci 2005;6:201–14.

68. Hirokawa N, Takemura R. Kinesin superfamily proteins and their various functions and dynamics. Exp Cell Res 2004;301:50–9.

69. Muresan V. One axon, many kinesins: What's the logic? J Neurocytol 2000;29:799–818.

70. Bridgman PC, Elkin LL. Axonal myosins. J Neurocytol 2000;29:831–41.

71. Vallee RB, Williams JC, Varma D, Barnhart LE. Dynein: an ancient motor protein involved in multiple modes of transport. J Neurobiol 2004;58:189–200.

72. Paschal BM, Vallee RB. Retrograde transport by the microtubule-associated protein MAP 1C. Nature 1987;330:181–3.

73. Susalka SJ, Pfister KK. Cytoplasmic dynein subunit heterogeneity: implications for axonal transport. J Neurocytol 2000;29:819–29.

74. Dillman JF III, Dabney LP, Pfister KK. Cytoplasmic dynein is associated with slow axonal transport. Proc Natl Acad Sci USA 1996;93:141–4.

75. Dillman JF III, Pfister KK. Differential phosphorylation in vivo of cytoplasmic dynein associated with anterogradely moving organelles. J Cell Biol 1994;127:1671–81.

76. Giuditta A, Kaplan BB, van Minnen J, et al. Axonal and presynaptic protein synthesis: new insights into the biology of the neuron. Trends Neurosci 2002;25:400–4.

77. Koenig E, Martin R, Titmus M, Sotelo-Silveira JR. Cryptic peripheral ribosomal domains distributed intermittently along mammalian myelinated axons. J Neurosci 2000; 20:8390–400.

78. Quigley HA, Anderson DR. Distribution of axonal transport blockade by acute intraocular pressure elevation in the primate optic nerve head. Invest Ophthalmol Vis Sci 1977;16: 640–4.

79. Quigley H, Anderson DR. The dynamics and location of axonal transport blockade by acute intraocular pressure elevation in primate optic nerve. Invest Ophthalmol 1976;15: 606–16.

80. Quigley HA, Flower RW, Addicks EM, McLeod DS. The mechanism of optic nerve damage in experimental acute intraocular pressure elevation. Invest Ophthalmol Vis Sci 1980;19:505–17.
81. Quigley HA, Guy J, Anderson DR. Blockade of rapid axonal transport. Effect of intraocular pressure elevation in primate optic nerve. Arch Ophthalmol 1979;97:525–31.
82. Minckler DS, Bunt AH, Johanson GW. Orthograde and retrograde axoplasmic transport during acute ocular hypertension in the monkey. Invest Ophthalmol Vis Sci 1977;16:426–41.
83. Gaasterland D, Tanishima T, Kuwabara T. Axoplasmic flow during chronic experimental glaucoma. 1. Light and electron microscopic studies of the monkey optic nerve head during development of glaucomatous cupping. Invest Ophthalmol Vis Sci 1978;17:838–46.
84. Quigley HA, Addicks EM. Chronic experimental glaucoma in primates. II. Effect of extended intraocular pressure elevation on optic nerve head and axonal transport. Invest Ophthalmol Vis Sci 1980;19:137–52.
85. Minckler DS, Spaeth GL. Optic nerve damage in glaucoma. Surv Ophthalmol 1981;26:128–48.
86. Quigley HA, Addicks EM, Green WR, Maumenee AE. Optic nerve damage in human glaucoma. II. The site of injury and susceptibility to damage. Arch Ophthalmol 1981;99:635–49.
87. Johnson EC, Deppmeier LM, Wentzien SK, et al. Chronology of optic nerve head and retinal responses to elevated intraocular pressure. Invest Ophthalmol Vis Sci 2000;41:431–42.
88. Pease ME, McKinnon SJ, Quigley HA, et al. Obstructed axonal transport of BDNF and its receptor TrkB in experimental glaucoma. Invest Ophthalmol Vis Sci 2000;41:764–74.
89. Martin KR, Quigley HA, Zack DJ, et al. Gene therapy with brain-derived neurotrophic factor as a protection: retinal ganglion cells in a rat glaucoma model. Invest Ophthalmol Vis Sci 2003;44:4357–65.
90. Minckler DS, Tso MO. Experimental papilledema produced by cyclocryotherapy. Am J Ophthalmol 1976;82:577–89.

2

Clinical Testing of Optic Nerve Function

LAWRENCE M. BUONO

Clinical testing of optic nerve function is a critical component of the ophthalmologic examination in determining the cause of visual loss. Characteristic features of an optic neuropathy include decreased visual acuity, visual field defect, decreased brightness sensation, relative afferent pupillary defect, and loss of color vision (acquired dyschromatopsia). This chapter focuses on relevant clinical tests used to assess the function of the optic nerve.

2-1 EVALUATION OF THE PATIENT

2-1-1 *History Taking.* Patients with optic nerve dysfunction typically present with complaints of diminished vision. The patient may sometimes be able to accurately describe the nature of the visual disturbance; more often, however, patients may describe only vague symptoms such as "something is wrong with my vision." Patients may not be aware of their visual loss and may report difficulty performing a task they were previously able to do. They may say that they bump into objects on one side or are having more difficulty driving. Often, patients with homonymous visual field loss localize the visual loss to the eye with the temporal hemianopic defect. Occasionally, patients are suddenly made aware of a monocular visual deficit that has been present for some time only after occluding the fellow eye. The history should help gather information defining the nature of the visual loss and assist with anatomic localization.

First, determine whether the visual loss is monocular or binocular. This information is critical to localization; therefore if the patient is not sure whether one or both eyes are affected, a cross-cover test to assess the vision in each eye should be performed before continuing with the history. Monocular visual loss localizes to structures of the eye and optic nerve. Binocular visual loss suggests disorders of the optic chiasm and retrochiasmal visual pathways.

Second, determine the onset and tempo of the visual loss. A sudden or acute onset is suggestive of vascular compromise, such as an ischemic optic neuropathy. Subacute visual decline over several days may be due to an inflammatory, infiltrative, or demyelinating cause. Gradual or slowly progressive visual loss occurring over weeks to months suggests a compressive optic neuropathy. Intermittent visual loss lasting seconds suggests transient visual obscurations due to papilledema, while intermittent visual loss lasting seconds to minutes may be due to embolic disease of the retinal circulation.

The third step is to inquire about associated symptoms and signs. Pain with eye movement is typical of optic neuritis. Headache, jaw claudication, scalp tenderness, weight loss, fever, or night sweats raises the suspicion of giant cell arteritis.

The fourth step is to perform a directed review of systems, including medication and family history. Much of this information may prove helpful in evaluating ischemic, toxic, and hereditary forms of optic nerve disease. History taking is an interactive, searching, and adaptive process, which, if done carefully, yields valuable information. "The patient will often tell us what is wrong if we have the patience to listen and the background to ask the proper questions at the appropriate times."[1]

2-1-2 *Visual Acuity.* Although one of the first measurements made, Snellen acuity is perhaps the least sensitive of all functions routinely measured in detecting a disturbance in optic nerve function. It is possible, for instance, to measure 20/20 acuity in an eye that has had optic neuritis, with an afferent pupillary defect, reduced color vision, and a significant visual field defect. The resolving power of such an eye may be excellent but vastly different from that of the normal eye.

Despite these limitations, Snellen acuity is still useful, and how it is obtained is also of importance. Aside from controlling the obvious factors (optimal refraction, good light, proper correction for near vision), the manner in which the patient reads may give clues to the type of field defect. For example, a patient who misses all the letters on the left side of the chart may have a homonymous defect; if the patient omits temporal letters on each side, a bitemporal or central defect may be present.

2-1-3 *Visual Field.* Visual field testing is essential in assessing optic nerve function. Of particular importance is the central 30 degrees of the visual field. Within this region, at least 95% of significant neuro-ophthalmologic lesions will cause visual field defects.[2,3] Visual field defects due to optic nerve disease conform to a limited number of patterns. Typically, disorders of the optic nerve may depress the function of fibers within the central core of the nerve (papillomacular bundle), leading to central, paracentral, pericentral, and centrocecal defects. The other major pattern of field loss also confroms to damage to the retinal nerve fiber bundle, and—depending on the pattern of damage—may result in generalized depression as well as altitudinal and arcuate defects. Visual field defects from optic nerve disease respect the horizontal meridian, and visual field defects from disorders of the optic chiasm and retrochiasmal pathways respect the vertical meridian.

The testing of confrontation visual fields is a valuable way of screening for defects in the central visual field. A basic technique works best and helps avoid confusing results. The examiner should sit approximately 1 m from the patient. With one of the patient's eyes occluded, the examiner presents fingers in one of the four quadrants of the central 30 degrees and asks the patient to count the number of fingers. Next, the examiner repeats the process in each of the successive three quadrants. The entire process is then repeated for the fellow eye. The results are documented by shading the quadrants identified incorrectly. If all of the quadrants were correctly identified, the documentation is simply "full confrontation visual fields."

The Amsler grid can be utilized as an additional screening tool to test the central 10 degrees of the visual field. Again, one eye is occluded and the Amsler grid is held at 14 inches. The patient is asked to fixate on the central point and describe areas of metamorphopsia or scotoma. Patients should be instructed to avoid scanning the grid while making the assessment, and appropriate presbyopic correction should be used.

The tangent screen was an early method used to examine the central visual field. With the advent of the manual bowl perimeter (Goldmann), it became possible to accurately evaluate the entire visual field. Automated bowl perimetry (e.g., Humphrey) has largley supplanted manual perimtery because of improved standardization, sensitivity, and reproducibility. Ideally, the method for evaluating the visual field should be tailored to the age, cooperation level, and attention span of the patient.

2-1-4 *Color Vision.* Loss of color vision is often present in the setting of optic nerve dysfunction and may precede the loss of visual acuity or field. Acquired dyschromatopsia must be distinguished from congenital dyschromatopsia in this setting. Clinical testing of color vision can be performed by a variety of methods. The Farnsworth-Munsell 100-hue test is a comprehensive color vision test in which the patient must arrange 84 colored disks. This test can identify a particular type of dyschromatopsia and help distinguish acquired from congenital loss. However, it is time-consuming to perform, thus limiting its clinical usefulness. The Farnsworth Panel D-15 is an abbreviated version of this test but is less sensitive for detecting color deficiency.

Pseudoisochromatic color-plate tests such as the *Ishihara* or *Hardy-Rand-Rittler* (HRR) tests are designed to assess congenital dyschromatopsia but can be used clinically as a screening test for a gross estimation of acquired dyschromatopsia. The patient is asked to identify the color plates one eye at a time and the number correctly identified over the number tested is documented.

Color desaturation relies on a relative loss of color vision in one eye. A brightly colored red test object (mydriatic bottle top) works best. The patient is asked to compare the saturation of the color as perceived in each eye. Patients with acquired dyschromatopsia will say that the color in the affected eye appears "washed out," or they may say that the red color appears "orange" or "pink."

2-1-5 *Brightness Comparison.* Comparing the sensation of brightness of a light source can be a useful subjective test in assessing afferent function of the optic nerve. This test is complementary to pupillary testing and is most useful in the setting of monocular disease. The test is performed by shining a bright light into the normal eye while the fellow eye is occluded, The patient is then asked to assign a numerical value to the degree of brightness perceived. The process is repeated in the contralateral eye, and the patient is again asked to assign a numerical value to the degree of brightness perceived. For example, in a patient with a left optic neuropathy, the degree of brightness perceived in the right eye might be 100% as compared with 75% on the left.

2-1-6 *Pupillary Testing.* The swinging-flashlight test (Fig 2–1) and detection of a relative afferent pupillary defect (RAPD) are important clinical tests of optic nerve function. Only one reactive pupil is required to detect a RAPD. The patient should fixate on a distant object (to avoid accommodation) and maintain his or her gaze during the test; the examiner should not obstruct the line of sight. The examiner should observe the pupil being directly stimulated and note the initial constriction, usually followed by a small amount of dilation (hippus). On swinging the light to the other side, the examiner should note a similar brisk constriction and dilation if the pupil is normal. A pupil with a RAPD will not react as briskly; after a weak initial constriction, it will dilate or "escape." Some experimentation with the movement, speed, and duration of the light stimulus is necessary to optimize the response. It is important to use a bright light, such as a bright penlight or the indirect ophthalmoscope. A RAPD is not typically seen with visual loss from other causes (e.g., cataract, corneal scarring, or macular degeneration). This pupillary abnormality is the single best objective test of optic nerve dysfunction. Neutral density filters (NDF) can be utilized to quantify the size of a RAPD and for following the degree of a RAPD over time. Additionally, NDF can be useful in detecting the presence of a small RAPD that may be difficult to detect otherwise (Fig. 2–2).[4]

2-1-7 *Photostress Recovery Test.* The photostress recovery test helps to distinguish visual loss caused by macular disease from that due to an optic neuropathy. The objective of the test is to determine the time required for recovery of photoreceptor function after exposure to a bright light. Initially the patient's best corrected visual acuity is obtained. The patient is asked to stare for 10 seconds at a bright light (the indirect ophthalmoscope) held approximately 2 cm from the eye. The number of seconds needed for the patient to recover the ability to read the same line or one line larger is recorded. The test is performed in one eye at a time with the fellow eye occluded. With an optic neuropathy, the time for recovery of vision is typically less than 60 seconds. However, with a maculopathy, the time for recovery of vision may be markedly prolonged, often to more than 90 seconds. This test is most reliable if the baseline visual acuity is 20/80 or better.[5]

2-1-8 *Contrast Sensitivity.* Resolution of contrast in the central area of the field, first by the standard optotypes used in measuring acuity and then by means of contrast sensitivity, provides another avenue for testing optic nerve function. Gradings or figures with a spectrum of spatial and temporal frequencies are presented to the patient. Contrast sensitivity is a broader test of visual function than is visual acuity, which measures spatial resolution only at high contrast. Thus, contrast-sensi-

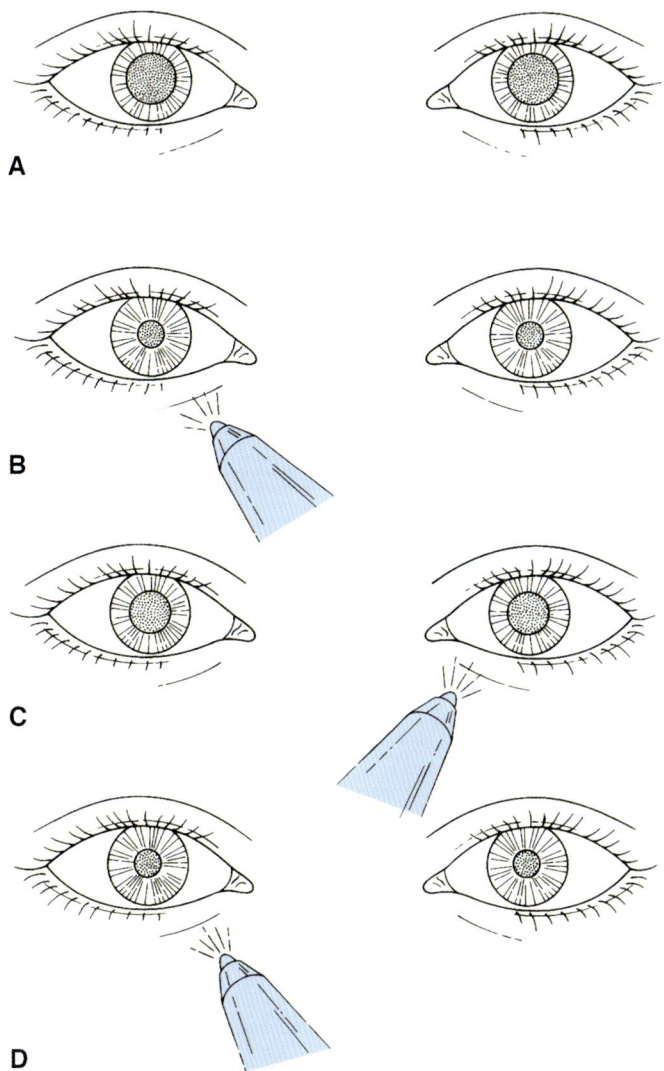

Figure 2–1. Relative afferent pupillary defect in left eye determined by swinging-flashlight test. (A) Pupils are equal in size in dim illumination. (B) When light is shined in right eye, pupils constrict. (C) However, when light is shined in left eye, both pupils dilate. (D) When light is swung back to right eye, both pupils again constrict.

tivity thresholds at various frequencies may be depressed in optic nerve disease despite normal visual acuity.[6] However, resolution of contrast is also affected by changes in ocular media and by macular disease. This lack of specificity has limited the role of this test in disorders of the optic nerve.

2-1-9 *Ophthalmoscopy.* Careful ophthalmoscopy is an essential part of evaluating the optic nerve. The clinician should assess the color, size, shape, contour, and extent of cupping of the optic nerve head, along with the clarity and quantity of the nerve fibers emanating from its borders. Careful inspection of the optic disc and adja-

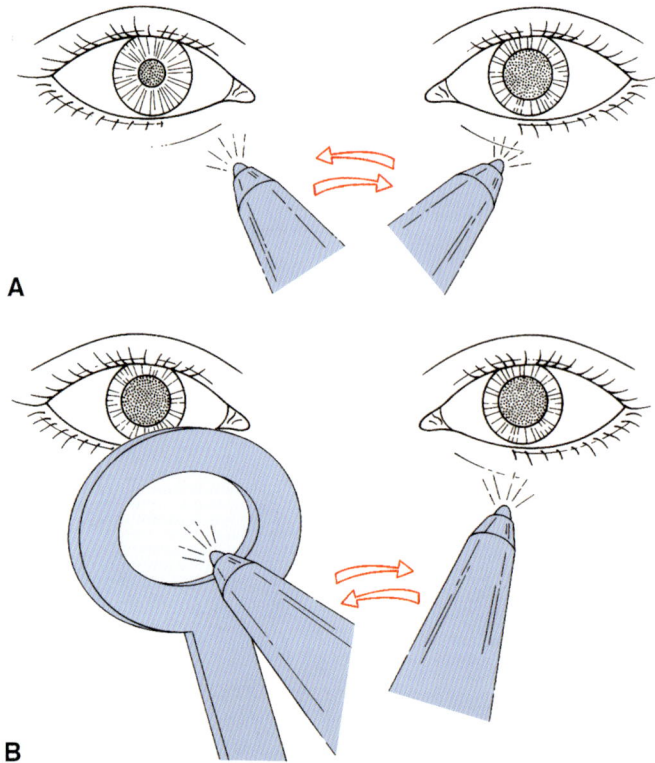

Figure 2–2. (A) Afferent pupillary defect in left eye is present when, during swinging-light ma-neuver, left pupil dilates and right pupil constricts. (B) After afferent pupillary defect is found by swinging-light technique, filter is placed before normal eye. By choosing appropriate amount of filter, examiner can neutralize afferent pupillary defect so that pupils constrict equally and reach the same final resting size.

cent nerve fiber layer requires use of an ophthalmoscope (direct, indirect) or a biomi-croscope coupled with an appropriate examining lens (contact, Hruby, 60, 78, or 90 diopters). Stereo photographs are also helpful for detailed study, with red-free and color slides. This last method is especially important in the fourth dimension of viewing optic nerve changes over time.

2-1-10 *Electrophysiology*. There are several methods of obtaining objective evidence of optic nerve function; these depend, for the most part, on electrophysiology. The visual evoked potential (VEP) compares visual impulse transmission along each optic nerve. Measurement of the latency of a major positive waveform produced at ap-proximately 100 milliseconds is used to assess optic nerve conduction. Limitations of pattern-reversal visual potentials are imposed by the need for accurate fixation, sharp imagery on the retina, and cooperation from the patient.[7] Pupillography can be used to measure pupillary responses, and a pupillographic swinging-light test is available in some centers for measuring afferent pupillary defects. While electrore-tinography measures the integrity of the outer retinal layers, pattern electroretin-ography is derived from the inner retinal layers, including the ganglion cells. This test may provide evidence of optic nerve dysfunction, particularly that due to involvement of inner retinal fiber projections.[8]

2-1-11 *Imaging Studies.* Current imaging techniques, including computed tomography (CT) and magnetic resonance imaging (MRI), provide detailed information of disease processes within the central nervous system. The neuro-ophthalmologist plays a critical role in detecting and interpreting clinical signs and correlating these findings with neuroimaging studies. For example, optic nerve enlargement, seen with CT or MRI, may be due to a variety of conditions, including optic neuritis, papilledema, or optic nerve neoplasm. Yet each of these entities is associated with different historical details and examination findings, and the clinician must correlate this information to arrive at the correct diagnosis.

Ultrasonography can supplement CT and MRI. One such example is enlargement of the orbital segment of the optic nerve. By measuring the thickness of the nerve and sheath as the nerve is put on stretch in lateral gaze ("30-degree test"), ultrasound can help distinguish fluid within the sheath from a solid mass within the nerve.[9] In addition, B-scan echography is a quick and sensitive method to detect optic disc drusen. Ultrasonographic techniques, which can detect blood flow into and out of the back of the eye, may be important in identifying circulatory disease of the eye and optic nerve.[10]

Color Doppler imaging is a noninvasive technique that allows for simultaneous two-dimensional structural imaging and Doppler evaluation of blood flow. Blood flow can be identified in the ophthalmic, central retinal, nasal, and temporal ciliary arteries and in the central retinal vein (Fig. 2–3).

2-2 ASSESSMENT OF THE FINDINGS

The value of the astute examiner lies in correlating the patient's history with the clinical findings. The clinician must be cautious in interpreting test results, remembering that most tests depend on the subjective responses of the patient. In optic nerve disease, the diagnosis may remain uncertain despite many clinical examinations and multiple ancillary studies. Patients in these circumstances are subject to the suggestions of previous examiners, to their own worries, and the concern generated by not knowing what is causing the trouble. The physician must also be alert to the patient who may have some secondary gain, either of a subconscious or monetary or legal nature, from a specific diagnosis. The clinician should be prepared to give the patient with functional visual loss a gentle way out if the symptoms do not fit the findings, because the findings may have been reinforced by the insecurity of other examiners. The patient may merely have been giving the answers expected by the examiners, so that the loss of function may actually have an iatrogenic component. This type of visual loss is more often seen with hysteria or malingering, but the symptoms are as real as those caused by optic atrophy.

Most of the time, optic nerve disorders are easy to localize because of the constellation of findings: decreased visual acuity, relative afferent pupillary defect,

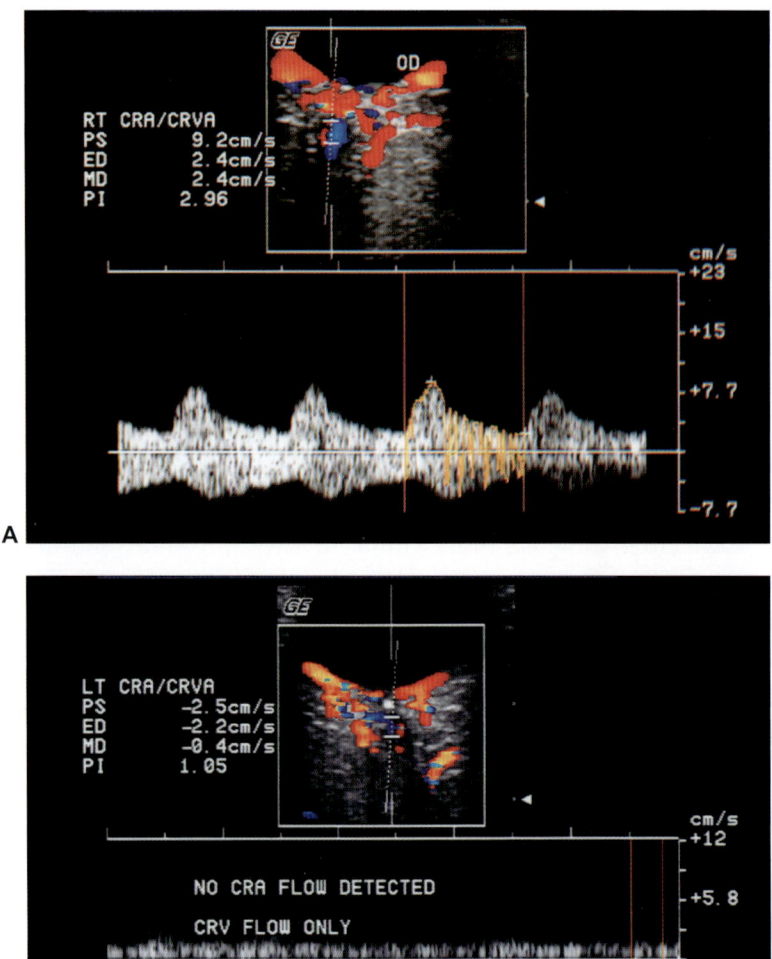

Figure 2–3. Color Doppler spectrum. (A) Normal perfusion through the central artery and vein. Red color indicates normal arterial flow in the ultrasonogram, while normal peak systolic velocity is demonstrated graphically above the x axis for the central retinal artery and below the x axis for the central retinal vein. (B) After central retinal artery occlusion, arterial flow is no longer detected on ultrasonogram or by Doppler analysis. (Courtesy of Robert C. Sergott, MD.)

diminished color vision, abnormal visual field, and altered appearance of the optic disc. Combining these with the patient's age, ocular and medical history, and concomitant illnesses, the clinician may establish the cause. In some instances, further diagnostic studies may be necessary to delineate the probable cause. In others, little hard evidence of optic nerve disease may be found; it may then be reasonable to let some time pass, because a change (either for the worse or for the better) may shed light on the cause. Even if no change occurs over time, the nonprogressive nature of the disorder may be reassuring.

2-2-1 *Clinical Examples.* The following clinical examples have particular teaching value in the assessment of optic nerve function as well as in methods of management.

2-2-1-1 *Optic Disc Drusen.* A 42-year-old woman was referred with the diagnosis of swollen optic nerves and a possible brain tumor. She reported a long history of headaches and poor side vision. She had 20/20 vision in both eyes and constricted visual fields. Funduscopic examination of the optic nerves revealed optic disc drusen with diffuse loss of the retinal nerve fiber layer and optic nerve pallor (Fig. 2–4A). The disc drusen were confirmed by reviewing her previously performed CT scan (Fig. 2–4B). She had pseudopapilledema from optic disc

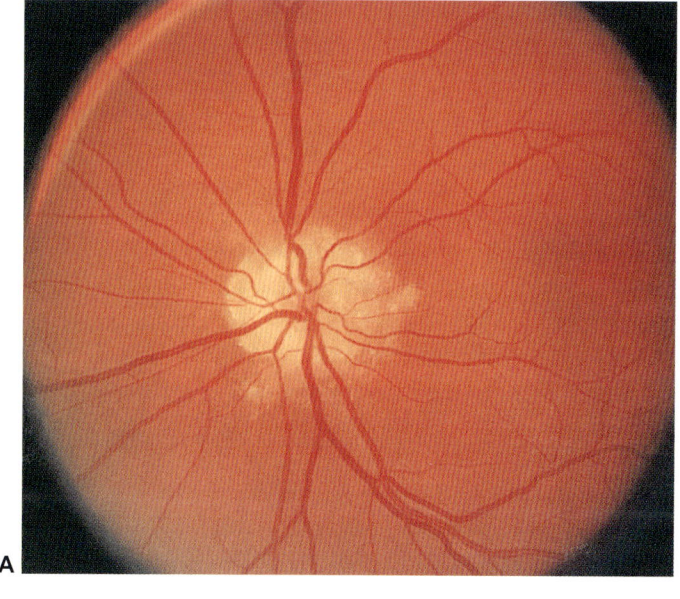

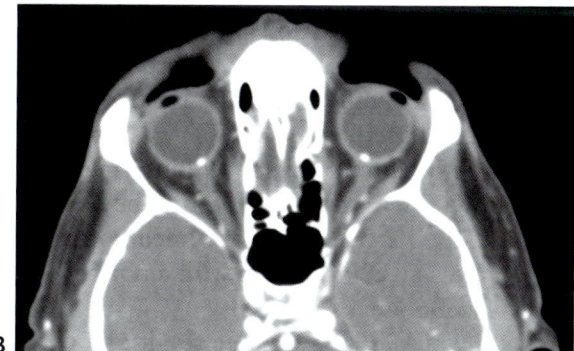

Figure 2–4. Optic disc drusen. (A) Fundus photograph shows drusen, loss of nerve fiber substance, and optic atrophy. Visual acuity is still normal at 20/20, but fields are constricted. (B) Cranial CT scan. Hyperradiodensity at junction of optic nerve and globe in each eye is due to calcified drusen.

drusen, and no further neuroimaging or surgery were warranted. Annual fundus-copic examination was planned to monitor for the development of juxtapapillary choroidal neovascularization.

2-2-1-2 *Optociliary Shunt Vessels.* A 42-year-old man presented with decreased vision in the left eye. He reported that his vision had been worsening slowly over the past several years. He did not have any associated symptoms. His visual acuity was 20/20 OD and 20/100 OS. Color vision was normal OD and absent OS. He had a relative afferent pupillary defect OS. Humphrey visual field testing was normal OD and generally depressed OS. The funduscopic examination showed a normal optic disc OD and diffuse optic nerve pallor with mild swelling of the nerve fiber layer and optociliary shunt vessels (Fig. 2–5A). Optic nerve compression was suspected and an MRI scan confirmed the presence of a meningioma of the optic nerve sheath (Fig. 2–5B). The patient was observed for more than 2 years without progression of visual loss. This case represents the classic presentation and fundu-scopic appearance of an optic nerve sheath meningioma.

2-2-1-3 *Optic Atrophy.* A 52-year-old man who had experienced meningitis earlier in life reported that his vision had never been "quite right" since this illness. He had been thoroughly investigated with neuroimaging and cerebral angiography, and all studies were unremarkable. His optic nerves were pale (Fig. 2–6), and his visual fields showed optic nerve–type defects (Fig. 2–7). For many years, his visual fields remained stable and he had no further loss of vision. The probable cause of his visual loss was either optic neuritis or chiasmatic arachnoiditis secondary to meningitis. It seemed unreasonable to subject him to further studies because his visual function remained stable and his neurologic function remained normal for 15 years.

2-2-1-4 *Functional Visual Loss.* An 11-year-old boy failed a vision screening test at school. He had recently complained of headaches and reported difficulty in "seeing things." He was an only child whose parents had recently divorced. Visual acuity could not be corrected beyond 20/400 OU, and the patient denied seeing any of the Ishihara color plates with either eye. Pupillary reactions, extraocular movements, slit-lamp examination, and fundus investigation yielded normal results. Visual fields were moderately constricted bilaterally. His pediatrician obtained a CT scan of the brain, which was normal. A pattern-reversal VEP was obtained and found to be normal (Fig. 2–8). The child and his parents were informed that the results of all studies were normal. During 2 months of follow-up, the boy's visual acuity spontaneously improved to 20/20 OU. The VEP confirmed normal function of the anterior visual pathway and this, in combination with a normal clinical examination, obviated the need for further testing.

In this patient, functional visual loss was the result of a conversion reaction to the stress in his life. The disproportionate decrease in visual acuity compared to objective findings on clinical examination was the clue to the diagnosis. A firm diagnosis early in the course eliminated continued reinforcement of symptoms by the troubled patient, his parents, and uncertain clinicians.

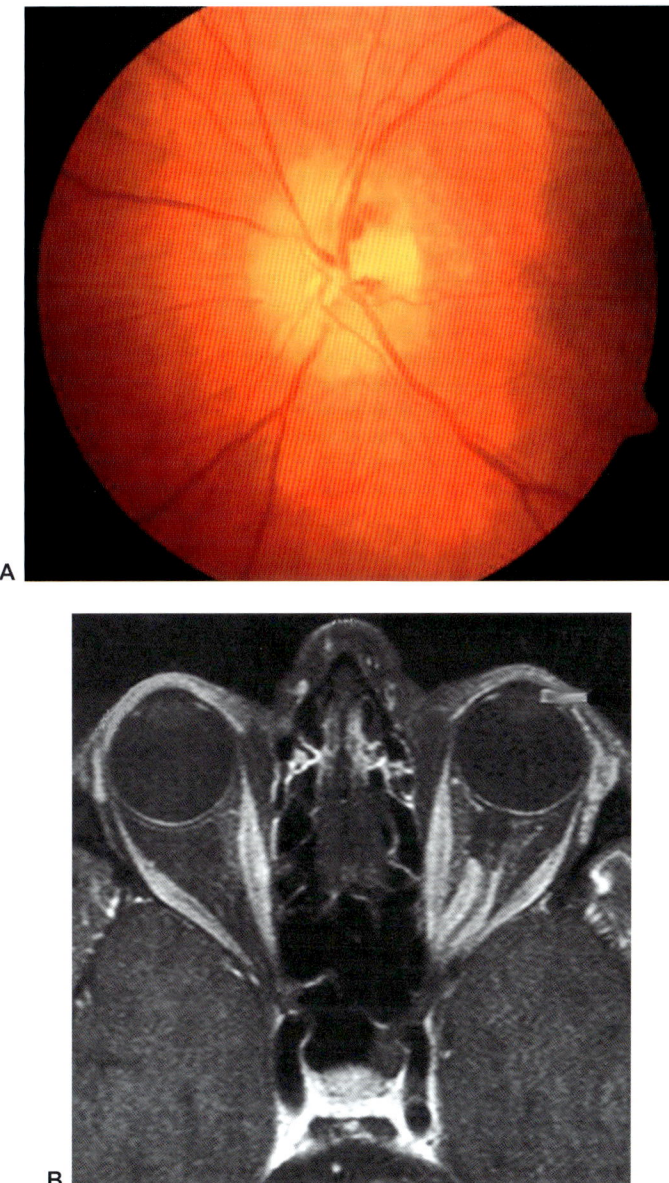

Figure 2–5. Optociliary shunt vessels. (A) Fundus photograph of the left eye shows diffuse optic nerve pallor with mild swelling of the nerve fiber layer and optic disc with optochoroidal shunt vessels. (B) Orbital MRI scan. Axial section shows an area of hyperintensity surrounding the left optic nerve adjacent to the optic canal, representing optic nerve sheath meningioma.

2-2-1-5 *Optic Neuritis.* A 23-year-old woman was referred because of severe loss of vision in her right eye, which had begun 1 week earlier. She had pain with eye movement, especially on upgaze. Her vision was light perception in the right eye and 20/15 in the left eye. She had a right relative afferent pupillary defect and mild swelling of the optic disc in the same eye (Fig. 2–9). She had no history of eye problems or neurologic disease. An MRI scan with gadolinium of the brain and orbits

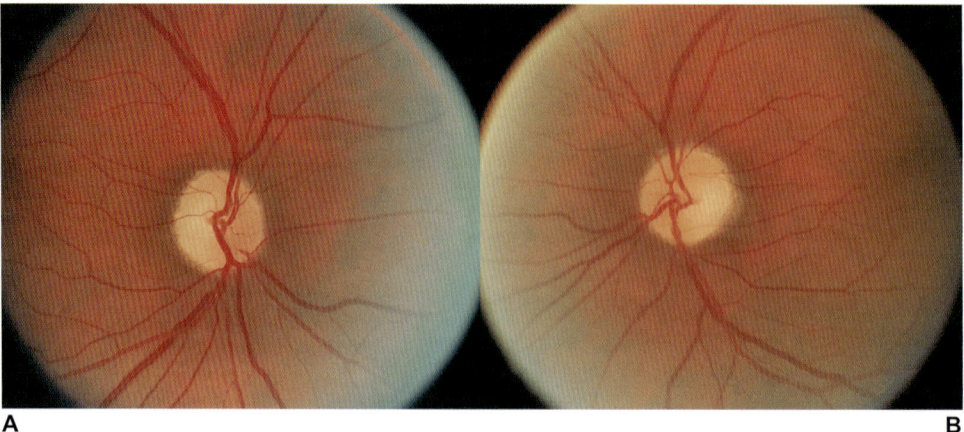

A   B

Figure 2–6. Optic atrophy. (A) Right eye. (B) Left eye. Showed no change over a follow-up period of 12 years.

was obtained, which showed enhancement of the right optic nerve and no other abnormalities. She began to recover vision in the right eye approximately 2 weeks later, and her visual deficit resolved completely by 6 months.

In this patient, optic neuritis was most likely caused by demyelination, and she is at increased risk for the development of multiple sclerosis. This patient should be followed closely for the development of a second demyelinating event, and a surveilance MRI scan may be performed at some point in the future.

2-2-1-6 *Craniopharyngioma*. A 48-year-old woman had noted dizziness and blurred vision in both eyes postoperatively after laser in situ keratomileusis (LASIK) sur-

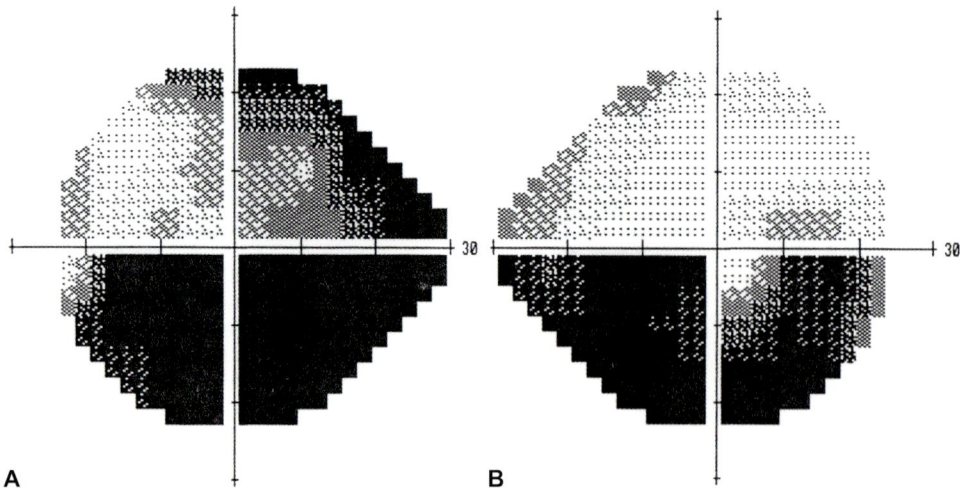

A   B

Figure 2–7. Automated visual fields of patient in Figure 2–6. (A) Left eye. (B) Right eye. Gray scales show optic nerve–type defects. Visual acuity has been stable at 20/30 in the right eye and 20/400 in the left eye.

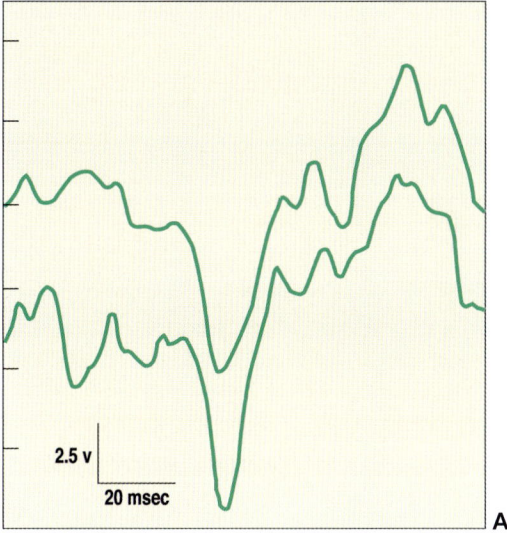

2.5 v

20 msec

A

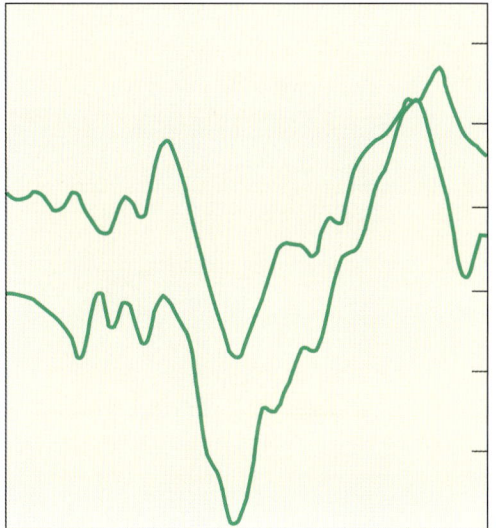

B

Figure 2–8. Functional visual loss. Pattern-reversal VEP demonstrates intact waveforms with latencies within normal limits. (A) Right eye, 103 milliseconds; (B) left eye, 106 milliseconds.

gery. The corneal flaps appeared to be distorted, and she was fitted with rigid gas-permeable contact lenses. These, however, failed to improve her vision. She was thought to have functional visual loss and was referred to neuro-ophthalmology for further evaluation. Her best corrected visual acuity was 20/30 on the right and 20/40 on the left. She correctly identifed all of the Ishihara pseudoisochromatic color plates with both eyes. She had red desaturation across fixation in the temporal hemifields in both eyes. Her pupils were normal, without a relative afferent pupillary defect. Her confrontation visual fields were normal bilaterally. Automated perimetry showed bilateral inferotemporal defects (Fig. 2–10A,B). An MRI scan showed chiasmal compression from a craniopharyngioma (Fig. 2–10C,D). She underwent tumor resection, with postoperative improvement of her visual acuity and visual fields.

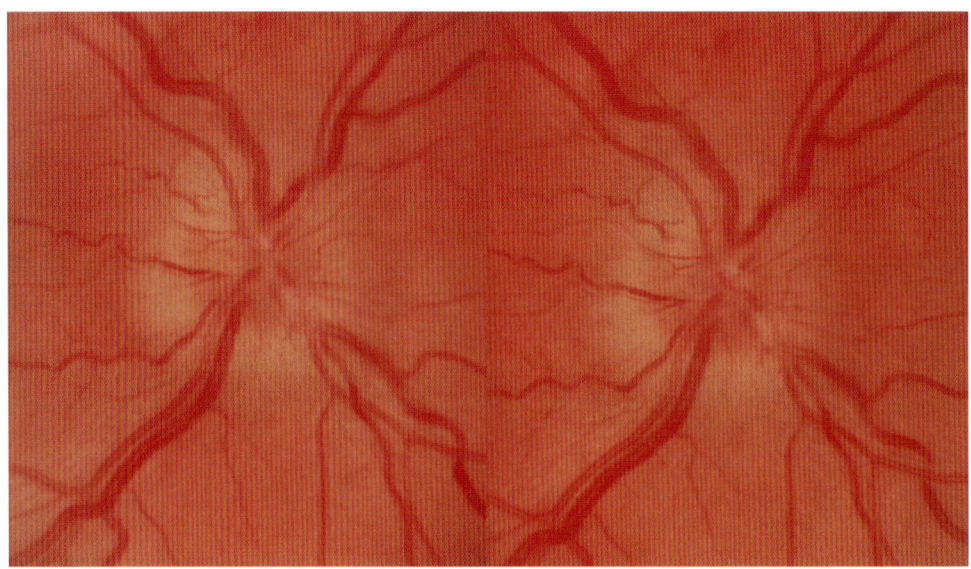

Figure 2–9. Optic neuritis. Stereo photographs showing swelling of right optic nerve head. These photos are best viewed by using the free stereo technique of crossing the eyes and fusing the central image.

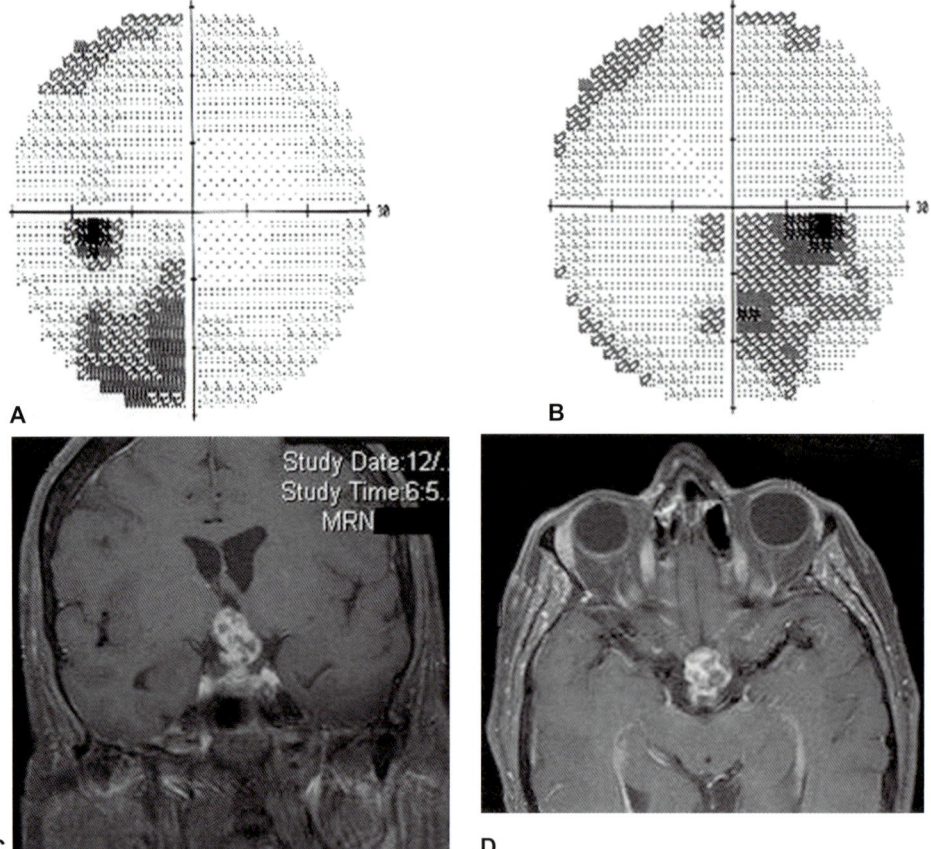

Figure 2–10. Craniopharyngioma. Humphrey visual field: (A) OS and (B) OD, showing subtle bilateral inferotemporal visual field defects consistent with chiasmal compression. (C) Cranial MRI scan, coronal section, showing a heterogeneous space-occupying mass in the sellar region (D) Cranial MRI scan, axial section, again showing a space-occupying mass lesion in the sellar region, most consistent with a craniopharyngioma.

References

1. Glaser J. Neuro-Ophthalmology. Hagerstown, MD: Harper & Row, 1978; 3–4.

2. Wirtschafter JD, Hard-Boberg AL, Coffman SM: Evaluating the usefulness in neuro-oph-thalmology of visual field examinations peripheral to 30 degrees. Trans Am Ophthalmol Soc 1984; 82:329–57.

3. Blum FG Jr., Gates LK, James BR: How important are peripheral fields? AMA Arch Ophthalmol 1959;61:1–8.

4. Fineberg ET. Quantification of the afferent pupillary defect. In: JL. S, ed. Neuro-ophthamology Focus. New York: Masson, 1979.

5. Glaser JS, Savino PJ, Sumers KD, et al. The photostress recovery test in the clinical assessment of visual function. Am J Ophthalmol 1977;83:255–60.

6. Mannis MZ, Johnson CA. Contrast sensitivity: a viewpoint for clinicians. In: Nadler MM, D. Nadler DJ., eds. Glare and Contrast Sensitivity for Clinicians. New York: Springer-Verlag, 1990.

7. Bumgartner J, Epstein CM. Voluntary alteration of visual evoked potentials. Ann Neurol 1982;12:475–8.

8. Nesher R, Trick GL. The pattern electroretinogram in retinal and optic nerve disease. A quantitative comparison of the pattern of visual dysfunction. Doc Ophthalmol 1991; 77:225–35.

9. Byrne SG. Ultrasound of the Eye and Orbit. St. Louis: Mosby–Year Book, 1992.

10. Aburn NS, Sergott RC. Orbital colour Doppler imaging. Eye 1993;7:639–47.

3

Papilledema

ROD FOROOZAN AND LANNING B. KLINE

The term *papilledema* has been applied to any type of swelling of the optic disc, with or without visual loss or other signs of optic neuropathy. However, most neuro-ophthalmologists reserve *papilledema* for optic disc swelling due to increased intracranial pressure and designate *optic disc edema* as a more general term to describe other forms of acquired disc swelling. Some of these forms may be further specified with respect to presumed causation; for example, anterior ischemic optic neuropathy (vascular infarction) or papillitis (demyelination or idiopathic inflammation). Throughout this chapter, *papilledema* is used only to describe optic disc swelling associated with elevated intracranial pressure.

3-1 PATHOGENESIS OF PAPILLEDEMA

The precise pathogenesis of papilledema remains unclear. The animal model of using inflatable balloons in the subarachnoid space of the monkey has furthered the understanding of papilledema dramatically.[1] After radioactive-labeled amino acids were injected into the vitreous cavity, the accumulation of both fast and slow components of axonal transport in the region of the lamina cribrosa was studied (Fig. 3–1). This accumulation of axoplasm results in the axonal swelling seen with electron microscopy. Nerve fibers within the optic nerve are compressed by elevated cerebrospinal fluid pressure in the subarachnoid space of the intraorbital portion of the optic nerve. The resultant axoplasmic stasis is seen ophthalmoscopically as optic disc swelling. Venous obstruction and dilation, hypoxia of the nerve fiber layer, and vascular telangiectasias of the optic discs are secondary events.

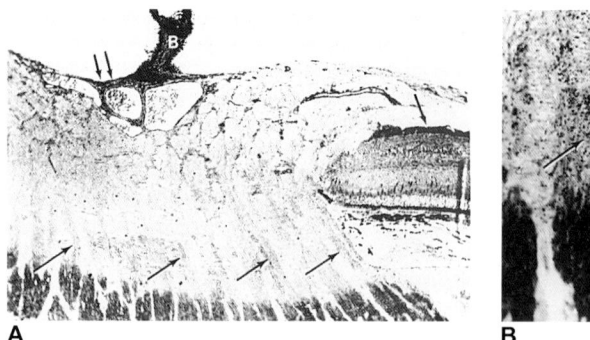 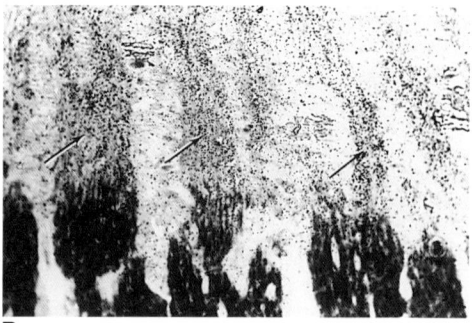

Figure 3–1. Papilledema secondary to elevated intracranial pressure. (A) Autoradiograph of optic nerve head of rhesus monkey. Eye was enucleated 6 h after intravitreous injection of tritiated leucine. Silver grains have accumulated in the retinal ganglion cells (single black arrow). Supporting meniscus tissue of Kuhnt (double black arrows). Bergmeister papilla (B). Perivascular glial tissue and axonal bundles in region of lamina choroidalis and lamina scleralis (black and white arrows). (Paraphenylenediamine, original magnification 80X.) (B) Lamina choroidalis and lamina scleralis under higher magnification. Silver grains have accumulated in axonal bundles (arrows). Few grains are present over connective tissue septa separating axonal bundles. (Paraphenylenediamine, original magnification 300X.)(Reproduced with permission from Tso MO, Hayreh SS. Optic disc edema in raised intracranial pressure: IV. Axoplasmic transport in experimental papilledema. Arch Ophthalmol 1977;95:1458–62. Copyright 1977, American Medical Association.)

3-1-1 *Ophthalmoscopic Findings.* In most patients, papilledema is bilateral and approximately equal in the two eyes. In some patients, papilledema may be asymmetric and rarely unilateral. Most patients with "unilateral" disc swelling in the setting of increased intracranial pressure actually have bilateral but asymmetric papilledema. Careful attention must be given to the "normal" disc in order to detect the early, subtle changes of papilledema. Table 3–1 summarizes the ophthalmoscopic findings of papilledema.

Bona fide unilateral papilledema may be due to a variety of mechanisms. Previous optic atrophy or a dysplastic disc are two possibilities. If there are not enough viable nerve fibers to swell (i.e., optic atrophy), papilledema cannot occur. When unilateral papilledema does occur in a patient with a truly normal disc on the opposite side, a congenital anomaly of the nerve sheaths may be suspected on the side where the papilledema is absent.

Table 3–1 Ophthalmoscopic Features of Papilledema

 1. Bilateral disc edema—may be asymmetric; rarely unilateral
 2. Opacification of peripapillary nerve fiber layer
 3. Hyperemia of disc
 4. Loss of spontaneous venous pulsations
 5. Venous distension
 6. Hemorrhages
 7. Exudates
 8. Cotton-wool spots
 9. Circumferential retinal folds (Paton's lines)—peripapillary region
10. Obliterated central cup—late finding

An increasing number of techniques have been used to study the retinal nerve fiber layer in patients with papilledema (Fig. 3–2), but thus far none has been proven to be a better predictor than ophthalmoscopy.[2]

3-2 CLASSIFICATION OF PAPILLEDEMA

Clinically, it is often helpful to stage papilledema ophthalmoscopically. As suggested by Hughlings Jackson in 1871, papilledema may be classified as (1) early, (2) fully developed, (3) chronic, and (4) atrophic.[3]

3-2-1 *Early Papilledema*. The early phase of papilledema is that during which incipient disc changes occur before the development of obvious disc swelling. Opacification of the peripapillary nerve fiber layer, leading to obscuration of the superior and inferior disc margins, is an early change that may precede venous engorgement (Fig. 3–3). Use of the red-free (green) filter in the ophthalmoscope may further delineate these early changes in the nerve fiber layer. Disc hyperemia, another early sign of papilledema, develops as a result of the dilation of capillaries on the disc surface (Fig. 3–4). The presence of a small hemorrhage in the nerve fiber layer may be a very important sign of early papilledema. These hemorrhages usually appear as thin radial streaks on the disc or near its margin and are due to the rupture of distended capillaries within or surrounding the disc.

The absence of spontaneous retinal venous pulsations has been described as an early sign of papilledema. According to several authorities, pulsations cease when intracranial pressure exceeds 200 ± 25 mm H_2O.[4,5] However, fluctuations in intracranial pressure occur, particularly in patients with elevated intracranial pressure. Thus, a patient with elevated intracranial pressure may be observed during a period of transient decrease in intracranial pressure and noted to have spontaneous venous pulsations. Furthermore, spontaneous venous pulsations occur in only 80% of eyes in normal subjects,[6] so that 20% of patients without increased intracranial pressure have no spontaneous venous pulsations. Therefore the absence of spontaneous venous pulsations does not necessarily indicate the presence of papilledema, and the presence of spontaneous venous pulsations indicates only that the intracranial pressure is below 200 mm H_2O at that point in time.[7]

The diagnosis of early papilledema cannot be made on the basis of a single ophthalmoscopic finding. Multiple factors should be looked for, and at times serial observations are required to ensure a correct diagnosis.

3-2-2 *Fully Developed Papilledema*. With fully developed papilledema, the surface of the disc lies above the plane of the retina. Swelling of the nerve fiber layer obscures the disc margins, with small and large vessels buried as they course off the disc (Fig. 3–5). At this stage, papilledema is usually accompanied by flame-shaped hemorrhages and infarcts, called cotton-wool spots, of the nerve fiber layer (Fig. 3–6). Circumferential retinal folds, known as Paton's lines, may be observed due to lateral displacement of the retina (Fig. 3–7). Exudates and hemorrhages may occur in the macula and, because of the radial fan-shaped arrangement of the papillomacular nerve fibers,

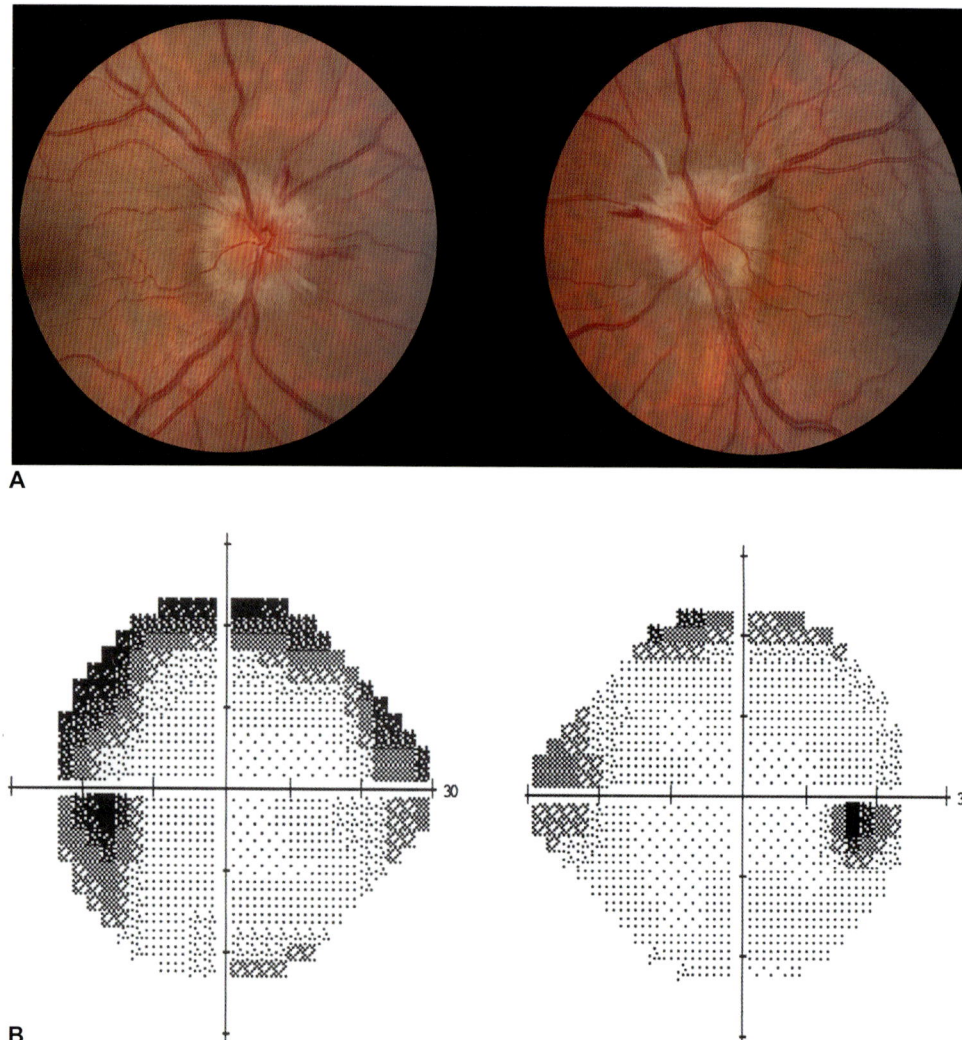

Figure 3–2. Elevation of the retinal nerve fiber layer in papilledema. (A) Papilledema with hemorrhages and cotton-wool spots within the retinal nerve fiber layer. (B) Automated perimetry shows nerve fiber bundle defects on each side. (C) (On facing page) Optical coherence tomography (OCT) measures reflected laser light within the eye. The measures of reflected light correlate with retinal thickness, including the thickness of the retinal nerve fiber layer, with the normal retinal nerve fiber layer thickest superiorly and inferiorly along the optic disc (see also Chapter 1, section 1–1). Normal retinal thickness for 95% of age-matched subjects is represented by the shaded green area. This OCT shows elevation of the retinal nerve fiber layer on each side (ar-

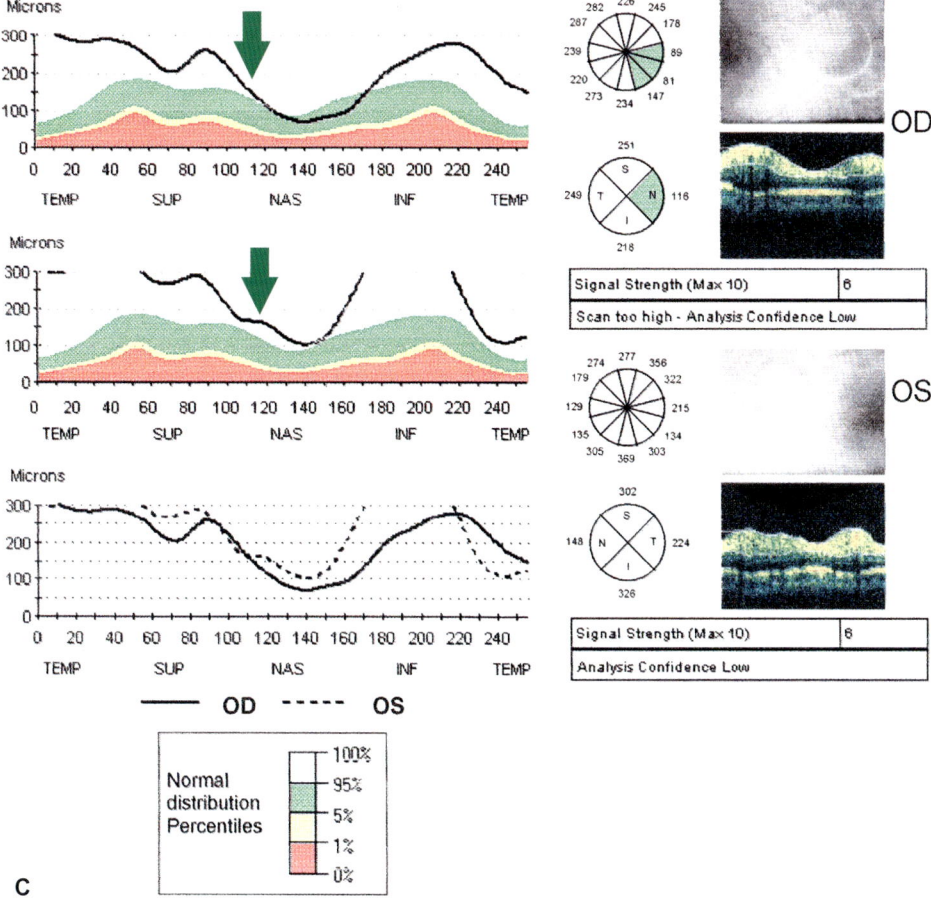

C

Figure 3–2 (continued)

these hemorrhages and exudates may take on a star shape (macular star). In some patients, if the rise in intracranial pressure has been rapid, subhyaloid hemorrhages may be present and blood may extend into the vitreous. Multiple posterior pole hemorrhages may be seen; these phenomena are believed to represent compromise of the central retinal vein due to edema of the optic disc.[8] Other rare associations described with papilledema include choroidal folds[9] and peripheral retinal hemorrhages.[10]

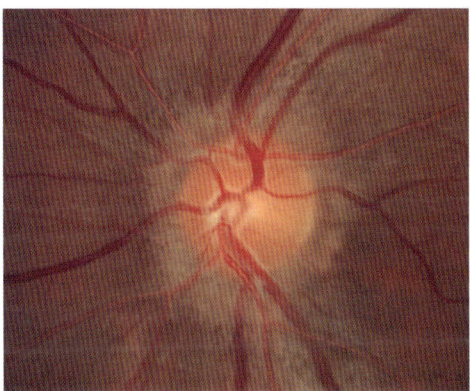

Figure 3–3. Opacification of the peripapillary nerve fiber layer.

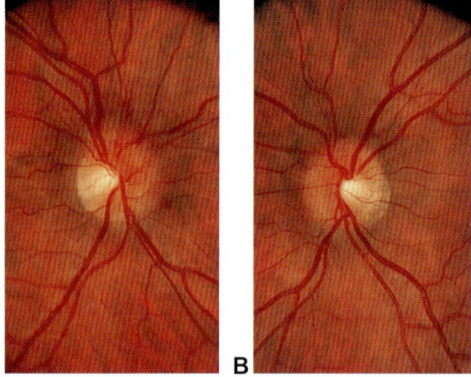

Figure 3–4. Early papilledema character-ized by hyperemia of nasal, superior, and inferior portions of optic discs. (A) Right eye. (B) Left eye.

3-2-3 *Chronic Papilledema.* With persistence of increased intracranial pressure over months, the hemorrhagic and exudative components of papilledema resolve. The disc develops a rounded "champagne cork" appearance, with obliteration of the central cup (Fig. 3–8). The optic nerve head assumes a milky gray appearance. Small, glistening hard exudates become apparent in the superficial disc substance, simulating buried drusen (Fig. 3–9). They may represent chronic axoplasmic sta-sis and signify the presence of papilledema for several months. There is loss of the retinal nerve fiber layer (Fig. 3–10) with progressive visual field loss. Both macular and peripapillary subretinal neovascularization have been associated with chronic papilledema.[11]

3-2-4 *Postpapilledema Optic Atrophy.* As chronic papilledema resolves, the disc be-comes atrophic, with narrowed, sheathed retinal vessels. Generally, the disc has a grayish-white appearance, although at times it may be diffusely white (Fig. 3–11). At this point, visual field loss, diminished color vision, and reduced Snellen acuity are significant. In some patients, as papilledema evolves from the chronic to the atrophic stage, optociliary shunt vessels may develop (Fig. 3–12). These vessels are presumably due to a chronic obstruction of central retinal venous

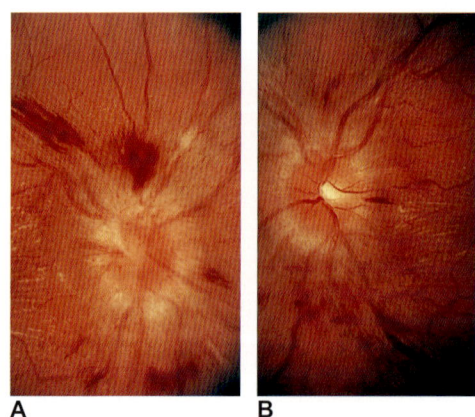

Figure 3–5. Fully developed asymmetric papilledema. (A) Right eye. (B) Left eye.

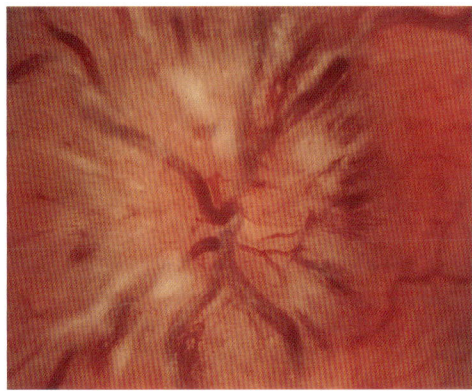

Figure 3–6. Cotton-wool spots accompanying papilledema.

drainage. With the resolution of increased intracranial pressure, these shunt vessels may regress as the papilledema resolves. At times, pigment epithelial changes are found in the peripapillary retina and macula (Figs. 3–13 and 3–14). The latter changes are thought to occur secondary to edema or subretinal hemorrhage.

3-3 ASSOCIATED CLINICAL FEATURES

3-3-1 *Visual Symptoms.* Patients with early papilledema and even those with fully developed papilledema are usually visually asymptomatic. Indeed, this fact is of great value in distinguishing papilledema from other forms of acquired disc swelling, particularly those due to inflammation or ischemia. At times, patients with well-developed papilledema may experience visual "grayouts" or "blackouts."[12] Typically, these events are reported with changes in posture, although they may occur spontaneously. Dimming of vision lasts a few seconds, usually involves one eye at a time, and clears completely. These transient obscurations should not necessarily be considered a warning of impending permanent visual failure.

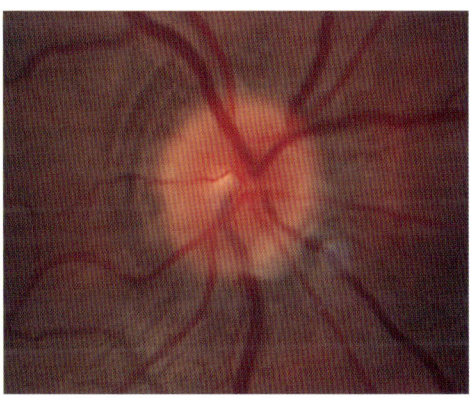

Figure 3–7. Paton's lines on the temporal side of the optic disc.

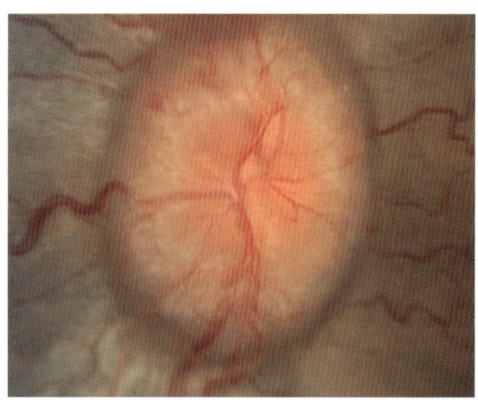

Figure 3–8. Chronic papilledema with obliteration of the central cup.

3-3-2 *Visual Acuity.* Loss of visual acuity is a late finding in papilledema, occurring in the chronic and atrophic stages. Acuity is usually lost gradually and only after extensive peripheral field loss. When blindness is rapid, it is generally due to local rather than intracranial causes, including vitreous hemorrhage, retinal hemorrhages involving the macular area, subretinal neovascular membrane formation, and, rarely, ischemic optic neuropathy.[13]

3-3-3 *Visual Field Defects.* Enlargement of the blind spot is the most common and frequently the only visual field defect in patients with papilledema. Yet enlargement of the blind spot is of no help in early diagnosis, because ophthalmoscopically visible disc swelling precedes and actually accounts for this field change.[14] In addition, congenitally anomalous optic discs may be associated with visual field defects, including an enlarged blind spot. With loss of the retinal nerve fiber layer, progressive field loss occurs in the form of peripheral constriction and nerve fiber bundle defects. As the chronic stages progress to optic atrophy, field loss occurs more rapidly on the nasal than on the temporal side. The inferonasal quadrant is particularly vulnerable (Fig. 3–15). A temporal island of vision may be preserved before progression to complete blindness (Fig. 3–16).

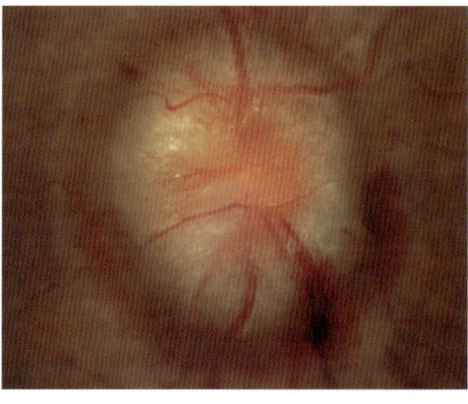

Figure 3–9. "Pseudodrusen" of chronic papilledema.

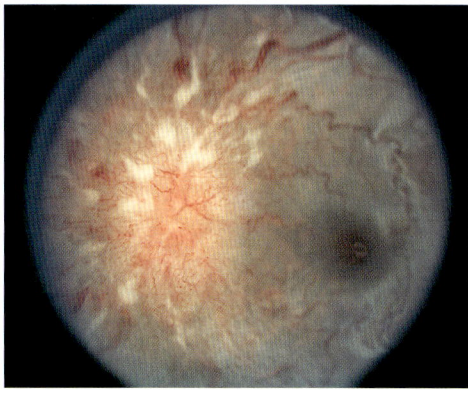

Figure 3–10. Chronic atrophic papilledema.

3-3-4 *Pupillary Function.* In early papilledema, the pupils react normally. With extensive asymmetric involvement of the visual field, pupillary reflexes are altered. An afferent pupillary defect may be found in the eye with the greater field loss.

3-3-5 *Diplopia.* Increased intracranial pressure may lead to abducens nerve palsies, either unilateral or bilateral. It has been postulated that these palsies are due to compression of the abducens nerve against the edge of the petrous temporal bone at the base of the skull. Rare reports have documented oculomotor[15] and trochlear[16] nerve palsies caused by increased intracranial pressure.

3-4 VISUAL PROGNOSIS

It is usually difficult to ascertain the visual prognosis in a patient with papilledema. Disc pallor and vascular sheathing signify irreversible changes in the optic nerve tissue. Extensive field loss, color vision abnormalities, and an afferent pupillary defect are also signs of at least some permanent visual impairment. The presence of severe venous engorgement, retinal hemorrhages, and exudates is of no prognostic significance.

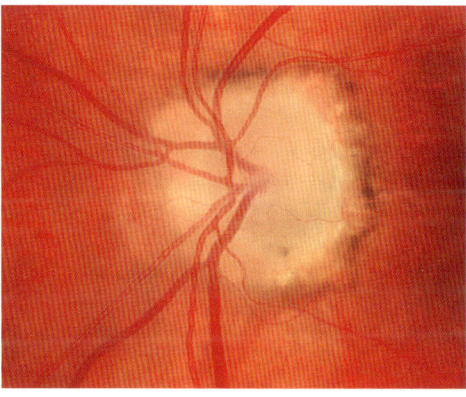

Figure 3–11. Postpapilledema optic atrophy.

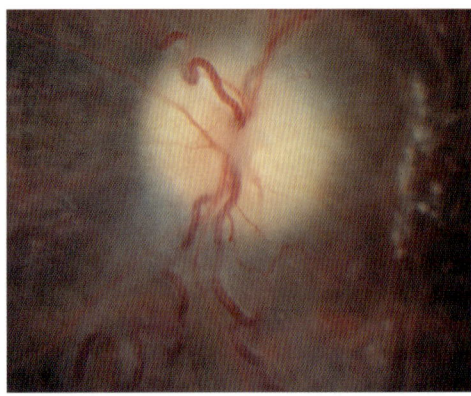

Figure 3–12. Optociliary shunt vessels with chronic atrophic papilledema. Exudates are present on the nasal side of the disc.

Rapid reduction of increased intracranial pressure by cranial surgery or cerebrospinal fluid diversion in the presence of chronic papilledema may rarely be followed by abrupt visual loss.[17] This outcome is neither predictable nor understood. Speculative mechanisms for postdecompression optic neuropathy include hypoperfusion of the prelaminar portion of the optic nerve, at times associated with a drop in systemic blood pressure during the operative procedure. An alternative explanation is that the reduction in intracranial pressure alters local regulatory factors within the optic nerve vasculature, thus reducing perfusion. Currently, there is no way to predict which patients with chronic papilledema will experience this devastating outcome following surgery.

3-5 FOSTER KENNEDY SYNDROME

A well-described but rare condition, the Foster Kennedy syndrome, is characterized by optic atrophy in one eye and papilledema in the other (Fig. 3–17).[18] This condition usually occurs in patients with subfrontal masses, such as frontal-lobe

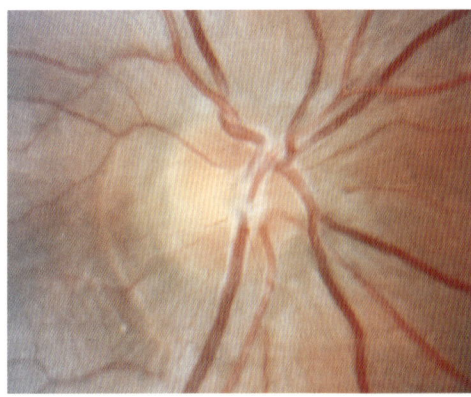

Figure 3–13. Depigmented line temporal to optic disc represents retinal pigment epithelial change due to previous papilledema.

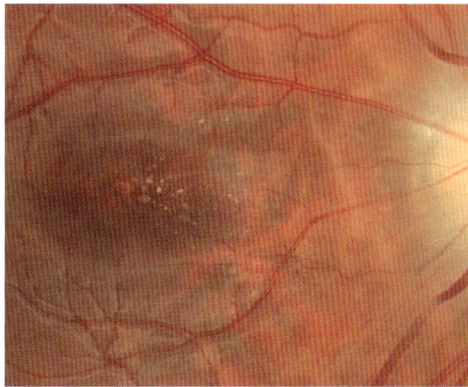

Figure 3–14. Macular pigmentary disturbance following resolution of papilledema.

or olfactory-groove tumors (masses of the anterior cranial fossa). The optic disc edema is caused by increased intracranial pressure. The optic atrophy in the fellow eye is caused by compression from the mass lesion. The lack of swelling of the atrophic disc is probably due to a combination of the absence of increased nerve sheath pressure and atrophy of nerve fibers (the lack of axoplasmic flow). In the Foster Kennedy syndrome, the eye with disc edema has good vision, which is typical of papilledema.

This is in contrast to the pseudo–Foster Kennedy syndrome, which occurs in bilateral sequential episodes of ischemic optic neuropathy.[19] In this condition, optic atrophy has developed in one eye previously involved with ischemic optic neuropathy, while the other eye is acutely affected, developing disc edema. In this case, the eye with disc edema generally has poor vision, which is typical of ischemic optic neuropathy.

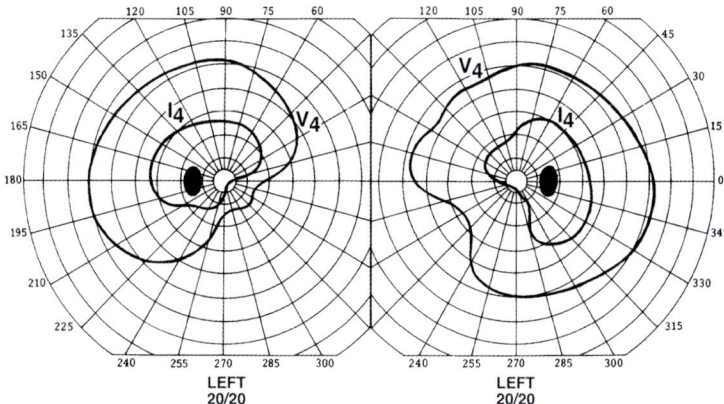

Figure 3–15. Visual fields of a patient with chronic papilledema, demonstrating generalized constriction and nasal field loss bilaterally.

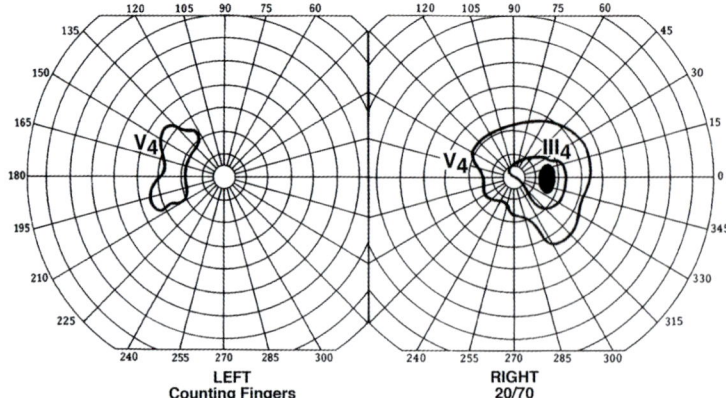

Figure 3–16. Extensive field loss bilaterally with only a temporal island remaining in the left eye.

3-6 NEUROLOGIC SYMPTOMS

To a large extent, signs and symptoms associated with papilledema are related to the pathologic process causing increased intracranial pressure. Usually, one of the earliest symptoms of intracranial hypertension is headache, although intracranial pressure may be elevated without headache. Classically, headache associated with raised intracranial pressure is worsened by the Valsalva maneuver (coughing, straining). The headache of increased intracranial pressure is believed to be due to stretching of the meninges.

Nausea and vomiting are frequent accompaniments of papilledema, particularly in the pediatric age group, and on occasion the vomiting may be projectile. Other neurologic findings—such as hemiparesis, hemisensory deficits, seizures, cerebellar signs, and ocular motility disturbances—all have localizing value. Knowledge of these findings by the radiologist is of great help in interpreting neuroimaging studies.

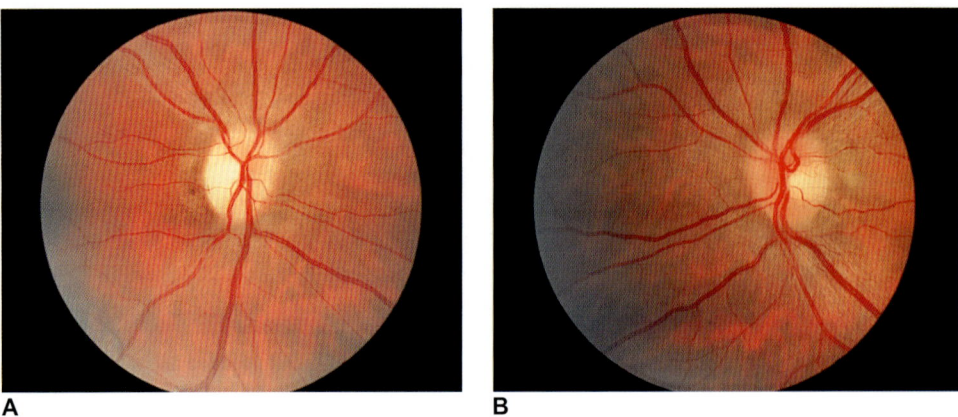

A   **B**

Figure 3–17. Foster Kennedy syndrome. (A) Optic atrophy of the right optic disc with visual acuity of 20/200. (B) Papilledema of the left eye with visual acuity of 20/20.

3-7 CAUSES OF PAPILLEDEMA

The compartment surrounding the brain and spinal cord is virtually a closed system; it is completely filled by neural tissue, cerebrospinal fluid, and circulating blood. Cerebrospinal fluid is constantly produced, primarily within the ventricular system and mainly by the activity of the choroid plexuses of the lateral, third, and fourth ventricles. The major route of absorption of cerebrospinal fluid is through the arachnoid granulations into the dural venous sinuses. Any alteration in the three components of the craniospinal compartment may lead to increased intracranial pressure.

Six potential mechanisms of increased intracranial pressure have been proposed[20]:

1. The total amount of intracranial tissue may be increased by a space-occupying lesion (Fig. 3–18).
2. The volume of intracranial tissue may be increased by focal or diffuse cerebral edema.
3. The total volume within the cranial vault may be reduced by thickening of the skull.
4. The flow of cerebrospinal fluid may be blocked either within the ventricular system (noncommunicating hydrocephalus) or within the arachnoid granulations (communicating hydrocephalus) (Fig. 3–19).
5. The rate of absorption of cerebrospinal fluid may be reduced by obstruction or compromise of the venous outflow both intra- and extracranially (Fig. 3–20 and 3–21).

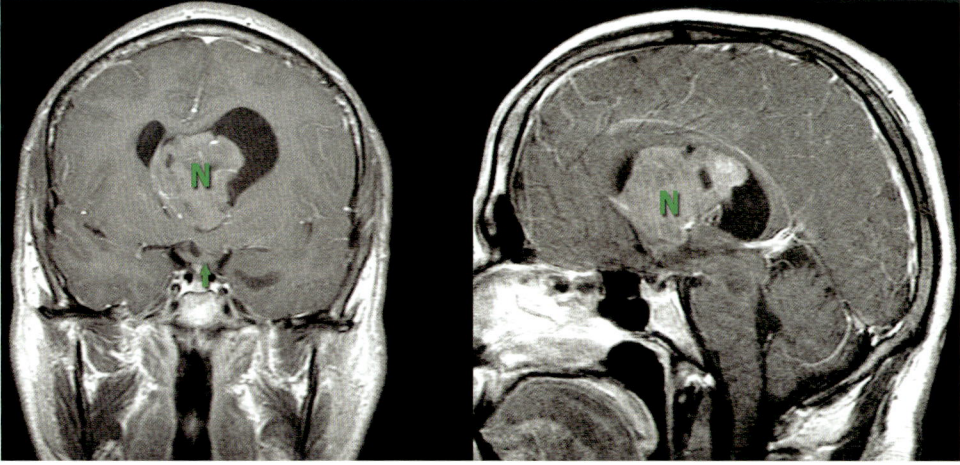

Figure 3–18. Papilledema from an intraventricular tumor. Coronal (left) and sagittal (right) T1–weighted MR images with contrast show a large intraventricular central neurocytoma (N) causing hydrocephalus. The tumor displaces the hypothalamus and left side of the optic chiasm (arrow). (Neuroimaging courtesy of Lisa Hinckley, MD.)

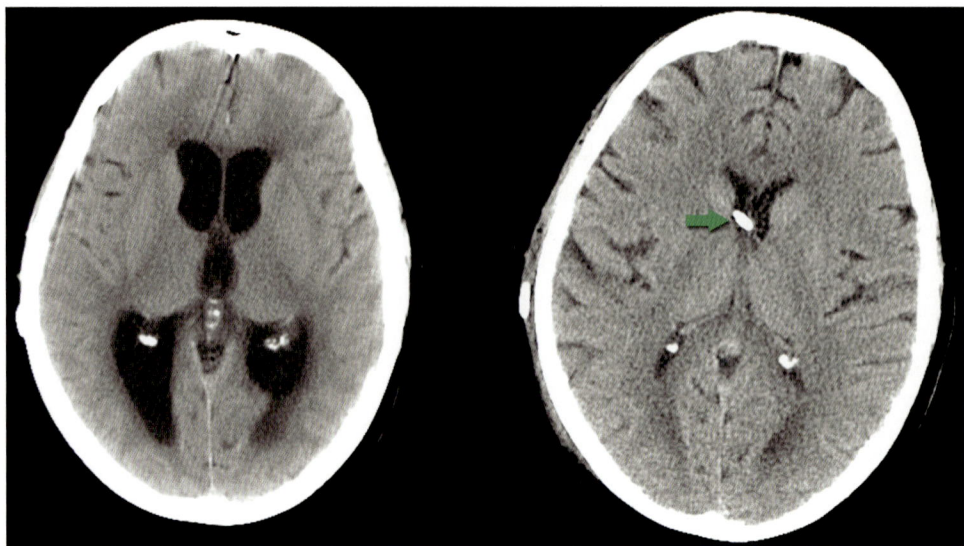

Figure 3–19. Hydrocephalus before and after neurosurgical shunting. Axial noncontrast CT scan shows dilation of the ventricular system (left) that is relieved (right) by a ventriculoperitoneal shunt (arrow). (Neuroimaging courtesy of Lisa Hinckley, MD.)

6. Tumors of the choroid plexus may rarely produce cerebrospinal fluid at a rate that exceeds adequate absorption for maintenance of normal intracranial pressure. The most common acquired causes of papilledema are listed in Table 3–2.

3-8 PATIENT EVALUATION

The finding of papilledema is an indication for prompt attention. The initial test obtained should be a cranial neuroimaging study. Currently, the procedure of choice is magnetic resonance imaging (MRI) with contrast enhancement. Orbital MRI may show increased cerebrospinal fluid signal around the optic nerves and flattening of the posterior aspects of the globes (Fig. 3–22).[21] Elevation of the optic nerve heads, with slight contrast enhancement, may be seen. Patients with idiopathic intracranial hypertension (see below) may have an enlarged and "empty sella" (Fig. 3–22). MRI allows not only visualization of the brain parenchyma and ventricular system but also assessment of flow in the dural venous sinuses. However, in some patients, cerebral venous sinus thrombosis (CVST) may not be visualized with MRI; magnetic resonance venography(MRV) (Figs. 3–20 and 3–21), computed tomographic (CT) venography, or catheter venography may be necessary.[22] False impressions of occlusions of the dural venous sinuses may arise from the use of flow-related unenhanced MRV. These misinterpretations can occasionally be avoided by using contrast-enhanced MRV.

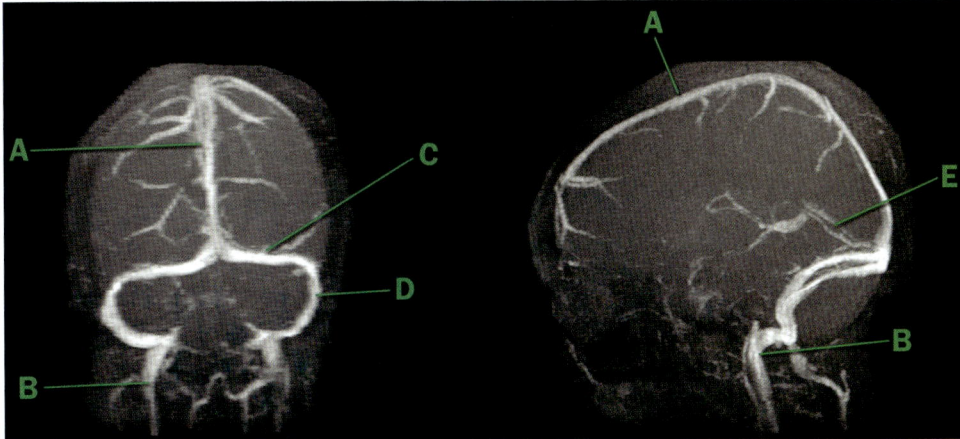

Figure 3–20. Normal cerebral venous sinuses. Anteroposterior (left) and sagittal (right) MRV show the anatomy of the normal cerebral venous sinuses. A, superior sagittal sinus; B, internal jugular vein; C, transverse sinus; D, sigmoid sinus; E, straight sinus. (Neuroimaging courtesy of Lisa Hinckley, MD.)

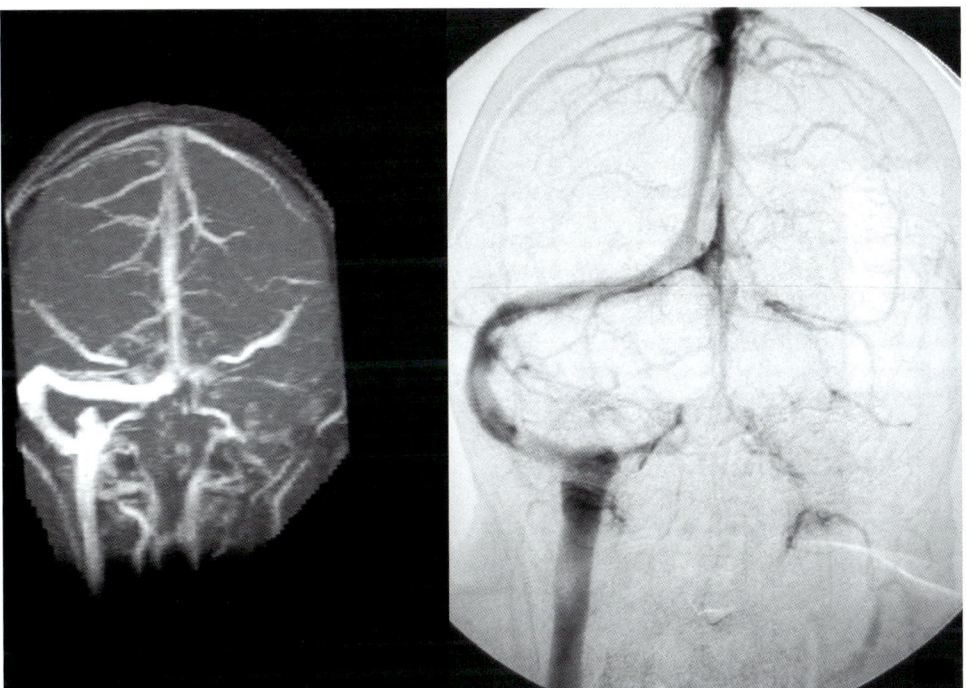

Figure 3–21. Venous sinus thrombosis. MRV (left) and cerebral angiography in the venous phase (right) showing absence of flow within the left (page right) transverse sinus, sigmoid sinus, and internal jugular vein. (Neuroimaging courtesy of Lisa Hinckley, MD.)

Table 3–2 Common Causes of Papilledema

Central nervous system mass lesion
Meningitis
Hydrocephalus
Cerebral venous sinus thrombosis
Idiopathic intracranial hypertension

An abnormal result dictates the appropriate medical or neurosurgical management. If the scanning reveals no abnormality, lumbar puncture is performed. The opening pressure should be carefully recorded, preferably with the patient relaxed and in the lateral decubitus position. Careful analysis of the cerebrospinal fluid is essential to exclude an infectious, inflammatory, or a neoplastic process. If the spinal

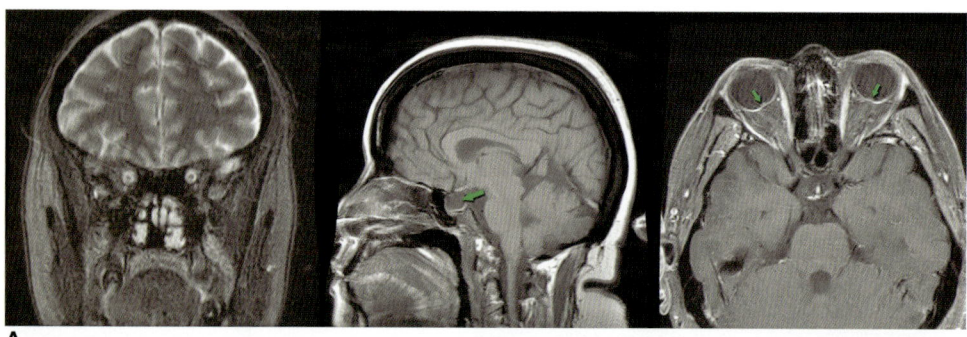

A

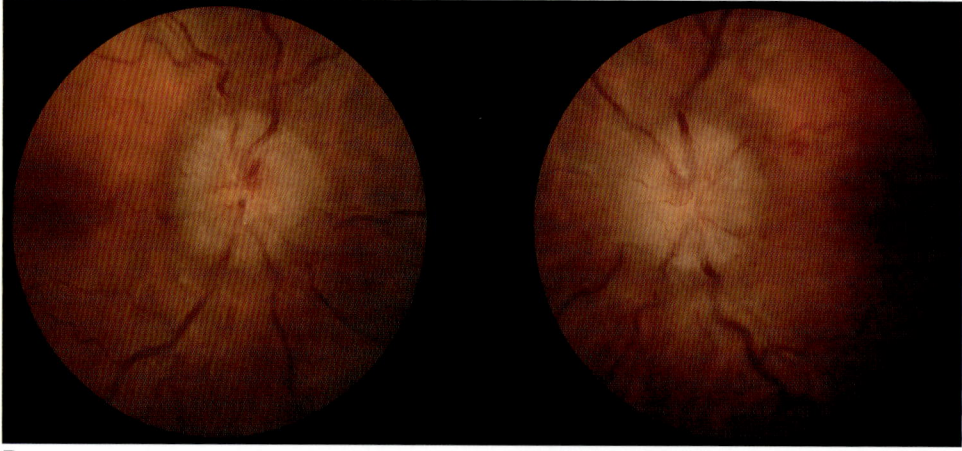

B

Figure 3–22. Papilledema from idiopathic intracranial hypertension. (A) Coronal (left) T2-weighted MRI shows increased cerebrospinal fluid signal around the optic nerves. Sagittal (center) T1-weighted MRI shows an "empty sella" (arrow). Axial (right) T1-weighted orbital MRI with contrast and fat suppression shows posterior bowing of the globes. There is enhancement and elevation in the region of the optic discs (arrows). (B) Bilateral papilledema. (C) (On opposite page) Automated perimetry showing enlargement of the blind spots and nerve fiber bundle defects. (D) (on opposite page) Despite maximum medical therapy, 1 week later there is progression of the visual field defects, which prompted neurosurgical shunting. (Neuroimaging courtesy of Lisa Hinckley, MD.)

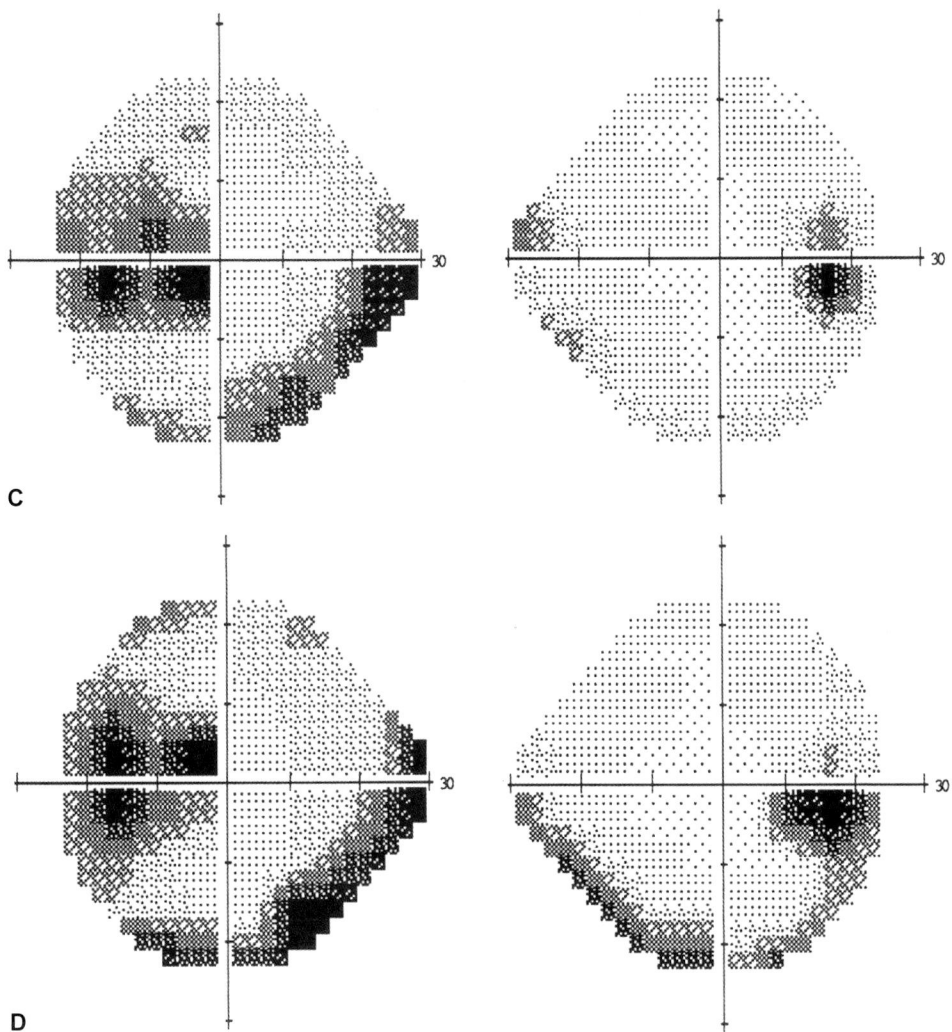

C

D

Figure 3–22 (continued)

fluid is normal except for increased pressure, the patient probably has idiopathic intracranial hypertension (also known as pseudotumor cerebri).

3-9 IDIOPATHIC INTRACRANIAL HYPERTENSION

Idiopathic intracranial hypertension (IIH) is characterized by (1) increased intracranial pressure, (2) normal or small-sized ventricles on neuroimaging studies, (3) normal cerebrospinal fluid composition, (4) papilledema, and (5) lack of any neurologic deficits that cannot be attributed to elevated intracranial pressure. On occasion papilledema may not be present despite elevated intracranial pressure. The diagnostic criteria for IIH continue to be modified (Table 3–3).[23] Although this condition may affect any age group, the peak incidence is in the third decade, occurring at least twice as frequently in females as males. The patient is often obese,

Table 3-3 Criteria for the Diagnosis of Idiopathic Intracranial Hypertension

1. If symptoms present, they may only reflect those of generalized intracranial hypertension or papilledema
2. If signs present, they may only reflect those of generalized intracranial hypertension or papilledema
3. Documented elevated intracranial pressure measured in the lateral decubitus position
4. Normal CSF composition
5. No evidence of hydrocephalus or of mass, structural, or vascular lesion on MRI or contrast-enhanced CT for typical patients and on MRI and MR venography for all others
6. No other cause of intracranial hypertension identified

Source: Modified from criteria established by W. E. Dandy, an American neurosurgeon. Reprinted with permission from Friedman DI, Jacobson DM. Diagnostic criteria for idiopathic intracranial hypertension. Neurology 2002; 59:1492–1495.

complaining of generalized headache made worse by Valsalva's maneuver. Other symptoms include nausea, vomiting, dizziness, and tinnitus. Visual complaints include transient visual obscurations (due to papilledema) and horizontal diplopia (from abducens nerve paresis). The degree of optic disc edema from papilledema in IIH generally correlates with the degree of visual dysfunction.[24]

Although the cause of IIH remains unknown, a wide variety of disorders can cause a clinically identical syndrome (Table 3–4). These disorders have been categorized as (1) obstructed or impaired intracranial venous drainage, (2) endocrine and metabolic dysfunction, (3) exogenous agent, (4) systemic illness, (5) central nervous system lesions, and (6) idiopathic condition.[20]

Table 3-4 Conditions Associated with Papilledema

Obstructed or Impaired Intracranial Venous Drainage

Dural sinus thrombosis
Radical neck surgery
Chronic respiratory insufficiency
Mediastinal mass
Cerebral or spinal arteriovenous fistula
Cerebral or spinal arteriovenous malformation

Endocrine and Metabolic Dysfunction

Eclampsia
Hypoparathyroidism
Addison's disease
Scurvy
Oral progestational agents
Diabetic ketoacidosis
Menarche
Obesity
Menstrual abnormalities

Table 3–4 (continued)

Pregnancy
Peripheral neuropathy, organomegaly, endocrinopathy,
monoclonal gammopathy, and skin changes (POEMS)

Exogenous Agents

Heavy metals (lead, arsenic)
Vitamin A
Tetracycline
Nalidixic acid
Prolonged corticosteroid therapy
Corticosteroid withdrawal

Systemic Illness

Chronic uremia
Infectious disease
Bacterial disease (subacute bacterial endocarditis, meningitis)
Viral disease (meningitis, Guillain-Barré syndrome)
Chronic inflammatory demyelinating polyneuropathy (CIDP)
Parasitic disease
Neoplastic disease
  Carcinomatous meningitis
  Leukemia
Hematologic disease
  Infectious mononucleosis
  Anemia
  Hemophilia
  Idiopathic thrombocytopenic purpura
Miscellaneous disease
  Systemic lupus erythematosus
  Sleep apnea
  Sarcoidosis
  Syphilis
  Paget's disease
  Whipple's disease

Central Nervous System Lesions

Gliomatosis cerebri
Chiari malformation
Spinal cord tumor

In the majority of patients, IIH is a self-limited condition that resolves within months, and the term *benign* has been applied in the past. Recurrence is experienced by up to 40% of patients.[25]

However, patients having a single episode or those experiencing recurrences may develop significant visual morbidity. The duration of papilledema does not appear to be a critical factor in the development of visual field loss. Progressive visual field defects may appear in weeks or may not appear even after years of chronic papilledema.[26] Nevertheless, patients with IIH must be monitored regularly during therapy to document any progression of field defects and avert blinding visual loss or severe visual impairment (Fig. 3–22).[27]

3-10 MANAGEMENT OF PAPILLEDEMA

Relief of papilledema requires long-term lowering of intracranial pressure. This goal entails neurosurgical intervention if cranial neuroimaging studies reveal a mass lesion. If the lesion cannot be removed or if the reabsorption of cerebrospinal fluid is reduced, then a procedure for the diversion of cerebrospinal fluid (including ventriculostomy, ventriculoperitoneal shunt, and lumboperitoneal shunt) is indicated. As noted above, some patients, despite normalization of intracranial pressure, experience postdecompression optic neuropathy, with progressive visual failure despite the resolution of papilledema. The cause of this complication is not completely understood.

Indications for treatment of patients with IIH include severe intractable headaches and evidence of progressive optic nerve dysfunction. Therapy includes a number of different modalities, such as weight loss (including that from gastric bypass surgery),[28] serial lumbar punctures, as well as treatment with dehydrating agents, diuretics, and corticosteroids. To date, there have been no controlled studies to compare the efficacy of these therapies.

Surgical management includes some type of procedure for the diversion of cerebrospinal fluid or decompression of the optic nerve sheath.[29] The frequency of surgical procedures for IIH has been reported to be increasing.[30] Since the ventricles are not enlarged, lumboperitoneal shunting has been the preferred neurosurgical approach and is effective in improving visual dysfunction.[31] These shunts may cease to function, and reoperation for shunt revision is often necessary.[32] Some authors feel that placement of a ventriculoperitoneal shunt may have a better long-term prognosis.[33]

Decompression of the optic nerve sheath may also provide relief of papilledema.[34] This procedure is accomplished by incision of the dura and arachnoid surrounding the intraorbital optic nerve (Fig. 3–23).[27,32,34,35] Although this intervention provides local decompression of the optic nerve, it does not lower intracranial pressure.[26] Nevertheless, improvement or resolution of headache has been reported in two-thirds of the patients who undergo this procedure.[27,32] Long-term improvements in visual function and optic disc swelling have been noted after decompression of the optic nerve sheath.[36–38] In addition, unilateral decompression may lead to bilateral resolution of papilledema in some patients (Figs. 3–24 and 3–25). There are few reports of serious complications following decompression of the optic nerve sheath,[39,40] although papilledema may recur (presumably due to closure of the fenestration sites) and reoperation may be necessary. There are no controlled studies comparing the efficacy of cerebrospinal fluid diversion procedures with fenestration of the optic nerve sheath. Decompression of the optic nerve sheath is sometimes favored over neurosurgical shunting when surgery is indicated for progressive visual loss or for papilledema in the absence of headaches in IIH.[41]

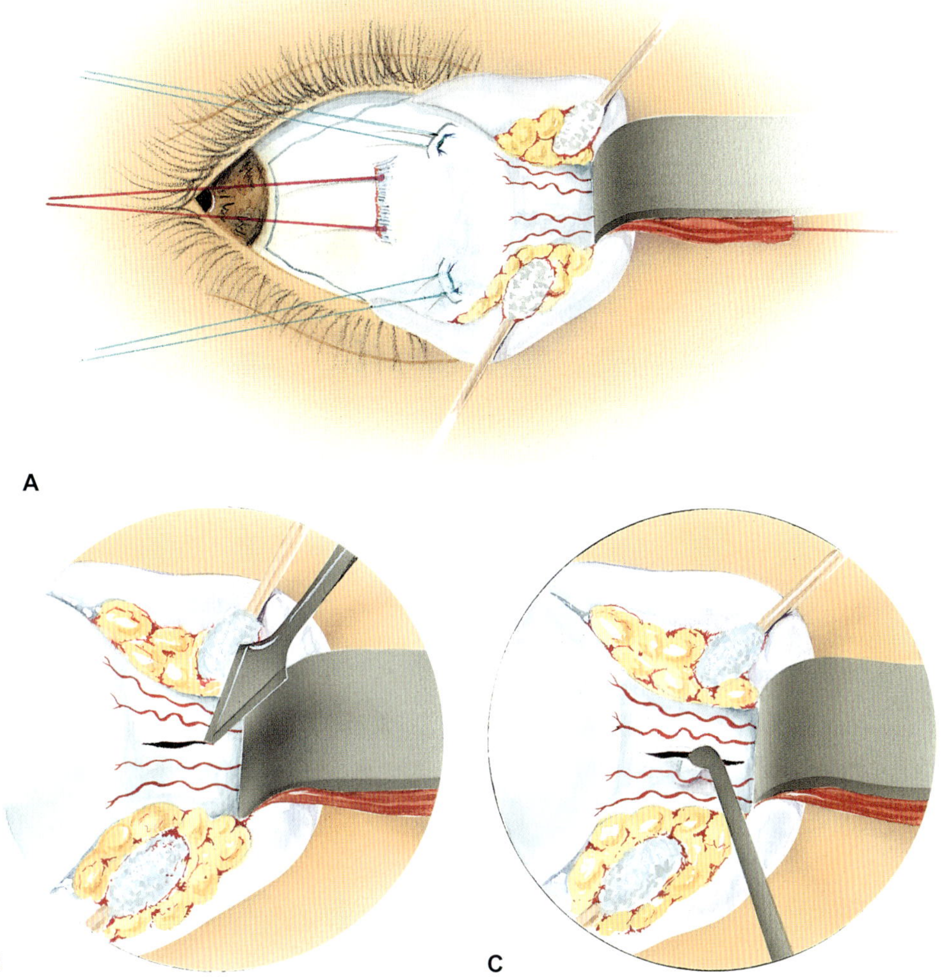

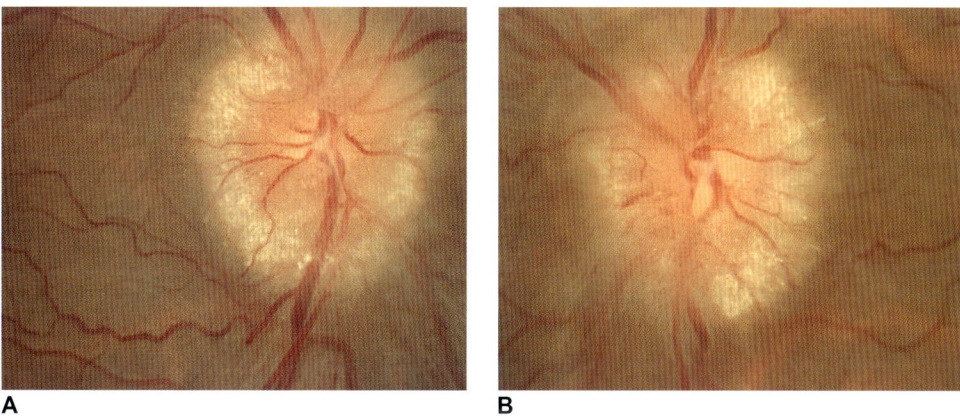

Figure 3–23. Medial orbital approach for decompression of the optic nerve sheath. (A) Eye firmly turned into abduction following disinsertion of medial rectus muscle and positioning of orbital retractor. (B) Optic nerve sheath incised with triangular blade. (C) Fisher tenotomy hook used to disrupt arachnoidal adhesions. For details of technique, see ref. 32.

Figure 3–24. Chronic papilledema. Appearance of (A) right disc and (B) left disc prior to surgery.

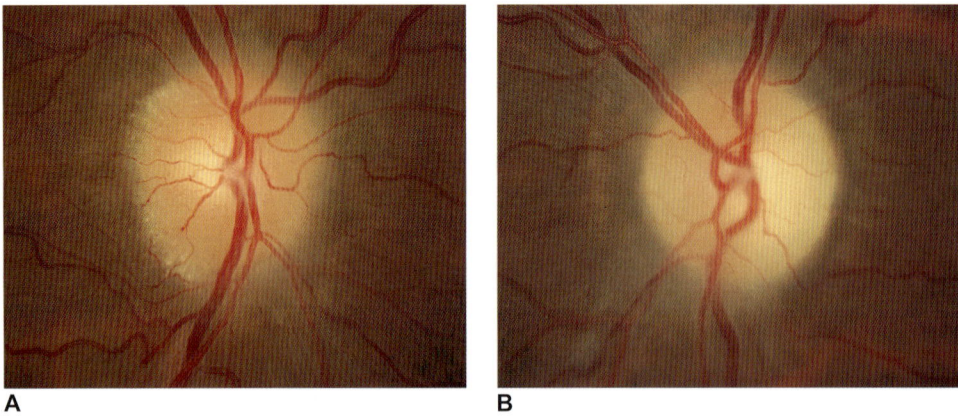

A   B

Figure 3–25. About 3 months after decompression of the optic nerve sheath in the left eye, there is bilateral improvement in papilledema. (A) Right eye. (B) Left eye.

References

1. Tso MO, Hayreh SS. Optic disc edema in raised intracranial pressure. IV. Axoplasmic transport in experimental papilledema. Arch Ophthalmol 1977;95:1458–62.
2. Karam EZ, Hedges TR. Optical coherence tomography of the retinal nerve fibre layer in mild papilloedema and pseudopapilloedema. Br J Ophthalmol 2005;89:294–8.
3. Jackson JH. On the routine use of the ophthalmoscope in cases of cerebral disease. Med Times Gaz 1871;1:627–9.
4. Williamson-Noble FA. Venous pulsations. Trans Ophthalmol Soc UK 1953;72:317–26.
5. Walsh TJ, Garden JW, Gallagher B. Obliteration of retinal venous pulsations during elevation of cerebrospinal-fluid pressure. Am J Ophthalmol 1969;67:954–6.
6. Lorentzen SE. Incidence of spontaneous venous pulsation in the retina. Acta Ophthalmol (Copenh) 1970;48:765–70.
7. Jacks AS, Miller NR. Spontaneous retinal venous pulsation: aetiology and significance. J Neurol Neurosurg Psychiatry 2003;74:7–9.
8. Keane JR. Papilledema with unusual ocular hemorrhages. Arch Ophthalmol 1981;99: 262–3.
9. Bird AC, Sanders MD. Choroidal folds in association with papilloedema. Br J Ophthalmol 1973;57:89–97.
10. Galvin R, Sanders MD. Peripheral retinal haemorrhages with papilloedema. Br J Ophthalmol 1980;64:262–6.
11. Morse PH, Leveille AS, Antel JP, Burch JV. Bilateral juxtapapillary subretinal neovascularization associated with pseudotumor cerebri. Am J Ophthalmol 1981;91: 312–7.
12. Cogan DG. Blackouts not obviously due to carotid occlusion. Arch Ophthalmol 1961;66: 180–7.
13. Green GJ, Lessell S, Loewenstein JI. Ischemic optic neuropathy in chronic papilledema. Arch Ophthalmol 1980;98:502–4.
14. Corbett JJ, Jacobson DM, Mauer RC, Thompson HS. Enlargement of the blind spot caused by papilledema. Am J Ophthalmol 1988;105:261–5.
15. McCammon A, Kaufman HH, Sears ES. Transient oculomotor paralysis in pseudotumor cerebri. Neurology 1981;31:182–4.

16. Halpern JI, Gordon WH, Jr. Trochlear nerve palsy as a false localizing sign. Ann Ophthalmol 1981;13:53–6.
17. Beck RW, Greenberg HS. Post-decompression optic neuropathy. J Neurosurg 1985;63:196–9.
18. Kennedy F. Retrobulbar neuritis as an exact diagnostic sign of certain tumors and abscesses in the frontal lobes. Am J Med Sci 1911;142:355–68.
19. Schatz NJ, Smith JL. Non-tumor causes of the Foster Kennedy syndrome. J Neurosurg 1967;27:37–44.
20. Friedman DI. Papilledema. In: Miller NR, Newman NJ, eds. Walsh and Hoyt's Clinical Neuro-ophthalmology, 6th ed. Philadelphia: Lippincott Williams & Wilkins, 2005:237–92.
21. Brodsky MC, Vaphiades M. Magnetic resonance imaging in pseudotumor cerebri. Ophthalmology 1998;105:1686–93.
22. Crassard I, Bousser MG. Cerebral venous thrombosis. J Neuroophthalmol 2004;24:156–63.
23. Friedman DI, Jacobson DM. Diagnostic criteria for idiopathic intracranial hypertension. Neurology 2002;59:1492–5.
24. Wall M, White WN II. Asymmetric papilledema in idiopathic intracranial hypertension: prospective interocular comparison of sensory visual function. Invest Ophthalmol Vis Sci 1998;39:134–42.
25. Rush JA. Pseudotumor cerebri: clinical profile and visual outcome in 63 patients. Mayo Clin Proc 1980;55:541–6.
26. Wall M, George D. Idiopathic intracranial hypertension. A prospective study of 50 patients. Brain 1991;114(Pt 1A):155–80.
27. Corbett JJ, Thompson HS. The rational management of idiopathic intracranial hypertension. Arch Neurol 1989;46:1049–51.
28. Sugerman HJ, Felton WL III, Sismanis A, Kellum JM, DeMaria EJ, Sugerman EL. Gastric surgery for pseudotumor cerebri associated with severe obesity. Ann Surg 1999;229:634–40; discussion 640–2.
29. Binder DK, Horton JC, Lawton MT, McDermott MW. Idiopathic intracranial hypertension. Neurosurgery 2004;54:538–51; discussion 551–2.
30. Curry WT, Jr., Butler WE, Barker FG II. Rapidly rising incidence of cerebrospinal fluid shunting procedures for idiopathic intracranial hypertension in the United States, 1988–2002. Neurosurgery 2005;57:97–108; discussion 97–108.
31. Burgett RA, Purvin VA, Kawasaki A. Lumboperitoneal shunting for pseudotumor cerebri. Neurology 1997;49:734–9.
32. Sergott RC, Savino PJ, Bosley TM. Modified optic nerve sheath decompression provides long-term visual improvement for pseudotumor cerebri. Arch Ophthalmol 1988;106:1384–90.
33. Bynke G, Zemack G, Bynke H, Romner B. Ventriculoperitoneal shunting for idiopathic intracranial hypertension. Neurology 2004;63:1314–6.
34. Galbraith JE, Sullivan JH. Decompression of the perioptic meninges for relief of papilledema. Am J Ophthalmol 1973;76:687–92.
35. Brourman ND, Spoor TC, Ramocki JM. Optic nerve sheath decompression for pseudotumor cerebri. Arch Ophthalmol 1988;106:1378–83.
36. Banta JT, Farris BK. Pseudotumor cerebri and optic nerve sheath decompression. Ophthalmology 2000;107:1907–12.
37. Goh KY, Schatz NJ, Glaser JS. Optic nerve sheath fenestration for pseudotumor cerebri. J Neuroophthalmol 1997;17:86–91.
38. Spoor TC, McHenry JG. Long-term effectiveness of optic nerve sheath decompression for pseudotumor cerebri. Arch Ophthalmol 1993;111:632–5.

39. Plotnik JL, Kosmorsky GS. Operative complications of optic nerve sheath decompression. Ophthalmology 1993;100:683–90.
40. Spoor TC, McHenry JG. Complications of optic nerve sheath decompression. Ophthalmology 1993;100:1432–3.
41. Keltner JL. Optic nerve sheath decompression. How does it work? Has its time come? Arch Ophthalmol 1988;106:1365–9.

4

Optic Neuritis

MICHAEL S. VAPHIADES AND LANNING B. KLINE

The term *optic neuritis* denotes primary inflammation of the optic nerve, usually from demyelinating disease. The term can also be used in describing an optic neuropathy due to the contiguous spread of inflammation from meninges, orbital tissues, or paranasal sinuses. When there is swelling of the optic disc, the term *papillitis* is sometmes used. When the clinical history and examination suggest optic neuritis but the optic disc appears normal, the term *retrobulbar optic neuritis* is used.

The diagnosis of optic neuritis is based on clinical criteria. Critical elements in establishing the diagnosis are a detailed history and an accurate examination. For this reason, the ophthalmologist must be familiar with the clinical profile of optic neuritis.

4-1 CLINICAL FEATURES

4-1-1 *Visual Symptoms.* Optic neuritis is the most common cause of acute visual loss from optic nerve disease in young and middle-aged adults. It has a peak incidence in the third and fourth decades and is more often seen in females.[1] The unilateral visual loss is rapid in onset and almost always accompanied by pain. The periocular pain may precede the visual loss by several days and is characteristically precipitated or aggravated by eye movement.[2] The acute visual loss in optic neuritis usually progresses for 1 to 2 weeks before steadily improving over the next 6 to 12 weeks. The range of visual reduction is variable, from minimal reduction in Snellen acuity to no light perception.

Ten years after an episode of optic neuritis, the visual acuity in affected eyes is better than 20/20 in 74%, 20/25–20/40 in 18%, 20/40–20/200 in 5%, and worse than 20/200 in 3% of patients. In general, visual function is worse for patients with multiple sclerosis (MS) than for patients without the disease.[3]

In addition to visual loss, patients with optic neuritis often report other visual aberrations. One is positive visual phenomena or phosphenes.[4] Descriptions of this visual disturbance include flashing black squares, flashes of light, and showers of sparks. Another complaint, difficulty with depth perception, may accompany an attack of optic neuritis or become apparent following recovery. This abnormality can be demonstrated by having the patient look at a linearly swinging pendulum with both eyes open. If an optic neuropathy exists in either eye, she or he will see the pendulum swinging in an ellipse, the direction of which is dependent upon which eye is affected. This is termed the *Pulfrich stereoillusion* (Fig. 4–1), which is caused by a relative delay in conduction along the impaired optic nerve.[5] More specifically, the effect is due to a disparity of intereye luminance. This binocular stereoillusion is generally seen only with monocular optic neuropathy.[6]

4-1-2 *Color Vision.* Deficits in color vision invariably accompany an attack of optic neuritis. Use of the Ishihara pseudoisochromatic color plates allows rapid detection of the acquired color deficit. Dyschromatopsia is a sensitive indicator of optic neuritis, and color vision is often more severely affected than Snellen visual acuity.

4-1-3 *Pupillary Function.* An afferent pupillary defect is almost always present in optic neuritis unless the other eye was previously involved; its detection provides objective evidence of optic nerve dysfunction. Although the afferent defect improves over time, it may not completely disappear.

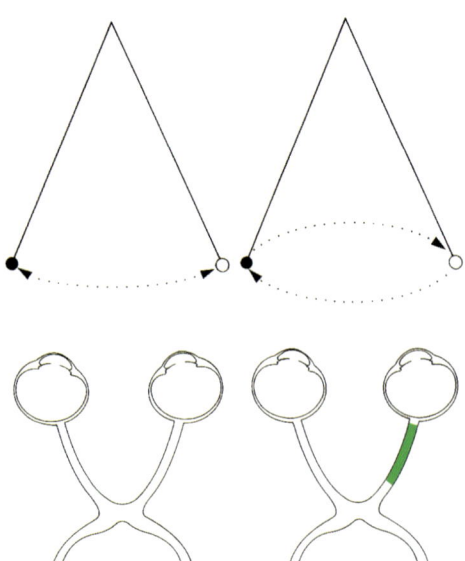

Figure 4–1. Clinical use of Pulfrich's phenomenon. (A) Normal appearance of pendular movement. (B) Apparent elliptical movement of pendulum with unilateral optic nerve damage. **A**   **B**

4-1-4 *Visual Field Defects.* Studies using manual techniques (tangent screen, bowl perimeter) have consistently demonstrated a central scotoma as the most common visual field abnormality in optic neuritis.[7] Recent analysis of visual field loss with optic neuritis comes from the Optic Neuritis Treatment Trial, using automated static threshold techniques.[8] The most common visual field abnormality, detected with the Humphrey 30-2 program, was a decrease in light sensitivity over the entire central visual field, as found in 48% of 448 patients presenting with acute optic neuritis. More localized depression confined to one quadrant, two quadrants (a hemifield), or three quadrants of the central visual field was seen in 17.3% of patients, altitudinal field defects in 14.9%, centrocecal scotomas in 4.5%, central scotomas in 3.8%, and arcuate scotomas in 4.5% (Fig. 4–2).

In addition, the data on automated visual field testing and optic neuritis gathered from the Optic Neuritis Treatment Trial demonstrate that visual field defects can be uncovered in up to one-third of the asymptomatic fellow eyes.[9] A history of an attack of optic neuritis in the fellow eye may not be elicited, and these field defects often improve or resolve, as documented by follow-up perimetry. In essence, optic neuritis does not have a predilection for any particular area of the visual field.[10]

Although automated perimetry has proven extremely useful in establishing the progression and recovery of visual field loss in optic neuritis, the patterns of visual field defects are not particularly helpful in distinguishing optic neuritis from any other form of optic nerve disease (e.g., ischemic, compressive).[11]

4-1-5 *Optic Disc Abnormalities.* Examination of the fundus may or may not reveal optic disc abnormalities. In the Optic Neuritis Treatment Trial, approximately one-third of patients with recent-onset optic neuritis demonstrated optic disc edema or papillitis (Fig. 4–3). Cells in the adjacent vitreous were usually not present; when seen, they were few in number. When the cellular reaction is extensive, the inflammatory process is usually intraocular and often associated with systemic disease. In addition, accompanying sheathing of the retinal veins is also suggestive of a systemic disorder (e.g., sarcoidosis, syphilis, MS). The optic disc initially appears normal in approximately two-thirds of patients with optic neuritis (retrobulbar neuritis). The presence of optic disc pallor does not invalidate the diagnosis of optic neuritis, but it does indicate that some form of optic neuropathy antedated any recent complaint of sudden visual loss.

4-1-6 *Uhthoff's Symptom.* Following an episode of optic neuritis, some patients describe visual blurring with activities that raise body temperature (e.g., exercise or a hot bath or shower).[12] This complaint, termed *Uhthoff's symptom,* is explained by two major theories: (1) that an elevation of body temperature interferes with axonal conduction and (2) that a rise in body temperature releases a chemical substance that interferes with conduction. Uhthoff's symptom occurs most commonly in patients with other evidence of MS, occasionally with Leber's hereditary optic neuropathy, or in otherwise healthy individuals.

4-1-7 *Visual Evoked Response.* Psychophysical tests, including contrast sensitivity and visual evoked responses, invariably yield abnormal results in patients with optic

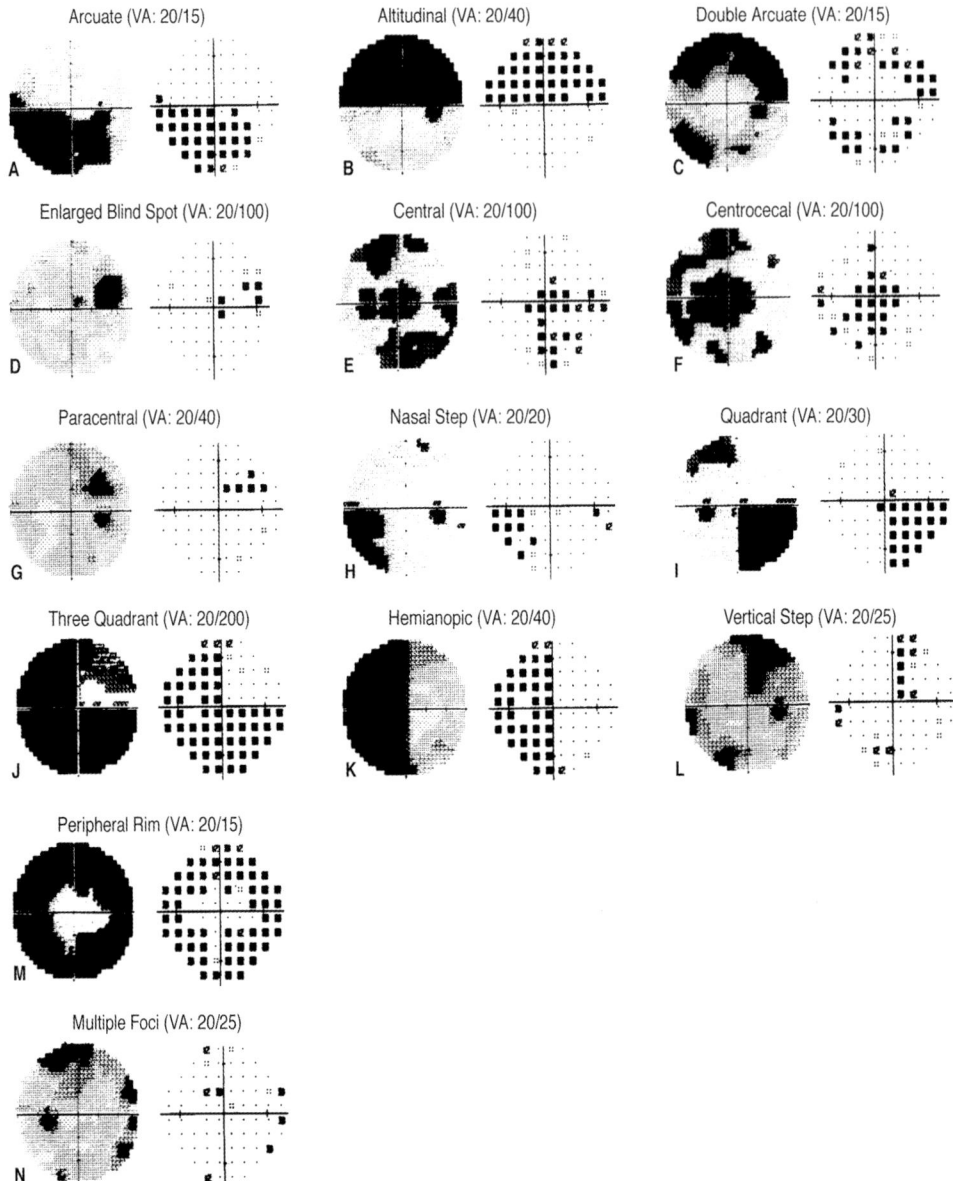

Figure 4–2. Examples of 14 categories of localized monocular visual field defects used in ONTT Visual Field Reading Center's classification system. Humphrey gray scale and pattern deviation are included for each example. Examples D, G, and N are considered minimal local defects; examples C and L are considered moderate defects; and examples A, B, E, F, H, I, J, K, and M are considered severe defects. Examples A and B may be superior or inferior, G is a cluster of points not located at a typical anatomic site and may be anywhere in the central 30 degrees, and N is not a trial-lens rim artifact because no lens correction was used. VA, visual acuity. (Reproduced with permission from Keltner JL, Johnson CA, Spurr JO, Beck RW. Baseline visual field profile of optic neuritis: the experience of the Optic Neuritis Treatment Trial. Arch Ophthalmol 1993;111:231–34. Copyright 1993, American Medical Association.)

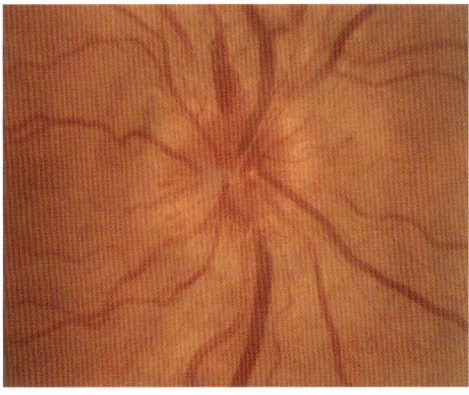

Figure 4–3. Disc edema due to papillitis.

neuritis. Such tests are not necessary to establish the diagnosis but may play a confirmatory role. For example, the pattern-reversal visual evoked response is abnormal in approximately 90% of patients in the acute stage of optic neuritis (Fig. 4–4).[13] In addition, after clinical recovery, only approximately 10% of patients reestablish normal pattern-reversal visual evoked responses.[14] Thus, this testing modality may serve as a permanent marker of a previous attack of optic neuritis.

4-1-8 *Neuroimaging Abnormalities.* Both computed tomography (CT)[15] and magnetic resonance imaging (MRI)[16] may reveal abnormalities along the course of the optic

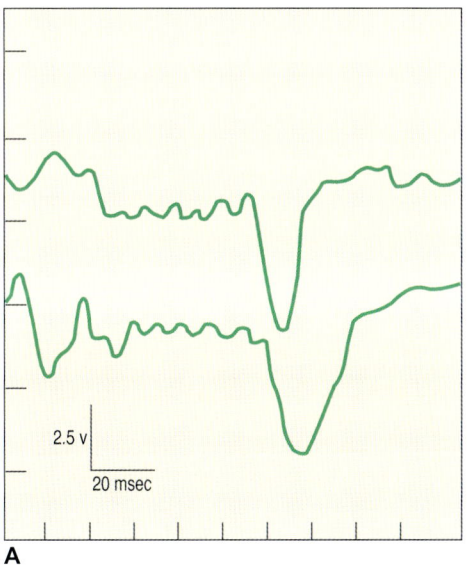

2.5 v

20 msec

A

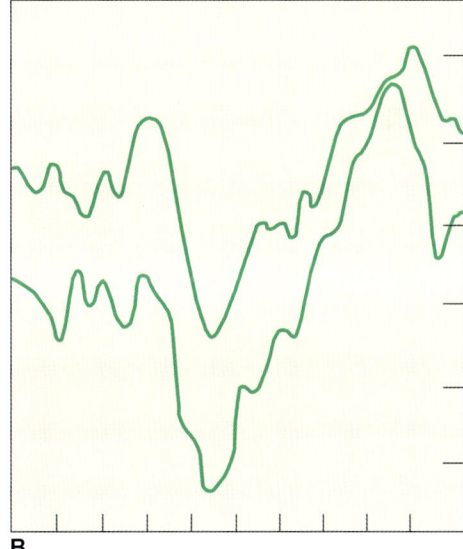

B

Figure 4–4. This 24-year-old woman experienced acute loss of vision in the right eye accompanied by ocular pain. Visual acuity: 20/70 right eye, 20/20 left eye. Diminished color vision and afferent pupillary defect were present in the right eye. Fundi were normal. A diagnosis of right retrobulbar optic neuritis was made; over 6 weeks, there was recovery of 20/20 acuity on the right. Pattern-reversal visual evoked response 5 days after onset of symptoms shows prolongation of latency on the right as compared with the left. (A) Right eye, 130 msec; (B) left eye, 91 msec.

nerve in patients with acute optic neuritis. However, MRI is far superior to CT in this regard. The frequency of positive MRI studies varies depending on the technique employed.[16,17] In retrospective observational series of patients with acute optic neuritis who had gadolinium-enhanced fat-suppressed cranial MRI scans within 20 days of the visual loss, enhancement of the orbital optic nerve occurred in 94% of patients.[18] This pattern of enhancement is compatible with disruption of the blood-brain barrier (Fig. 4–5). This abnormality is not specific for demyelinating optic neuritis, since various other diseases such as sarcoidosis and radiation optic neuropathy (discussed in Chapter 10) can produce a similar appearance on MRI.

4-2 OPTIC NEURITIS AND MULTIPLE SCLEROSIS

Up to one-third of patients who experience optic neuritis have a history or neurologic findings consistent with MS.[1] A related clinical question concerns the frequency with which MS follows an attack of monosymptomatic optic neuritis. The answers vary widely, depending on the series reported. A British study included 66 patients with a mean follow-up of 10.2 years (range of 6 months to 20 years).[19] Approximately 20% developed definite MS, all but 1 patient within 4 years of the attack of optic neuritis. Another group reported the results of a prospective study conducted in the northeastern United States.[20] Over a 15-year follow-up, these investigators found that 74% of women and 34% of men with isolated optic neuritis developed MS. In a population-based study, other researchers found that 39% of 95 patients with isolated optic neuritis progressed to clinically definite MS by 10 years of follow-up, 49% by 20 years, 54% by 30 years, and 60% by 40 years.[21] There was no

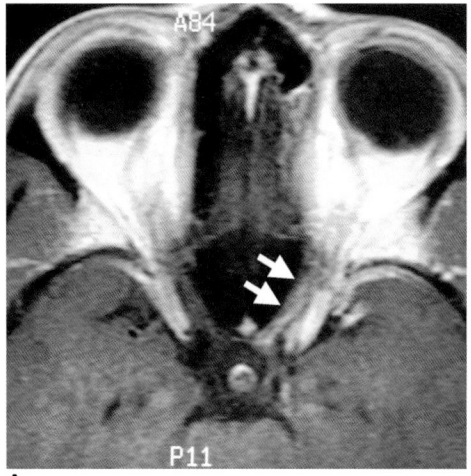
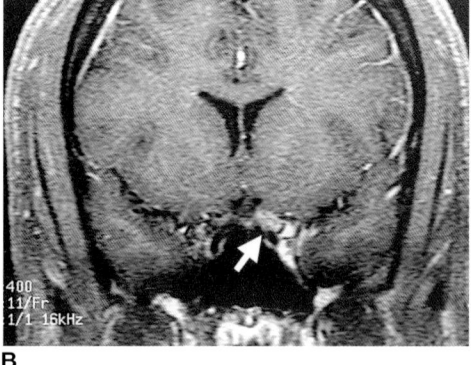

A   **B**

Figure 4–5. This 30-year-old woman reported acute visual loss in the left eye accompanied by pain with eye movement. Visual acuity: 20/20 right eye, 20/100 left eye. A left afferent pupillary defect and swollen left optic disc were found on examination. Gadolinium-enhanced T1-weighted (A) axial and (B) coronal MRI scans demonstrate swelling and enhancement of the intracranial portion of the left optic nerve (arrows).

difference in the risk of developing MS between men and women. An assessment of these studies and others would lead to the conclusion that at least half of those who develop MS show clinical signs within 3 years of an optic neuritis attack, and thereafter 2%–5% per year continue to develop demyelinating disease.[22,23]

From the Optic Neuritis Treatment Trial (see below), the 10 year risk of developing MS based on clinical criteria is 38%. Patients who had one or more typical brain lesions (at least 3 mm in diameter) on baseline cranial MRI had a 56% risk of developing clinically definite MS at 10 years (Fig. 4–6). Those with no lesions on cranial MRI had a 22% risk of developing MS at 10 years. The 10-year risk of MS following an initial episode of acute optic neuritis was significantly higher if there was a single brain MRI lesion at outset. The greater number of lesions did not increase the risk for clinically definite MS.[24]

4-3 OPTIC NEURITIS TREATMENT TRIAL

A national collaborative study, the Optic Neuritis Treatment Trial (ONTT), has provided a wealth of information regarding the natural history of this condition, the need for patient evaluation, and potential forms of therapy. To be eligible for the study, the patient had to be between 18 and 45 years of age, have a history compatible with acute optic neuritis, and have visual symptoms lasting 8 days or less. In addition, patients were required to have a relative afferent pupillary defect and a visual field defect in the affected eye.

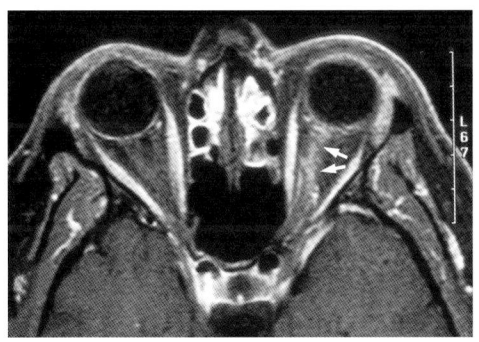

A

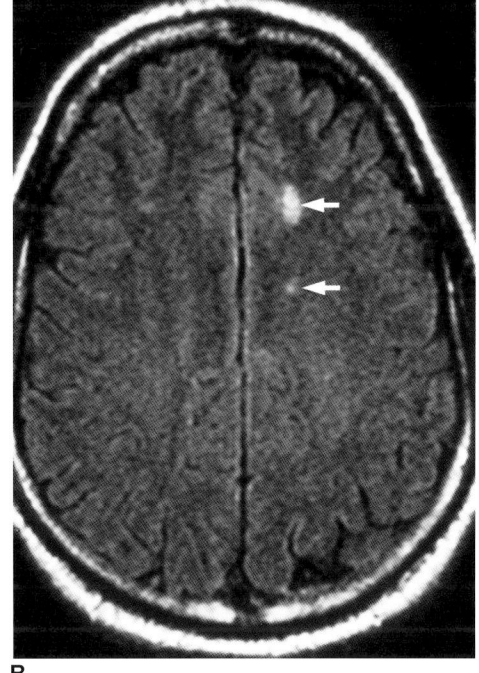

B

Figure 4–6. 39-year-old man developed left optic neuritis. (A) (above) Axial MRI with fat suppression following intravenous gadolinium demonstrates enhancement (arrows) of orbital portion of left optic nerve. (B) (right) Axial FLAIR MRI reveals two white-matter lesions (arrows), consistent with MS.

A total of 457 patients were admitted to the study; 77% were women, and the mean age was 32 years. Patients were randomized to three clinical treatment arms:

1. Oral prednisone (1 mg/kg/day for 14 days)
2. Intravenous methylprednisolone (250 mg qid, 1000 mg/day) for 3 days, followed by oral prednisone (1 mg/kg/day) for 11 days
3. Oral placebo for 14 days

There were no serious side effects in any of the groups. In all three groups, the vast majority of patients experienced excellent visual recovery. Most of the visual improvement occurred within the first 15 days, with the median acuity being 20/25 in the placebo group and 20/20 in the two groups receiving treatment.[25] The speed of recovery was greatest during this period for the patients treated with the intravenous regimen. After 1 year of follow-up, no statistically significant difference was noted among the groups in visual acuity, contrast sensitivity, color vision, or visual field.[26] At 1 year, Snellen acuity was 20/40 or better in 95% of the placebo group, 94% of the intravenous/oral corticosteroid group, and 91% of those given oral prednisone alone. The failure of steriod therapy to improve visual outcome following an attack of optic neuritis has been confirmed in up to 10 years of follow-up.[24]

The regimen of oral prednisone alone not only failed to improve vision but also was associated with an increased rate of new attacks of optic neuritis in both the initially affected eye and the fellow eye.[25,26] Within the first 2 years of follow-up, new attacks of optic neuritis in either eye occurred in 30% of the patients in the oral-prednisone-only group, compared with 16% in the placebo group and 14% in the intravenous/oral prednisone group. Even without this finding, which is unexplained, the ONTT results indicate that oral prednisone alone in the dosage used in this study should not be prescribed for acute demyelinative optic neuritis, since it showed no benefit compared with placebo.

Additional clinical data obtained on patient entry into the ONTT included the following studies: antinuclear antibody (ANA), fluorescent treponemal antibody (FTA) absorption test, chest radiograph, and MRI brain scan. These studies were of no value in establishing the correct diagnosis of optic neuritis, nor did they provide any prognostic data to help determine visual recovery. In the few patients with a positive ANA, there was no difference in the course of the disease or the response to treatment. The ONTT emphasizes the fact that optic neuritis is a clinical diagnosis, established by the history and the physical examination.

In addition, the ONTT found that cranial MRI was a powerful predictor of the 2-year risk of MS.[27,28] Patients with two or more typical white-matter lesions (≥ 3 mm, periventricular, and ovoid shape) had a 2-year risk of MS of 36%, whereas patients with normal scan results had a risk of about 3%. With longer follow-up (mean of 5.5 years), a study from England reported that 82% of patients who had abnormal MRI results at the time they presented with clinically isolated optic neuritis went on to develop MS.[29] As mentioned above, the 10-year risk of developing MS after an attack of optic neuritis rises to 56% with one or more white-matter lesions on MRI.[24]

Unexpectedly, the ONTT found that the group receiving the intravenous/oral corticosteroid regimen had a lower rate of development of MS within the first 2 years of follow-up than did the placebo or oral-prednisone-alone group.[27] Among the patients in the intravenous/oral group, definite MS developed within 2 years in only 7.5%, compared with 16.7% of the placebo group and 14.7% of the oral-prednisone-alone group. Most of the treatment effect was observed in the patients with abnormal MRI results at study entry. These data demonstrate that the intravenous therapy provided a statistically significant delay in the clinical expression of MS during the first 2 years after an attack of optic neuritis. However, by 3 years of follow-up, this "protective effect" could no longer be demonstrated.[30]

In summary, it seems appropriate to obtain a cranial MRI scan in all patients experiencing acute optic neuritis. Subjects with scans showing abnormalities consistent with MS should be considered for treatment with intravenous corticosteroids to retard the development of MS during the ensuing 2 years. Treatment with intravenous corticosteroids should also be considered in all patients with acute optic neuritis, whether or not the cranial MRI scan reveals an abnormality, as this medical management can lead to a more rapid improvement of visual function as compared with no treatment. However, in making treatment decisions, the clinician should bear in mind that data from the ONTT demonstrate that the visual outcome remains the same whether or not the patient received intravenous corticosteroid therapy.

4-4 THE CHAMPS TRIAL

The CHAMPS (Controlled High-Risk Subjects Avonex MS Prevention study) trial was a double-blind study evaluating patients who had a first clinical demyelinating event (optic neuritis, incomplete transverse myelitis, or brainstem/cerebellar syndrome) and evidence of two or more clinically silent lesions at least 3 mm in diameter on cranial MRI scan characteristic of MS. In this trial, 383 patients, all of whom received initial treatment of intravenous corticosteroids, were randomized to either weekly intramuscular injections of 30 µg of interferon beta-1a (Avonex) or placebo. At 3 years of follow-up, the cumulative probability of developing clinically definite MS was significantly lower in the interferon beta-1a group than in the placebo group.

The results of this study justify obtaining a brain MRI at the time of the first demyelinating event. They further support treatment with interferon beta-1a if the MRI scan shows two or more clinically silent lesions at least 3 mm in diameter.[31]

4-5 OPTIC NEURITIS IN CHILDREN

Several clinical differences exist between the pediatric and adult populations. One study of 30 children (mean age 9.5 years) with optic neuritis found disc swelling in 70% and bilateral involvement in 50%.[32] Similarly, a study from the United Kingdom reported on 39 children with isolated optic neuritis who were observed for a period of from 3 months to 29 years (mean follow-up of 8.8 years). Ages ranged from 3–15 years (mean 8.6 years). In 46% of the patients, there was an associated febrile prodrome. Furthermore, 74% had bilateral optic neuritis (in 25 of the 39 patients, onset was simultaneous; in 4, it was sequential) and swollen discs at onset.[33] These clinical features are much more prominent than in the adult population. Yet, as in the adult group, children developing optic neuritis experience acute, rapid decline in visual acuity associated with an afferent pupillary defect and visual field abnormalities.

The literature documents a favorable visual outcome for pediatric optic neuritis.[33–35] One study reported that 70% of patients recovered acuity of 20/20 or better.[33] In addition, long-term outcome studies of bilateral optic neuritis in children (less than 15 years of age) show only a 6%–12% incidence of MS,[32–35] or a lower incidence than in the adult population. Lucchinetti and colleagues showed that 13% of patients with isolated optic neuritis had progressed to clinically or laboratory-supported MS at 10 years, 19% at 20 years, 22% at 30 years, and 26% at 40 years. Also, the presence of bilateral sequential or recurrent optic neuritis increased the MS risk.[36]

One consistent finding in optic neuritis of childhood is the higher frequency of normal visual evoked responses (50%–70%) compared with adults (10%) after recovery from optic neuritis.[33,34] The reason for this difference is unclear: possibly a greater potential for remyelination exists in childhood and, conceivably, the primary pathologic process of optic neuritis in children differs from that in adults.

Acute disseminated encephalomyelitis (ADEM) is an inflammatory, often parainfectious syndrome affecting the central nervous system. It is more commonly seen in the pediatric population. Optic neuritis occurs with ADEM, yet there has been a paucity of publications regarding an association between the two. Kotlus and coworkers performed a retrospective study of pediatric patients presenting with ADEM from 1996 to 2003. Of 10 patients, six presented with optic neuritis, and 5 of those had bilateral disease associated with optic disc edema. A preceding viral syndrome was identified in 8 of 10 patients. All patients were treated with high-dose intravenous corticosteroids, with favorable visual outcomes.[37] Currently, no controlled studies exist.

4-6 NEUROMYELITIS OPTICA

Also known as *Devic's disease*, neuromyelitis optica (NMO) is the clinical syndrome of bilateral optic neuritis in association with transverse myelitis.[38,39] In all likelihood, it is a variant of MS, with a propensity for occurrence in children and young adults. Devic's disease is characterized by severe visual loss, with a less predictable course for good visual recovery. Patients may also be left with paraplegia as a permanent sequela of this disorder. Yet the neurologic prognosis is more favorable than once believed, primarily due to advances in supportive care and in the recognition of mild cases.[40] NMO may be monophasic or relapsing. Patients with a monophasic course usually presented with rapidly sequential events and moderate recovery. Those with a relapsing course had an extended interval between events (median 166 days) followed by severe disability in a stepwise manner.[41] Recent data suggest that an NMO-IgG autoantibody may play a role in distinguishing NMO from MS.[42]

4-7 CHIASMAL AND OPTIC TRACT NEURITIS

Occasionally, demyelination may affect other portions of the anterior visual pathways. Chiasmal neuritis is surprisingly uncommon clinically, given the frequency with which typical lesions of MS are found within the chiasm in autopsy studies. Patients typically present with bilateral (often asymmetric) reduced acuity and visual field loss of a junctional or bitemporal hemianopic pattern.[43–45] Pathologic study in patients with acute onset has confirmed the presence of demyelination, gliosis, and chronic meningeal inflammation.[46] Both CT and MRI have documented abnormalities, including swelling of the chiasm and contrast enhancement (Fig. 4–7).[45] As with optic neuritis, the prognosis for functional recovery is generally good.

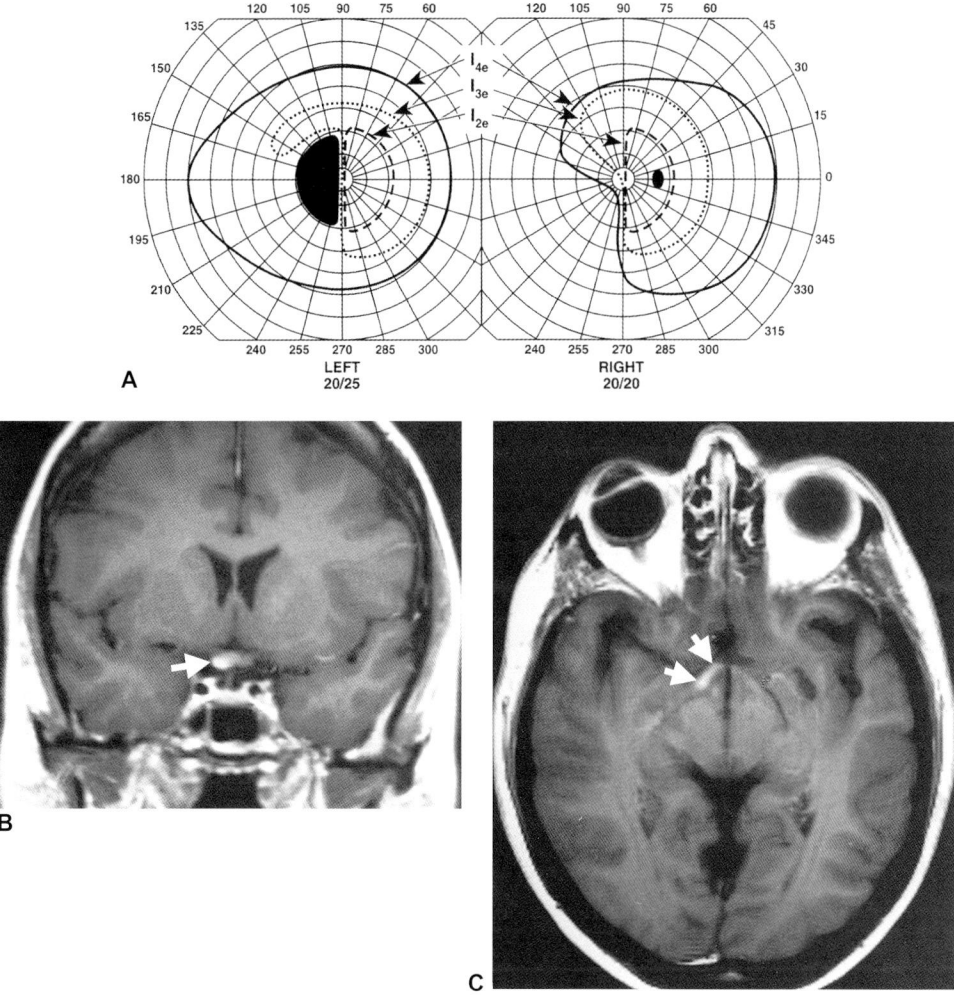

Figure 4–7. This 40-year-old woman experienced the sudden onset of a visual field defect in the left eye. Visual acuity: 20/20 right eye, 20/25 left eye. Pupils, color vision, and fundi were normal. (A) Visual field testing revealed an incongruous left homonymous hemianopia. Gadolinium-enhanced T1-weighted MRI revealed (B) enhancement and swelling (arrow) of the right side of chiasm and (C) enhancement of the right optic tract (arrows).

Optic tract neuritis is rare. It is characterized by a homonymous hemianopia, usually incongruous, and normal Snellen acuity unless there is concurrent chiasmal or optic nerve involvement. A report of two patients with optic tract neuritis illustrates the reversible nature of the visual field loss and documented contrast-enhancing lesions of the optic tract with MRI (see Fig. 4–7).[47]

Just as optic neuritis is often the initial manifestation of MS, chiasmal and optic tract neuritis can also be the first indication of more extensive demyelinating disease. Alternatively, the disturbance of the anterior visual pathways may be an isolated, often transient clinical finding.

4-8 DIFFERENTIAL DIAGNOSIS

The Optic Neuritis Treatment Trial has presented compelling evidence that a systemic workup is not necessary to diagnose typical optic neuritis. Questions then arise as to which patients should be evaluated for systemic disease and when this evaluation should be done. The following criteria have been offered:[48]

1. The optic neuritis occurs in a patient outside the 20- to 50-year age range.
2. The optic neuritis is bilateral and simultaneous.
3. The progressive visual loss endures beyond 14 days after onset.
4. If optic neuritis is accompanied by abnormalities in the patient's history or examination that cannot be attributed to MS, then three possible explanations for the optic neuropathy exist:
   a. The patient has an atypical clinical course of optic neuritis.
   b. Optic neuritis occurs in the context of a systemic disease other than MS.
   c. The patient's optic neuropathy mimics optic neuritis but is occurring on another basis (see section 4-9).

Table 4–1 summarizes the clinical settings in which optic neuritis may occur. Although not exhaustive, the list covers those conditions the practicing ophthalmologist encounters most frequently.

4-8-1 *Demyelinating Disorders.* Multiple sclerosis is by far the most common known cause of optic neuritis. Adrenoleukodystrophy is characterized by severe cerebral demyelination associated with Addison's disease. This demyelinating disease is inherited as an X-linked disorder, and patients demonstrate extensive white-matter changes on MRI. The condition follows a relentless, progressive course of generalized neurologic deterioration. Adrenomyeloneuropathy is a milder, more slowly progressive form of this disorder, with later onset.

4-8-2 *Infectious Agents.* The most frequent infectious cause of optic neuritis is viral and may occur in three clinical settings:

1. Direct viral infection of the central nervous system, particularly in children, seen in conditions such as measles, rubella, mumps, chickenpox, influenza,

Table 4-1 Causes of Optic Neuritis

Demyelinating Disorders

Multiple sclerosis
Devic's disease
Adrenoleukodystrophy (Schilder's disease)

Infectious Agents

Viral
  Paraviral neuritis
  Postviral neuritis
  Postvaccination neuritis
Fungal
  Histoplasmosis
  Cryptococcosis
  Aspergillosis
  Mucormycosis
Bacterial
  Sinusitis
  Spirochetal infection
  Syphilis
  Lyme disease

Association With Intraocular Inflammation

Infection
  Nematode infection
  Herpes zoster
  Toxoplasmosis
  Cat-scratch disease
Noninfectious uveitis

and cytomegalovirus. Typically, the patient presents with bilateral papillitis and may have other neurologic findings of an encephalitic illness.

2. Postviral syndrome either as isolated optic neuritis or accompanied by a postinfectious encephalomyelitis. Adverse neurologic reactions occur 1–3 weeks after the onset of the illness and usually resolve as a monophasic illness.

3. Postvaccination (mumps, measles, rubella) optic neuritis following a course similar to that of the postviral syndrome.

All three presentations are regarded as demyelinating disorders due to either direct viral invasion or an immune-mediated attack on specific neural antigens including those within the optic nerve.

Fungal infections of the optic nerve are unusual and generally occur in immuno-compromised individuals, including transplant patients and those with acquired immunodeficiency syndrome (AIDS) (Fig. 4–8). Mucormycosis must always be kept in mind in the poorly controlled diabetic patient presenting with painful ophthal-moplegia and sudden visual loss.

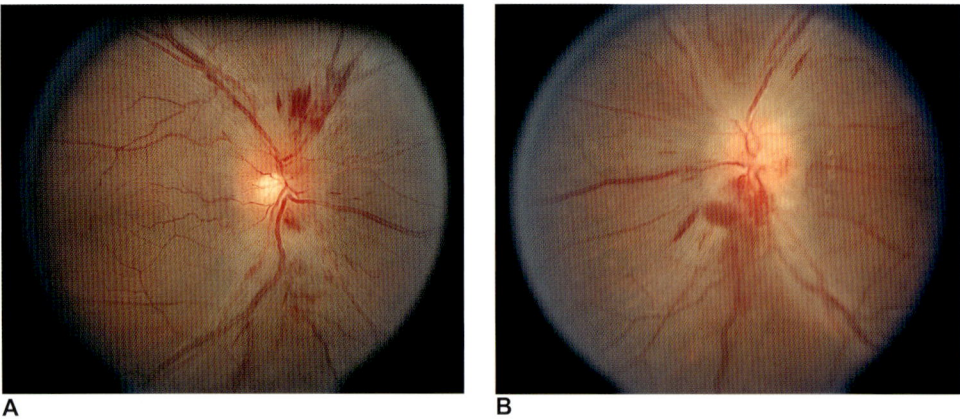

A   B

Figure 4–8. This 37-year-old man with AIDS developed cryptococcal meningitis with bilateral optic neuritis. Visual acuity: 20/70 right eye, 20/100 left eye. Visual fields show bilateral centro-cecal scotomas. (A) Right eye. (B) Left eye.

At one time, infection of the contiguous paranasal sinuses was thought to be a frequent cause of optic neuritis. With more sophisticated patient evaluation for demyelinating disease and better imaging techniques of the sinuses, the relationship between sinusitis and optic neuritis has become more tenuous.[49] However, there are clear instances when paranasal sinusitis spreads to the orbit and causes an inflammatory optic neuritis.[50] In these cases, aggressive therapy including antibiotics and/or surgical drainage may be necessary to save sight.

In addition, mucoceles of the ethmoid and sphenoid sinuses may lead to optic nerve compression and can mimic optic neuritis.[51]

Spirochetes, both of historical and recent vintage, may lead to inflammatory optic neuritis. Syphilis is a well-known cause of optic neuritis and has become more prevalent with the increase of the AIDS population. Optic perineuritis, a variant of optic neuritis that may be caused by syphilis, is characterized by optic disc edema and peripheral visual field loss with preservation of central acuity (Fig. 4–9). Syphilitic leptomeningitis leads to inflammation of the peripheral portions of the optic nerve, while the axial fibers are spared. Lyme neuroborreliosis may occasionally cause optic neuritis.[52,53] Besides hematologic and serologic studies, the diagnosis of optic neuritis due to Lyme disease should be confirmed with a lumbar puncture, demonstrating a pleocytosis and a *Borrelia burgdorferi* antibody titer higher than that in serum.

4-8-3 Intraocular Inflammation. Intraocular inflammation, including some of the entities that commonly cause uveitis, may lead to an associated optic neuritis. Toxoplasmosis may cause an inflammatory neuritis[54] with or without the typical fundus lesions of retinochoroiditis. Less common infectious agents include nematodes and varicella zoster virus. If the fundus findings include a macular star (Fig. 4–10), the designation *neuroretinitis* is applied (see Chapter 10).

4-8-4 Systemic Diseases. A variety of systemic diseases may cause optic neuritis. Two deserve special mention, as they may be responsive to appropriate treatment. Sar-

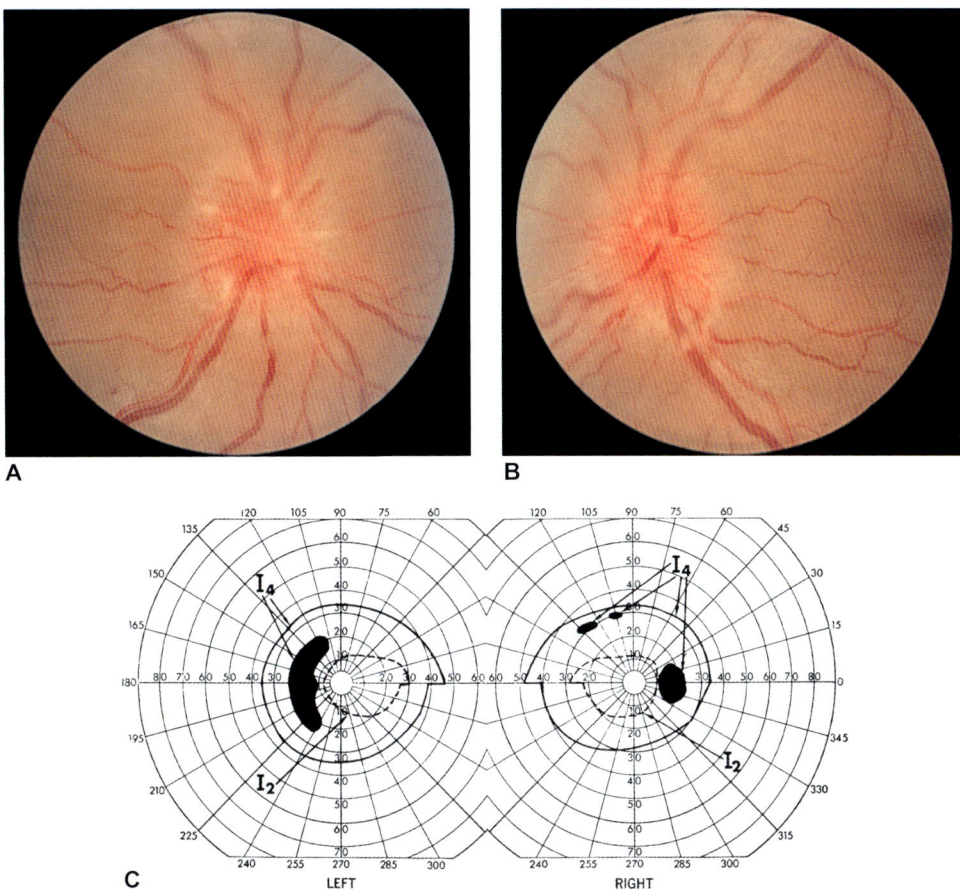

Figure 4–9. This 51-year-old man reported blurred vision and was found to have bilateral uveitis and optic neuritis. Evaluation was consistent with neurosyphilis. Both optic discs are edematous. (A) Right eye. (B) Left eye. (C) Visual fields demonstrate bilateral nerve fiber bundle defects.

coidosis involves the central nervous system in about 5% of patients.[55] The most common ocular manifestation of the posterior segment is retinal vasculitis, but the optic nerve may become inflamed without other signs. Swelling of the optic disc may or may not be present (Fig. 4–11). Visual loss may be acute or subacute and is often responsive to systemic corticosteroid treatment, which may be required for an extended period. Tapering should be very gradual, and cytotoxic agents may be required as an adjunctive therapy in patients who do not recover with corticosteroid treatment.[56]

The second systemic disease that may respond to treatment is an autoimmune optic neuritis that has been described in patients who manifest some clinical and serologic features of connective tissue disease but do not fulfill the criteria for a named condition.[57,58] The age range is 17–60 years, yet this condition can also occur in children as young as 4 years of age.[59] On laboratory testing, patients often exhibit abnormalities typical of autoimmune diseases, such as positive antinuclear antibodies (ANA). Anticardiolipin antibodies may be present, and biopsies

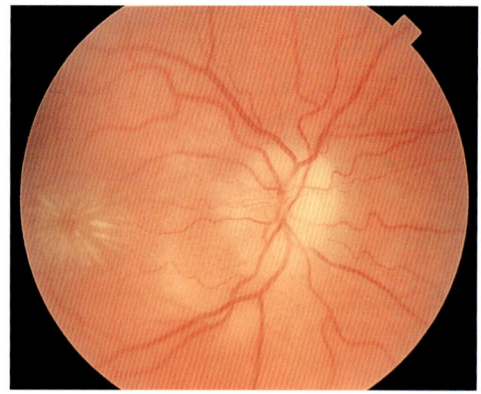

Figure 4–10. Toxoplasmosis optic neuritis with optic disc edema and macular star.

of skin not exposed to the sun, processed with direct immunofluorescent staining, may show immune-complex deposition.[60] Patients with autoimmune optic neuritis may have visual acuity worse than 20/200. Dramatic improvement after corticosteroid therapy can occur with either an intravenous or high-dose oral regimen. This entity should be considered whenever a patient with optic neuritis has a recurrent course.[61] The disease tends to recrudesce when immunosuppressive therapy is withdrawn too soon.

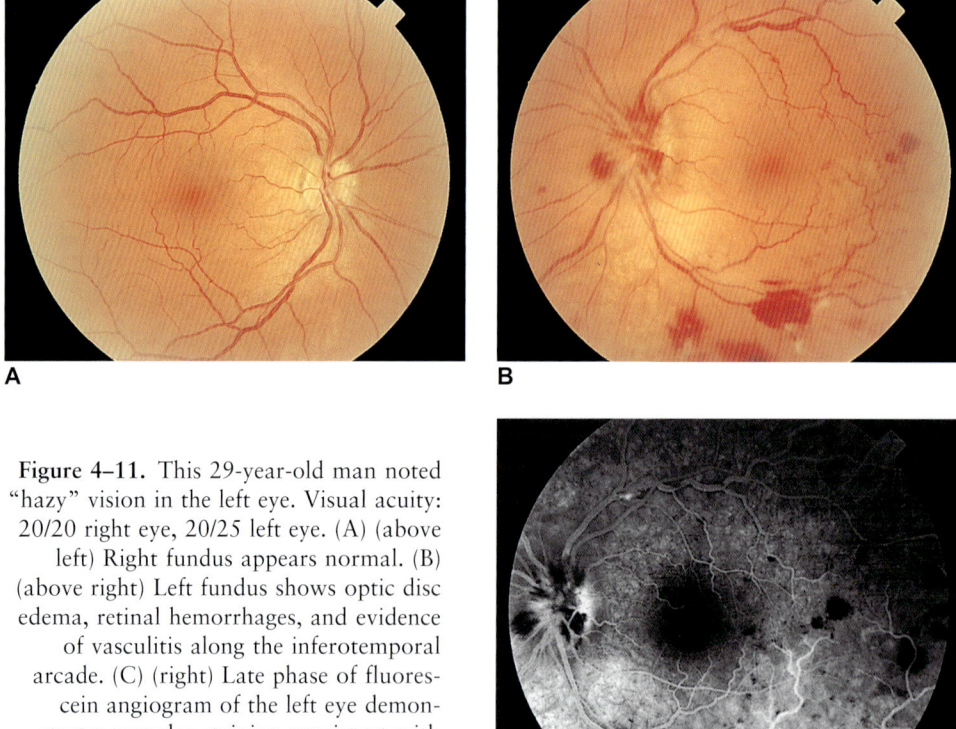

A

B

C

Figure 4–11. This 29-year-old man noted "hazy" vision in the left eye. Visual acuity: 20/20 right eye, 20/25 left eye. (A) (above left) Right fundus appears normal. (B) (above right) Left fundus shows optic disc edema, retinal hemorrhages, and evidence of vasculitis along the inferotemporal arcade. (C) (right) Late phase of fluorescein angiogram of the left eye demonstrates vascular staining consistent with vasculitis. Hilar lymph node biopsy provided pathologic evidence of sarcoidosis.

4-9 MIMICKERS OF OPTIC NEURITIS

Nonarteritic anterior ischemic optic neuropathy (NAION) may present with a similar clinical picture as optic neuritis: abrupt onset, visual acuity and field loss, and optic disc edema. However, in the majority of cases, patients with optic neuritis are younger (< 50 years), have ocular/orbital pain accompanying visual loss (92%), and demonstrate significant visual recovery. Fluorescein angiography often shows delayed optic disc filling with ischemia, while filling is normal with optic neuritis (papillitis). Typically there is enhancement of the optic nerve on MRI early in the course of optic neuritis, which is rarely seen in NAION.[62,63] In addition, optic neuritis is associated with periventricular white-matter lesions typical of MS.

Leber's hereditary optic neuropathy (LHON) may mimic optic neuritis, both clinically and on MRI (see Chapter 7). Both conditions tend to affect young adults in the second to fourth decades with abrupt visual loss. In contrast to optic neuritis, patients with LHON lack pain at onset of visual loss and only rarely experience significant visual recovery. MRI in LHON may demonstrate optic nerve enhancement similar in appearance to that of optic neuritis.[64] To add further difficulty in distinguishing the two entities, LHON may be associated with an MS-like illness.[65] These patients demonstrate signs and symptoms of demyelinating disease combined with non-remitting visual loss typical of LHON. It remains unclear whether this is a distinct entity or the association is no greater than the prevalence of the two diseases.

Optic nerve sheath meningioma (ONSM) can mimic optic neuritis both clinically and on enhanced orbital fat-suppressed MRI. With ONSM, the visual field defects include central scotomas, enlarged blind spots, and generalized constriction. The optic nerve is swollen in approximately 60% of patients, and one-quarter have retinochoroidal shunt vessels on the optic nerve. If the disc edema persists for more than 6–8 weeks, ONSM should be considered.[66] Contrasted orbital fat-suppressed MRI can usually distinguish optic neuritis from intrinsic optic nerve disease.

Other inflammatory optic neuropathies including optic perineuritis[67] as well as carcinomatous and immune-mediated optic neuropathy (see Chapter 10) may also simulate demyelinating optic neuritis.

4-10 CONCLUSION

Optic neuritis is a clinical diagnosis established only after careful patient evaluation. In the vast majority of cases, it is a primary demyelinative disorder that may, in some cases, be the harbinger of MS. The ophthalmologist must be familiar with the typical clinical profile of optic neuritis and be alert to secondarily demyelinative processes from infectious or non-MS autoimmune inflammation. In addition, some of the atypical cases may not represent a demyelinative process at all but rather another form of optic nerve disease simulating optic neuritis, like NAION, LHON, or neuroretinitis. As the late David Cogan cautioned: "Probably no branch of neuro-ophthalmology has to its discredit the abundance of erroneous diagnoses as has optic neuritis."[68]

References

1. Beck RW. The clinical profile of optic neuritis: experience of the Optic Neuritis Treatment Trial. Arch Ophthalmol 1991;109:1673–78.
2. Fazzone HE, Lefton DR, Kupersmith MJ. Optic neuritis. Correlation of pain and magnetic resonance imaging. Ophthalmology 2003;110:1646–49.
3. Optic neuritis study group. Visual function more than 10 years after optic neuritis: experience of the optic neuritis treatment trial. Am J Ophthalmol 2004:137;77–83.
4. Davis FA, Bergen D, Schauf C, et al. Movement phosphenes in optic neuritis: a new clinical sign. Neurology 1976;26:1100–4.
5. Sokol S. The Pulfrich stereo-illusion as an index of optic nerve dysfunction. Surv Ophthalmol 1976;20:432–34.
6. Vaphiades, MS and Eggenberger, E. The Pulfrich effect in its relationship to retinal illumination. J Neuro-ophthalmol 1997:17:240–42.
7. Perkin GD, Rose FC. Visual signs at presentation. In: Optic Neuritis and Its Differential Diagnosis. New York: Oxford University Press; 1979:43–73.
8. Keltner JL, Johnson CA, Spurr JO, Beck RW. Baseline visual field profile of optic neuritis: the experience of the Optic Neuritis Treatment Trial. Arch Ophthalmol 1993;111:231–34.
9. Beck RW, Kupersmith MJ, Cleary PA, Katz B. Fellow eye abnormalities in acute unilateral optic neuritis: experience of the Optic Neuritis Treatment Trial. Ophthalmology 1993;100:691–98.
10. Fang JP, Donahue SP, Lin RH. Global visual field involvement in acute unilateral optic neuritis. Am J Ophthalmol 1999;128(5):554–65.
11. Rizzo JF III, Lessell S. Optic neuritis and ischemic optic neuropathy: overlapping clinical profiles. Arch Ophthalmol 1991;109:1668–72.
12. Goldstein JE, Cogan DC. Exercise and the optic neuropathy of multiple sclerosis. Arch Ophthalmol 1964;72:168–70.
13. Halliday AM, McDonald WI. Visual evoked potentials. In: Stalberg E, Young RR, eds. Clinical Neurophysiology. London: Butterworths, 1981:228–58.
14. Halliday AM, ed. Evoked Potentials in Clinical Testing. Edinburgh: Churchill Livingstone; 1982.
15. Howard CW, Osher RH, Tomsak RL. Computed tomographic features in optic neuritis. Am J Ophthalmol 1980;89:699–702.
16. Miller DH, Newton MR, van der Poel JC, et al. Magnetic resonance imaging of the optic nerve in optic neuritis. Neurology 1988;38:175–79.
17. Merandi SF, Kudryk BT, Murtagh FR, Arrington JA. Contrast-enhanced MRI imaging of optic nerve lesions in patients with acute optic neuritis. Am J Neuroradiol 1991;12:923–26.
18. Kupersmith MJ, Alban T, Zeiffer B, Lefton D. Contrast-enhanced MRI in acute optic neuritis: relationship to visual performance. Brain 2002;125:812–22.
19. Bradley WG, Whitty CW. Acute optic neuritis: prognosis for development of multiple sclerosis. J Neurol Neurosurg Psychiatry 1968;31:10–8.
20. Rizzo JF III, Lessell S. Risk of developing multiple sclerosis after uncomplicated optic neuritis: a long-term prospective study. Neurology 1988;38:185–90.
21. Rodriguez M, Siva A, Cross SA, et al. Optic neuritis: a population-based study in Olmsted County, Minnesota. Neurology 1995;45:244–50.
22. Hutchinson WM. Acute optic neuritis and the prognosis for multiple sclerosis. J Neurol Neurosurg Psychiatry 1976;39:283–89.
23. Francis DA, Compston DA, Batchelor JR, McDonald WI. A reassessment of the risk of

multiple sclerosis developing in patients with optic neuritis after extended follow-up. J Neurol Neurosurg Psychiatry 1987;50:758–65.

24. Optic neuritis study group. High-and low-risk profiles for the development of multiple sclerosis within 10 years after optic neuritis. Experience of the optic neuritis treatment trial. Arch Ophthalmol 2003:121;944–49.

25. Beck RW, Cleary PA, Anderson MM, et al. A randomized, controlled trial of corticosteroids in the treatment of acute optic neuritis. N Engl J Med 1992;326:581–88.

26. Beck RW, Cleary PA. Optic Neuritis Treatment Trial: one-year follow-up results. Arch Ophthalmol 1993;111:773–75.

27. Beck RW, Cleary PA, Trobe JD, et al. The effect of corticosteroids for acute optic neuritis on the subsequent development of multiple sclerosis. N Engl J Med 1993;329:1764–69.

28. Beck RW, Arrington J, Murtagh FR, et al. Brain magnetic resonance imaging in acute optic neuritis: experience of the Optic Neuritis Study Group. Arch Neurol 1993;50:841–46.

29. Morrissey SP, Miller DH, Kendall BE, et al. The significance of brain magnetic resonance imaging abnormalities at presentation with clinically isolated syndromes suggestive of multiple sclerosis: a 5-year follow-up study. Brain 1993;116:135–46.

30. Beck RW. The Optic Neuritis Treatment Trial: three-year follow-up results. Arch Ophthalmol 1995;113:136–37.

31. Jacobs LD, Beck RW, Simon JH, et al. Intramuscular interferon beta–1a therapy initiated during the first demyelinating event in multiple sclerosis. N Engl J Med 2000: 343;898–904.

32. Kennedy C, Carroll FD. Optic neuritis in children. Arch Ophthalmol 1960;63:747–55.

33. Kriss A, Francis DA, Cuendet F, et al. Recovery after optic neuritis in childhood. J Neurol Neurosurg Psychiatry 1988;51:1253–58.

34. Parkin PJ, Hierons R, McDonald WI. Bilateral optic neuritis: a long-term follow-up. Brain 1984;107:951–64.

35. Brady KM, Brar AS, Lee AG, et al. Optic neuritis in children: clinical features and visual outcome. J AAPOS 1999;3:98–103.

36. Lucchinetti CF, Kiers L, O'Duffy A, et al. Risk factors for developing multiple sclerosis after childhood optic neuritis. Neurology 1997;49:1413–18.

37. Kotlus BS, Slavin ML, Guthrie DS, et al. Ophthalmic manifestations in pediatric patients with acute disseminated encephalomyelitis. J AAPOS 2005;9:179–83.

38. Allbutt TC. On the ophthalmoscopic signs of spinal disease. Lancet 1870;1:76–8.

39. Gault F. De la neuromyelité optique aigue. Thèse de Lyon. 1894; serre 1, no 981.

40. Whithan RH, Brey RL. Neuromyelitis optica: two new cases and review of the literature. J Clin Neuro-ophthalmol 1985;5:263–69.

41. Wingerchuk DM, Hogancamp WF, O'Brien PC, et al. The clinical course of neuromyelitis optica (Devic's syndrome). Neurology 1999;53:1107–14.

42. Lennon VA, Wingerchuk DM, Kryzer TJ, et al. A serum autoantibody marker of neuromyelitis optica: distinction from multiple sclerosis. Lancet 2004;364:2106–12.

43. Spector RH, Glaser JS, Schatz NJ. Demyelinative chiasmal lesions. Arch Neurol 1980;37: 757–62.

44. Reynolds WD, Smith JL, McCrary JA III. Chiasmal optic neuritis. J Clin Neuro-ophthalmol 1982;2:93–101.

45. Newman NJ, Lessell S, Winterkorn JM. Optic chiasmal neuritis. Neurology 1991;41: 1203–10.

46. Bell RA, Robertson DM, Rosen DA, Kerr AW. Optochiasmatic arachnoiditis in multiple sclerosis. Arch Ophthalmol 1975;93:191–93.

47. Rosenblatt MA, Behrens MM, Zweifach PH, et al. Magnetic resonance imaging of optic tract involvement in multiple sclerosis. Am J Ophthalmol 1987:104:74–9.

48. Burde RM, Savino PJ, Trobe JD. Prechiasmal visual loss. In: Clinical Decisions in Neuro-Ophthalmology. 3rd ed. St Louis: Mosby–Year Book; 2002:chap 2.

49. Smith CH. Optic neuritis. In: Walsh and Hoyt's Clinical Neuro-Ophthalmology. Baltimore: Lippincott Williams & Wilkins; 2005:chap 6.

50. Slavin ML, Glaser JS. Acute severe irreversible visual loss with sphenoethmoiditis—"posterior" orbital cellulitis. Arch Ophthalmol 1987;105:345–48.

51. Slavin ML, Liebergall DA. Acute visual loss in the elderly due to retrobulbar optic neuropathy. Surv Ophthalmol 1996;41:261–67.

52. Winward KE, Smith JL, Culbertson WW, Paris-Hamelin A. Ocular Lyme borreliosis. Am J Ophthalmol 1989;108:651–57.

53. Lesser RS, Kornmehl EW, Pachner AR, et al. Neuro-ophthalmologic manifestations of Lyme disease. Ophthalmology 1990;97:699–706.

54. Fish RH, Hoskins JC, Kline LB. Toxoplasmosis neuroretinitis. Ophthalmology 1993;100:1177–82.

55. Stern BJ, Krumholz A, Johns C, et al. Sarcoidosis and its neurological manifestations. Arch Neurol 1985;42:909–17.

56. Gelwan MJ, Kellen RI, Burde RM, Kupersmith MJ. Sarcoidosis of the anterior visual pathway: successes and failures. J Neurol Neurosurg Psychiatry 1988;51:1473–80.

57. Dutton JJ, Burde RM, Klingele TG. Autoimmune retrobulbar optic neuritis. Am J Ophthalmol 1982;94:11–7.

58. Kupersmith MJ, Burde RM, Warren FA, et al. Autoimmune optic neuropathy: evaluation and treatment. J Neurol Neurosurg Psychiatry 1980;51:1381–86.

59. Frohman L, Turbin R, Bielory L, Wolansky L, Lambert WC, Cook S. Autoimmune optic neuropathy with anticardiolipin antibody mimicking multiple sclerosis in a child. Am J Ophthalmol 2003;136:358–60.

60. Frohman L, Bielory L, Warren F, Kupersmith MJ. Skin biopsies in the evaluation of atypical optic neuropathies. Invest Ophthalmol Vis Sci 1991(suppl 32):951.

61. Riedel P. Wall M. Grey A. Cannon T. Folberg R. Thompson HS. Autoimmune optic neuropathy. Arch Ophthalmol 1998;116:1121–24.

62. Lessell S. Nonarteritic anterior ischemic optic neuropathy. Arch Ophthalmol 1999;117:386–88.

63. Rizzo JF, Andreoli CM, Rabinov JD. Use of magnetic resonance imaging to differentiate optic neuritis and nonarteritic anterior ischemic optic neuropathy. Ophthalmology 2002;109:1679–84.

64. Vaphiades MS, Newman NJ. Optic nerve enhancement on the orbital magnetic resonance imaging and Leber's hereditary optic neuropathy. J Neuro-ophthalmol 1999;19:238–39.

65. Bhatti, MT, Newman NJ. A multiple sclerosis-like illness in a man harboring the mtDNA 14484 mutation. J Neuro-ophthalmol 1989;19:20–33.

66. Vaphiades MS. Disk edema and cranial MRI optic nerve enhancement: how long is too long? Surv Ophthalmol 2001;46:56–8.

67. Purvin V, Kawasaki A, Jacobson DM. Optic perineuritis: clinical and radiographic features. Arch Ophthalmol . 2001;119:1299–306.

68. Glaser JS. Neuro-Ophthalmology. Philadelphia, PA: Lippincott, Williams & Wilkins, 1999.

5

Ischemic Optic Neuropathy

LAWRENCE M. BUONO

*I*schemic optic neuropathy is the most common nonglaucomatous optic nerve disorder encountered in patients above 50 years of age.[1] This disorder has been classified by the presence (anterior ischemic optic neuropathy) or absence (posterior ischemic optic neuropathy) of optic disc edema at the onset of visual loss. The former is common, while the latter is rare and established only as a diagnosis of exclusion. This chapter focuses primarily on anterior ischemic optic neuropathy, emphasizing current thinking on diagnosis, patient evaluation, and management.

Anterior ischemic optic neuropathy (AION) is characterized by a sudden onset of visual loss affecting visual acuity, visual field, or both. The visual loss is typically painless.[2] A relative afferent pupillary defect is present unless there is bilateral symmetric optic nerve dysfunction. The funduscopic appearance includes sectoral or generalized optic disc swelling, which may be hyperemic or pale, with hemorrhages of the nerve fiber layer.

Anterior ischemic optic neuropathy can occur in association with a systemic arteritis, most commonly giant cell arteritis, and is termed *arteritic AION*. Anterior ischemic optic neuropathy occurring in the absence of systemic arteritis is termed *nonarteritic anterior ischemic optic neuropathy* (NAION) and may occur in association with an identifiable disease process but is most often idiopathic. Table 5–1 outlines some conditions associated with ischemic optic neuropathy.

5-1 NONARTERITIC ANTERIOR ISCHEMIC OPTIC NEUROPATHY

NAION is thought to occur from an ischemic process of the anterior portion of the optic nerve; however, the exact pathophysiologic mechanism remains unknown.

85

Table 5–1 Conditions Associated
with Ischemic Optic Neuropathy

Arterial Disease

Arteriosclerosis
Inflammatory disease
  Giant cell (temporal) arteritis
  Polyarteritis nodosa
  Systemic lupus erythematosus
Vasospastic disease (migraine)
Postradiation

Hypovolemia/Hypotension

Severe anemia
Shock/blood loss
Hypotension, surgical or spontaneous

Mechanism Not Clear

Postcataract extraction
Amiodarone

There have been some histopathologic reports of NAION supporting arteriosclerosis as an underlying mechanism, but conclusive evidence has not been established.[3–5] Other evidence suggests that the anatomic configuration of the optic nerve head is a contributing factor and that NAION may represent a form of compartment syndrome causing tissue ischemia.[6] In most circumstances, NAION is idiopathic but has been associated with several risk factors. Occasionally NAION will occur in association with an easily identifiable cause or in a clinical setting suggesting the underlying etiology. These entities appear to be distinct from the idiopathic form.

5-1-1 *Idiopathic* NAION. The incidence of NAION is between 2.3 and 10.2 per 100,000 patients above 50 years of age, with a prevalence of 0.54 per 100,000 for all age groups.[1,7,8] Typically patients are above age 50, although NAION may occur at any age.[1,9] In a large study of 406 patients with NAION, the mean age was 60 ± 14 years and the range was 11–91 years.[9] The data from the Ischemic Optic Neuropathy Decompression Trial (IONDT) showed a higher mean age of 66.0 ± 8.7 years, with a range of 50 to 89 years. The prevalence among men and women appears to be equivalent. There is a racial predilection, as NAION affects Caucasian patients in approximately 95% of cases.[1,9–11]

5-1-1-1 *Risk Factors.* Several risk factors for the development of idiopathic NAION have been identified. Perhaps the most significant is the structural morphology of the optic disc. Several studies have shown that a small or absent central physiologic cup (small cup-to-disc ratio) and overall optic disc size (optic disc diameter) are more frequently found patients with NAION than in controls.[12–15] Systemic vasculopathic risk factors including hypertension, diabetes mellitus, and hypercholesterolemia have been associated with NAION. Systemic hypertension has been found in up to 49% and diabetes mellitus in up to 26% of patients with NAION.[9] Hypercholesterolemia has also been found in patients with NAION, especially in those under age 50 who develop this disorder.[16] Other less common risk factors include cardiac disease, cerebrovascular disease, hyperhomocystinemia, and sleep apnea.[9–11,17,18]

5-1-1-2 *Clinical Characteristics.* The typical presenting symptom of NAION is sudden loss of visual acuity or visual field. Patients may report periocular discomfort associated with the visual loss, but they do not typically have ocular pain. Patients may also report the onset of visual loss shortly after awakening. The IONDT reports that 42% of patients recalled that the onset of the visual loss was within 2 hours of awakening.[10] The level of visual acuity is variable and ranges from 20/20 to no light perception (NLP).[10,19–21] The IONDT showed that visual acuity was better than 20/64 in 49% and 20/64 or worse in 51% of 420 patients.[10] The visual field patterns are also variable (Fig. 5–1). In one study of 169 patients with NAION, 46% had an inferior altitudinal defect, 20% had a central defect, 17% had a superior altitudinal defect, 8% had an inferior arcuate defect, 8% had an inferior quadrantic defect, and 1% had an unclassified defect.[19]

Loss of color vision is variable; the degree of dyschromatopsia can be assessed with pseudoisochromatic plates and often coincides with the loss of central acuity. Patients with unilateral NAION will as a rule have a relative afferent pupillary defect. Optic disc swelling is a requirement for the diagnosis of NAION (Fig. 5–2). The swelling may be either sectoral or diffuse. The swollen area is most often hyperemic

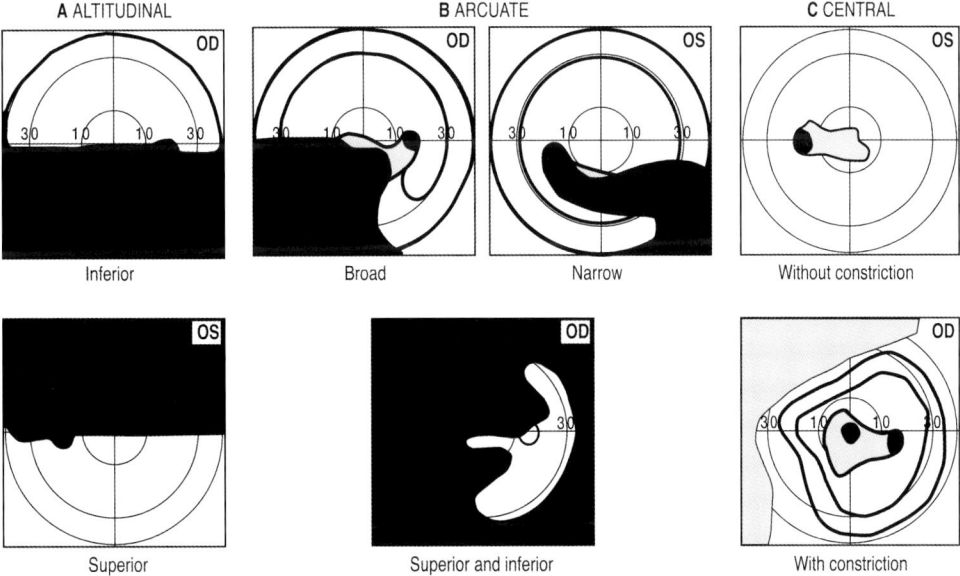

Figure 5–1. Types of visual field defects in nonarteritic ischemic optic neuropathy. (A) Altitudinal: inferior and superior. (B) Arcuate: broad, narrow, and superior/inferior. (C) Central: with and without constriction.(Redrawn with permission of Oxford University Press from Boghen DR, Glaser JS. Ischaemic optic neuropathy: the clinical profile and natural history. Brain 1975;98: 689–708.)

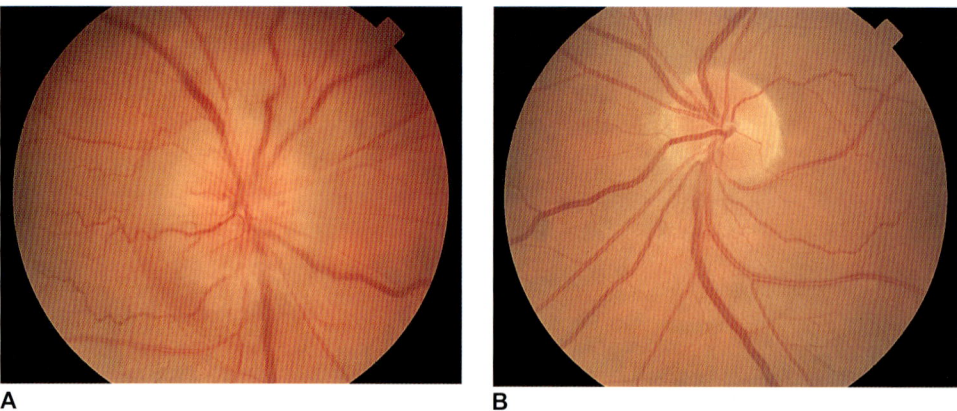

A   B

Figure 5–2. Typical clinical presentation of anterior ischemic optic neuropathy. (A) Right optic disc demonstrates diffuse edema. (B) Left optic disc is congenitally full, with no physiologic cup.

but may be mildly pale. Rarely is the optic disc markedly pale, raising the suspicion of arteritic AION. Focal hemorrahges of the nerve fiber layer are common and can be seen on the neuroretinal rim or on the margin of the optic disc. Occasionally, focal areas of telangiectasia can be seen. Infrequently, hard exudates can be seen in the parapapillary and macular region,[9] simulating neuroretinitis. Within 2–3 months of onset, optic disc edema resolves and the disc becomes pale, either diffusely or segmentally, typically without cupping of the optic disc (Fig. 5–3).

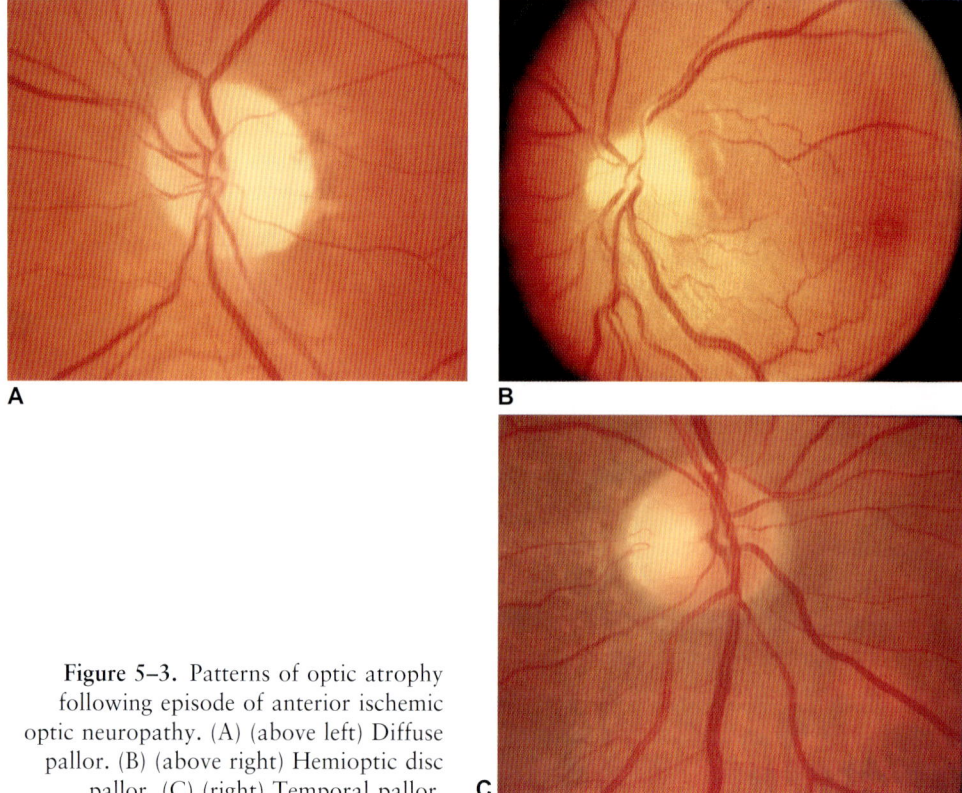

A   B

Figure 5–3. Patterns of optic atrophy following episode of anterior ischemic optic neuropathy. (A) (above left) Diffuse pallor. (B) (above right) Hemioptic disc pallor. (C) (right) Temporal pallor.   C

Retinal emboli occasionally may be found in the peripapillary retinal vasculature and should serve to exclude the idiopathic form of NAION and prompt an evaluation for the source of emboli (see section 5-1-2-4). The optic disc swelling typically resolves in 4–12 weeks. If the swelling persists, an alternative diagnosis should be considered.

5-1-1-3 *Progressive Disease.* For a small subgroup of patients, the visual acuity or visual field may continue worsen over several days to weeks.[22,23] This subgroup has been classfied as having "progressive" NAION.

5-1-1-4 *Recurrent and Sequential Disease.* Recurrent disease should be distinguished from progressive disease. Recurrent NAION is a second and separate ischemic event in the same eye after resolution of the first episode. The rate of recurrent NAION is low and ranges from 3.6%–6.4%.[19,24] Sequential NAION refers to the development of NAION in the fellow eye. The rate of involvement appears to increase over time. In one series, 20 of 83 patients (24%) developed NAION in the fellow eye. with a mean time interval of 2.9 years.[19] Some reports have documented sequential involvement as high as 40%. In one of the largest series of 431 patients with NAION, the probability of developing NAION in the fellow eye was 15% at 2 years and 20% at 5 years.[25]

5-1-1-5 *Visual Acuity Outcome.* The patient can be told that vision may improve in up to 43% of cases[26] with no further deterioration, as recurrent attacks of ischemic optic neuropathy in the same eye are uncommon.[27]

5-1-1-6 *Treatment.* Prior to 1989, no treatment was demonstrated to be effective in restoring vision to patients with ischemic optic neuropathy. In that year, the results of performing decompression of the optic nerve sheath on patients with NAION, both the progressive and nonprogressive forms, were reported.[28] The 3 patients with nonprogressive ischemic optic neuropathy had no improvement in visual function postoperatively; however, the patients who had a progressive loss of vision over 1–4 weeks after onset of their initial visual loss had, in 12 of 14 cases, a remarkable increase in visual function (visual acuity and field) postoperatively compared with a control group of 12 patients with progressive ischemic optic neuropathy who did not undergo surgery.

These results spurred other investigators to evaluate this surgical procedure for progressive ischemic optic neuropathy, with varying degrees of success.[29–32] In 1992, this led to creation of the Ischemic Optic Neuropathy Decompression Trial, involving 26 clinical centers in the United States, with a goal of recruiting 300 patients.[33] Of 244 patients with NAION and visual acuity of 20/64 or worse, 125 were randomized to careful follow-up and 119 to surgery, with 91 and 95, respectively, having completed 6 months of follow-up. Patients undergoing surgery did no better than patients assigned to careful follow-up regarding improved visual acuity of three or more lines at 6 months: 32.6% of the surgery group improved compared with 42.7% of the group that was carefully followed up. Patients undergoing surgery had a significantly greater risk of losing three or more lines of vision at

6 months: 23.9% in the surgery group worsened compared with 12.4% in the group that was carefully followed up. In addition, no benefit from surgery was found in those patients who experienced a progressive course of NAION. At present, there is no proven treatment for NAION.

5-1-1-7 *Atypical Features.* The diagnosis of the idiopathic form of NAION is based on the typical clinical presentation. When a patient presents with atypical features, the clinician should be mindful of other possible diagnoses. Atypical features include patients younger than 50 years of age and an absence of typical risk factors, especially a small or absent physiologic cup. Additionally no light perception vision, anterior or posterior vitreous cells, failure of the visual deficit to stabilize, and failure of the optic disc swelling to resolve within 3 months of the onset of symptoms should also raise the possibility of another cause of the optic neuropathy.

5-1-1-8 *Differential Diagnosis.* If atypical features are present, alternative diagnoses should be considered. Some optic neuropathies that may mimic NAION include arteritic AION (vasculitis), optic neuritis, Leber's hereditary optic neuropathy, infiltrative optic neuropathy (leukemia and lymphoma), sarcoidosis, and compressive optic neuropathy (optic nerve sheath meningioma).

On occasion, optic neuritis can be confused clinically with ischemic optic neuropathy. One helpful feature is the peak age of incidence, with optic neuritis usually occurring in the 20- to 40-year-old age group and ischemic optic neuropathy in those 55 years of age and above. A retrospective study of 81 patients with optic neuritis and 58 with NAION revealed an overlap in the rate of visual decline and range of visual acuities.[20] Pain with eye movement was reported by two-thirds of the patients with optic neuritis and by only 8% of those with ischemic optic neuropathy. Visual field defects were more likely to include central scotomas with optic neuritis and altitudinal defects with ischemic optic neuropathy. Not surprisingly, return of vision was better in patients with optic neuritis, with 65% showing improved visual function, while only 16% of patients with ischemic optic neuropathy improved. Neuroimaging can also be helpful as orbital magnetic resonance imaging (MRI) shows optic nerve enhancement in patients with optic neuritis but is typically normal in patients with NAION.[34]

Following is a clinical example:

A 54-year-old woman noted painless loss of vision over several days in her right eye. She had a history of mild amblyopia of the left eye. Best-corrected visual acuity was 20/30 on the right, with normal color vision, a right afferent pupillary defect, a right inferior arcuate visual field defect (Fig. 5–4), and right optic disc edema. Visual acuity on the left was 20/30, with a normal visual field and funduscopy. Several months later, her condition was unchanged, with persistence of the right disc edema. MRI revealed enlargement and enhancement of the right optic nerve sheath, consistent with a meningioma of the optic nerve sheath (Fig. 5–5A). Computed tomographic scanning confirmed this clinical impression (Fig. 5–5B). During 3 years of follow-up, visual function has remained unchanged except for slight progression of peripheral visual field loss on the right. Subsequent MRI has shown no change in the appearance of the meningioma.

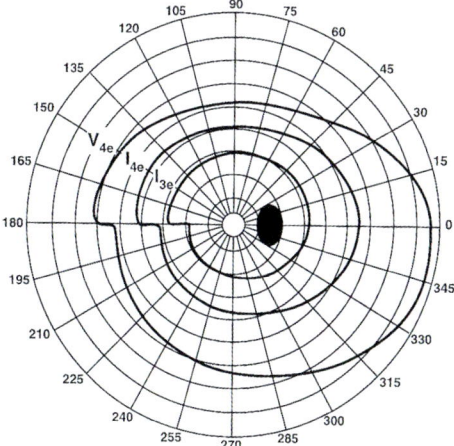

Figure 5–4. Inferior nerve fiber bundle defect detected in right visual field.

5-1-2 Nonarteritic Anterior Ischemic Optic Neuropathy. *Attributable to a Specific Condition.* Occasionally, NAION will occur in a clinical setting that may be related to an underlying cause.

5-1-2-1 Postcataract Extraction. Ischemic optic neuropathy may occur in the postoperative period following cataract surgery. A number of such patients have been reported, especially in the era of intracapsular lens removal.[35] It is recommended that any cataract patient who has suffered ischemic optic neuropathy be treated prophylactically with agents to lower the intraocular pressure (timolol maleate, acetazolamide) before and immediately after cataract surgery in the fellow eye.[36] Unfortunately, this regimen is not always protective,[37] and patients who have experienced ischemic optic neuropathy after cataract surgery have traditionally been warned that the risk to the other eye may be as high as 50%.

5-1-2-2 Amiodarone Toxicity. The existence of amiodarone-induced optic neuropathy is controverisal.[38]

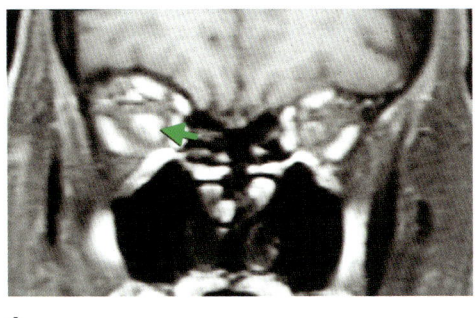
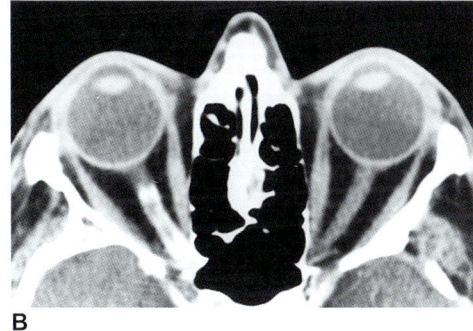

A   B

Figure 5–5. Optic nerve tumor. (A) Coronal MRI following intravenous gadolinium demonstrates enlargement and enhancement of right intraorbital optic nerve (arrow). (B) Axial CT study reveals "tram-track" calcification of right optic nerve, typical of optic nerve sheath meningioma.

Some feel that it is a form of ischemic optic neuropathy.[39] The clinical picture can be similar to that in ischemic optic neuropathy; however, more typically the onset of visual loss is more insidious, with a slow progression, and it is more often bilateral.[40] Visual function may improve in some of these patients if amiodarone is discontinued.

5-1-2-3 *Sildenafil Toxicity*. The use of sildenafil (Viagra) and tadalafil (Cialis) for erectile dysfunction has been associated with the development of NAION.[41–43] A plausible explanation may be on the basis of altered ocular blood flow resulting from the vasodilatory effect of this class of medications. However, a clear cause-and-effect relationship has not been established, and patients using this class of medications have many of the same risk factors as those who develop idiopathic NAION. Therefore some feel that the association may be coincidental.

5-1-2-4 *Embolic Occlusion*. Occasionally, a patient presents with emboli elsewhere in the fundus and ischemic optic neuropathy (Fig. 5–6).[44,45] The presumption is that embolic occlusion of the posterior ciliary arteries led to infarction of the optic disc. Such patients require an evaluation of the heart and internal carotid arteries for potential sources of emboli.

5-1-2-5 *Hypotension*. Another infrequent but important setting in which ischemic optic neuropathy can occur is that associated with acute blood loss or hypotension. A well-studied patient with anemia who was blind after repeated gastrointestinal bleeding and acute hypotension demonstrated, at autopsy, torpedo-shaped infarctions in the orbital section of both optic nerves.[46] The patient had no light perception vision bilaterally and only mild disc edema, which was consistent with the retrobulbar nature of her optic nerve infarctions. Another report described 4 similar patients in the setting of intentionally maintained hypotension during lumbar spine surgery, 3 with disc edema and 1 with initially normal-appearing optic discs.[47] Similar episodes have occurred after other operative procedures.[48] In these patients, spontaneous visual recovery is usually limited; but if prompt measures are taken to reverse the hypotension or hypovolemia, some feel that vision can sometimes be salvaged.[49]

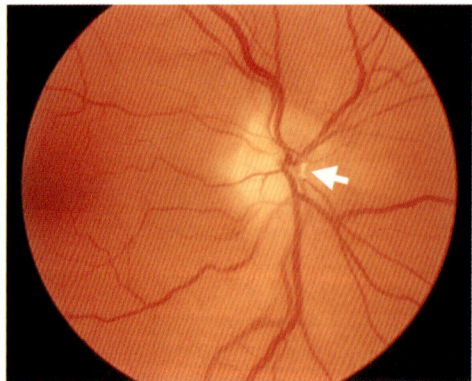

Figure 5–6. Emboli associated with ischemic optic neuropathy. Arrow demonstrates embolus on optic disc surface. (Reproduced from Tomsak RL. Ischemic optic neuropathy associated with retinal embolism. Am J Ophthalmol 1985;99:590–92. Published with permission from The American Journal of Ophthalmology. Copyright by The Ophthalmic Publishing Company.)

5-1-2-6 U*remia*. Several articles have described bilateral disc edema associated with rapid visual loss in patients known or found to be uremic.[50,51] In some, the presentation is indistinguishable from ischemic optic neuropathy. Some of the reported patients had elevated blood pressure as well, and many had visual improvement with dialysis, blood pressure reduction, and/or systemic corticosteroid therapy. Whether this optic neuropathy is truly ischemic is not known, but it resembles ischemic optic neuropathy clinically.

5-1-2-7 D*iabetic* P*apillopathy*. The condition known as *diabetic papillopathy* occurs in patients with both adult- and juvenile-onset diabetes in whom unilateral or bilateral prolonged optic disc edema may develop, with variable visual loss. Controversy exists as to whether this condition represents an unusual, mild form of ischemic optic neuropathy or a localized vasculopathy of the optic nerve head (see Chapter 10).

5-1-2-8 M*igraine*. Rarely, patients with migraine may develop ischemic optic neuropathy during a migrainous headache episode.[52,53] The diagnosis of migrainous ischemic optic neuropathy is based on the following:

1. A typical history of vascular headaches
2. The occurrence of unilateral visual loss during one of the headaches
3. Clinical findings consistent with optic nerve dysfunction causing the visual loss
4. The exclusion of other potential causes of optic neuropathy

Vasospasm of the optic nerve vessels may be the cause of the vaso-occlusion in these patients, although other possible causes include abnormal platelet aggregability, plasma hypercoagulability, and arteriovenous shunting. This rare form of ischemic optic neuropathy is a diagnosis of exclusion.

5-2 ARTERITIC ANTERIOR ISCHEMIC OPTIC NEUROPATHY

Arteritic AION results from infarction of the anterior optic disc due to occlusion of the posterior ciliary arteries. Giant cell arteritis is the most common systemic vasculitis responsible. It is critical to recognize this form of AION and distinguish it from NAION, because early treatment with corticosteroids may stabilize the visual deficit and prevent visual loss in the contralateral unaffected eye.

5-2-1 G*iant* C*ell* A*rteritis*. Giant cell arteritis (GCA) is a systemic vasculitis affecting large and medium-sized blood vessels. The incidence of GCA is estimated to be between 0.49 and 23.3 cases per 100,000 in patients above 50 years of age.[54–57] The pathogenesis is not completely understood; however a T cell–mediated immune response is thought to play a crucial role in the development of the vasculitis.[58] There is a greater prevalence of the disease among patients above 55 years of age, women, and those of northern European descent.

5-2-1-1 *Clinical Features.* The clinical presentation of GCA is variable. Patients often have systemic symptoms, which may be present in advance of visual loss and prompt the patient to seek relief from an internist. These symptoms include headache, jaw claudication, scalp tenderness, polymyalgia, anorexia, weight loss, and fever. The incidence of ocular involvement ranges between 14% and 70%.[59] The visual complications include central retinal and branch artery occlusion, ciliary artery occlusion, posterior ischemic optic neuropathy, and diplopia from ocular dysmotility. However, the most common ocular manifestation is AION.[60]

With arteritic AION, the optic disc often has a more ischemic appearance than in NAION, with more prominent pallid swelling (Fig. 5–7). The visual loss is typically more severe than with NAION at the onset; often, there is simultaneous bilateral optic nerve involvement, an unusual presentation for NAION. Table 5–2 outlines some important clinical features of NAION and arteritic AION. With resolution of the optic disc edema, optic disc cupping occurs in arteritic AION; however, this is an uncommon finding in NAION.[61]

5-2-1-2 *Serologic Markers.* With GCA, serologic inflammatory markers are typically elevated. The Westergren erythrocyte sedimentation rate (ESR) should be obtained if GCA is suspected. An ESR above 40 mm/h is generally considered elevated; however, the upper limit of normal is influenced by age.[62] Caution should be observed, because a normal ESR has been reported to occur in up to 22% of patients with GCA.[63] Conversely, the ESR can be elevated in the absence of GCA from several causes, including age, anemia, malignancy, and infection. Additionally, C-reactive protein (CRP), another inflammatory marker, and the platelet count can also be elevated in GCA.[64,65]

5-2-1-3 *Treatment.* The treatment of GCA consists of immediate corticosteroid therapy. The goal of therapy is to prevent visual loss and treat the systemic vasculitis. Once visual loss has occurred from arteritic AION, treatment is generally aimed at preventing occurrence in the fellow eye. The exact dose and route of corticosteroids remain controversial. If visual loss has not occurred, oral prednisone (at least 1mg/kg/day) appears to be adequate; however, once arteritic AION has developed, high-dose intravenous methylprednisolone (1 g/day for at least 3 days) followed by

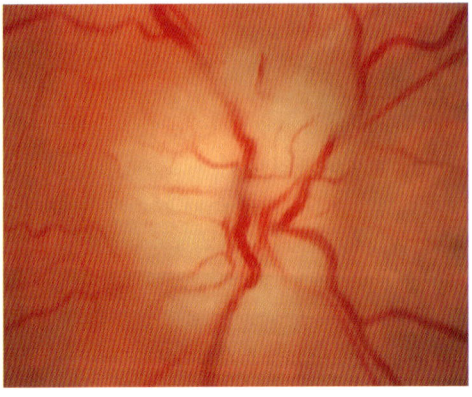

Figure 5–7. Pallid disc edema in arteritic ischemic optic neuropathy. Visual acuity was tested by counting fingers.

Table 5–2 Comparison of NAION With Arteritic ION due to Giant Cell Arteritis

	NAION	*Arteritic* ION
Usual age at presentation	55 to 70 yr	70+
Gender	Equal	Female > male
Fellow eye optic disc characteristics	Small or absent cup	No distinguishing optic disc characteristics; may have bilateral ischemic neuropathy
Systemic symptoms	None	Jaw claudication, headache, polymyalgia rheumatica, scalp tenderness, anorexia, weight loss, fever
Erythrocyte sedimentation rate (Westergren)	Normal	Usually elevated (>40 mm/h)
Temporal artery biopsy	May show arteriosclerotic change	Multinucleated giant cells, disruption of internal elastic membrane, granulomatous inflammation (acute and chronic)
Treatment	None	Corticosteroids, acutely may consider intravenous corticosteroids; oral dose 60 to 100 mg/day prednisone with slow taper; follow symptoms and sedimentation rate (may take 1+ years to taper off completely)

oral prednisone (1 mg/kg/day) is generally suggested, although there is no definitive evidence that the intravenous route is better than oral. The duration of treatment is variable and should be based on the clinical response. The dose of the corticosteroids should titrated down based in part on the serum inflammatory markers. Patients may need treatment for approximately 6–12 months or more.

5-2-1-4 *Temporal Artery Biopsy.* A temporal artery biopsy (TAB) should be performed in any patient in whom GCA is suspected. Initiation of corticosteroid therapy should not be delayed for the TAB. The biopsy should be performed as soon as possible, preferably within 2 weeks after initiating corticosteroid therapy, because the results may be altered by treatment.[66] Because of the possibility of "skip lesions" in a biopsy specimen,[67] a temporal artery biopsy should be a minimum of 2 cm and should be cross-sectioned into 1 mm segments, with a minimum of 9 sections per segment, to provide a high likelihood that active arteritis will be detected.[68]

5-3 POSTERIOR ISCHEMIC OPTIC NEUROPATHY

Compared with AION, posterior ischemic optic neuropathy (PION) is uncommon and can be classified into three subtypes: nonarteritic, arteritic, and perioperative.[69]

It is thought to be caused by the occlusion of one or more of the pial branches perfusing the posterior part of the optic nerve.[70] As in anterior ischemic optic neuropathy, patients with posterior ischemic optic neuropathy experience acute loss of visual acuity and visual field, with a relative afferent pupillary defect if the visual loss is asymmetric yet the fundus initially appears normal. Over the next 1–2 months, optic disc pallor becomes evident.

Posterior ischemic optic neuropathy attributable to arteriosclerosis is a diagnosis of exclusion. The diagnosis should be made with caution, even in patients with systemic vasculopathic risk factors such as hypertension and diabetes. A compressive, inflammatory, or infiltrative cause of optic nerve dysfunction must first be investigated. Posterior ischemic optic neuropathy has also been reported in the setting of giant cell arteritis,[71] herpes zoster ophthalmicus,[72] and connective tissue disorders such as systemic lupus erythematosus, Wegener's granulomatosis, and polyarteritis nodosa.[73] Infarction of the posterior portion of the optic nerve is also believed to be responsible for visual loss from invasive fungal disease and may occur as a complication of intracranial surgery and radiation therapy (see Chapter 10). Perioperative PION occurs in the setting of a surgical procedure under general anesthesia, often in association with acute blood loss and hypotension.[74]

REFERENCES

 1. Johnson LN, Arnold AC. Incidence of nonarteritic and arteritic anterior ischemic optic neuropathy. Population-based study in the state of Missouri and Los Angeles County, California. J Neuroophthalmol 1994;14:38–44.
 2. Swartz NG, Beck RW, Savino PJ, et al. Pain in anterior ischemic optic neuropathy. J Neuroophthalmol 1995;15:9–10.
 3. Ellenberger C Jr, Netsky MG. Infarction in the optic nerve. J Neurol Neurosurg Psychiatry 1968;31:606–11.
 4. Knox DL, Duke JR. Slowly progressive ischemic optic neuropathy. A clinicopathologic case report. Trans Am Acad Ophthalmol Otolaryngol 1971;75:1065–8.
 5. Lieberman MF, Shahi A, Green WR. Embolic ischemic optic neuropathy. Am J Ophthalmol 1978;86:206–10.
 6. Tesser RA, Niendorf ER, Levin LA. The morphology of an infarct in nonarteritic anterior ischemic optic neuropathy. Ophthalmology 2003;110:2031–5.
 7. Hattenhauer MG, Leavitt JA, Hodge DO, et al. Incidence of nonarteritic anterior ischemic optic neuropathy. Am J Ophthalmol 1997;123:103–7.
 8. Group TIONDTR. Optic nerve decompression surgery for nonarteritic anterior ischemic optic neuropathy (NAION) is not effective and may be harmful. JAMA 1995;273:625–32.
 9. Hayreh SS, Joos KM, Podhajsky PA, Long CR. Systemic diseases associated with nonarteritic anterior ischemic optic neuropathy. Am J Ophthalmol 1994;118:766–80.
10. Group TIONDTR. Characteristics of patients with nonarteritic anterior ischemic optic neuropathy eligible for the Ischemic Optic Neuropathy Decompression Trial. Arch Ophthalmol 1996;114:1366–74.
11. Guyer DR, Miller NR, Auer CL, Fine SL. The risk of cerebrovascular and cardiovascular disease in patients with anterior ischemic optic neuropathy. Arch Ophthalmol 1985;103:1136–42.
12. Beck RW, Servais GE, Hayreh SS. Anterior ischemic optic neuropathy. IX. Cup-to-disc ratio and its role in pathogenesis. Ophthalmology 1987;94:1503–8.

13. Feit RH, Tomsak RL, Ellenberger C, Jr. Structural factors in the pathogenesis of ischemic optic neuropathy. Am J Ophthalmol 1984;98:105–8.
14. Doro S, Lessell S. Cup-disc ratio and ischemic optic neuropathy. Arch Ophthalmol 1985;103:1143–4.
15. Jonas JB, Gusek GC, Naumann GO. Anterior ischemic optic neuropathy: nonarteritic form in small and giant cell arteritis in normal sized optic discs. Int Ophthalmol 1988;12 :119–25.
16. Deramo VA, Sergott RC, Augsburger JJ, et al. Ischemic optic neuropathy as the first manifestation of elevated cholesterol levels in young patients. Ophthalmology 2003;110 :1041–6; discussion 6.
17. Mojon DS, Hedges TR III, Ehrenberg B, et al. Association between sleep apnea syndrome and nonarteritic anterior ischemic optic neuropathy. Arch Ophthalmol 2002; 120:601–5.
18. Pianka P, Almog Y, Man O, et al. Hyperhomocystinemia in patients with nonarteritic anterior ischemic optic neuropathy, central retinal artery occlusion, and central retinal vein occlusion. Ophthalmology 2000;107:1588–92.
19. Repka MX, Savino PJ, Schatz NJ, Sergott RC. Clinical profile and long-term implications of anterior ischemic optic neuropathy. Am J Ophthalmol 1983;96:478–83.
20. Rizzo JF III, Lessell S. Optic neuritis and ischemic optic neuropathy. Overlapping clinical profiles. Arch Ophthalmol 1991:109:1668–72.
21. Sawle GV, James CB, Russell RW. The natural history of non-arteritic anterior ischaemic optic neuropathy. J Neurol Neurosurg Psychiatry 1990;53:830–3.
22. Kline LB. Progression of visual defects in ischemic optic neuropathy. Am J Ophthalmol 1988;106:199–203.
23. Borchert M, Lessell S. Progressive and recurrent nonarteritic anterior ischemic optic neuropathy. Am J Ophthalmol 1988;106:443–9.
24. Hayreh SS, Podhajsky PA, Zimmerman B. Ipsilateral recurrence of nonarteritic anterior ischemic optic neuropathy. Am J Ophthalmol 2001:132:734–42.
25. Beck RW, Hayreh SS, Podhajsky PA, et al. Aspirin therapy in nonarteritic anterior ischemic optic neuropathy. Am J Ophthalmol 1997;123:212–7.
26. Arnold AC, Hepler RS. Natural history of nonarteritic anterior ischemic optic neuropathy. J Neuroophthalmol 1994;14:66–9.
27. Beck RW, Savino PJ, Schatz NJ, et al. Anterior ischaemic optic neuropathy: recurrent episodes in the same eye. Br J Ophthalmol 1983;67:705–9.
28. Sergott RC, Cohen MS, Bosley TM, Savino PJ. Optic nerve decompression may improve the progressive form of nonarteritic ischemic optic neuropathy. Arch Ophthalmol 1989;107: 1743–54.
29. Kelman SE, Elman MJ. Optic nerve sheath decompression for nonarteritic ischemic optic neuropathy improves multiple visual function measurements. Arch Ophthalmol 1991: 109:667–71.
30. Spoor TC, McHenry JG, Lau-Sickon L. Progressive and static nonarteritic ischemic optic neuropathy treated by optic nerve sheath decompression. Ophthalmology 1993;100:306–11.
31. Yee RD, Selky AK, Purvin VA. Outcomes of optic nerve sheath decompression for nonarteritic ischemic optic neuropathy. J Neuroophthalmol 1994;14:70–6.
32. Glaser JS, Teimory M, Schatz NJ. Optic nerve sheath fenestration for progressive ischemic optic neuropathy. Results in second series consisting of 21 eyes. Arch Ophthalmol 1994;112:1047–50.
33. Kelman SE. The ischemic optic neuropathy decompression trial. Arch Ophthalmol 1993;111:1616–8.

34. Rizzo JF, Andreoli CM, Rabniov JD. Use of magnetic resonance imaging to differentiate optic neuritis and nonarteritic anterior ischemic optic neuropathy. Ophthalmology. 2002;109(9):1679–84.

35. McCulley TJ, Lam BL, Feuer WJ. Incidence of nonarteritic anterior ischemic optic neuropathy associated with cataract extraction. Ophthalmology 2001:108:1275–8.

36. Hayreh SS. Anterior ischemic optic neuropathy. IV. Occurrence after cataract extraction. Arch Ophthalmol 1980;98:1410–6.

37. Serrano LA, Behrens MM, Carroll FD. Postcataract extraction ischemic optic neuropathy. Arch Ophthalmol 1982;100:1177–8.

38. Murphy MA, Murphy JF. Amiodarone and optic neuropathy: the heart of the matter. J Neuroophthalmol 2005;25:232–6.

39. Gittinger JW, Jr., Asdourian GK. Papillopathy caused by amiodarone. Arch Ophthalmol 1987;105:349–51.

40. Macaluso DC, Shults WT, Fraunfelder FT. Features of amiodarone-induced optic neuropathy. Am J Ophthalmol 1999;127:610–2.

41. Pomeranz HD, Smith KH, Hart WM Jr, Egan RA. Sildenafil-associated nonarteritic anterior ischemic optic neuropathy. Ophthalmology 2002;109:584–7.

42. Pomeranz HD, Bhavsar AR. Nonarteritic ischemic optic neuropathy developing soon after use of sildenafil (Viagra): a report of seven new cases. J Neuroophthalmol 2005;25: 9–13.

43. Escaravage GK Jr, Wright JD Jr, Givre SJ. Tadalafil associated with anterior ischemic optic neuropathy. Arch Ophthalmol 2005;123:399–400.

44. Tomsak RL. Ischemic optic neuropathy associated with retinal embolism. Am J Ophthalmol 1985;99:590–2.

45. Portnoy SL, Beer PM, Packer AJ, Van Dyk HJ. Embolic anterior ischemic optic neuropathy. J Clin Neuroophthalmol 1989;9:21–5.

46. Johnson MW, Kincaid MC, Trobe JD. Bilateral retrobulbar optic nerve infarctions after blood loss and hypotension. A clinicopathologic case study. Ophthalmology 1987;94: 1577–84.

47. Katz DM, Trobe JD, Cornblath WT, Kline LB. Ischemic optic neuropathy after lumbar spine surgery. Arch Ophthalmol 1994;112:925–31.

48. Rizzo JF III, Lessell S. Posterior ischemic optic neuropathy during general surgery. Am J Ophthalmol 1987;103:808–11.

49. Connolly SE, Gordon KB, Horton JC. Salvage of vision after hypotension-induced ischemic optic neuropathy. Am J Ophthalmol 1994;117:235–42.

50. Knox DL, Hanneken AM, Hollows FC, et al. Uremic optic neuropathy. Arch Ophthalmol 1988;106:50–4.

51. Saini JS, Jain IS, Dhar S, Mohan K. Uremic optic neuropathy. J Clin Neuroophthalmol 1989;9:131–3; discussion 4–5.

52. Weinstein JM, Feman SS. Ischemic optic neuropathy in migraine. Arch Ophthalmol 1982;100:1097–100.

53. O'Hara M, O'Connor PS. Migrainous optic neuropathy. J Clin Neuroophthalmol 1984;4: 85–90.

54. Smith CA, Fidler WJ, Pinals RS. The epidemiology of giant cell arteritis. Report of a ten-year study in Shelby County, Tennessee. Arthritis Rheum 1983;26:1214–9.

55. Huston KA, Hunder GG, Lie JT, et al. Temporal arteritis: a 25-year epidemiologic, clinical, and pathologic study. Ann Intern Med 1978;88:162–7.

56. Machado EB, Gabriel SE, Beard CM, et al. A population-based case-control study of temporal arteritis: evidence for an association between temporal arteritis and degenerative vascular disease? Int J Epidemiol 1989;18:836–41.

57. Nordborg E, Bengtsson BA. Epidemiology of biopsy-proven giant cell arteritis (GCA). J Intern Med 1990;227:233–6.
58. Weyand CM, Goronzy JJ. Medium- and large-vessel vasculitis. N Engl J Med 2003;349: 160–9.
59. Ghanchi FD, Dutton GN. Current concepts in giant cell (temporal) arteritis. Surv Ophthalmol 1997;42:99–123.
60. Hayreh SS, Podhajsky PA, Zimmerman B. Ocular manifestations of giant cell arteritis. Am J Ophthalmol 1998;125:509–20.
61. Danesh-Meyer H, Savino PJ, Spaeth GL, Gamble GD. Comparison of arteritic and nonarteritic anterior ischemic optic neuropathies with the Heidelberg Retina Tomograph.Ophthalmology 2005;112:1104–12.
62. Miller A, Green M, Robinson D. Simple rule for calculating normal erythrocyte sedimentation rate. Br Med J (Clin Res Ed) 1983;286:266.
63. Salvarani C, Hunder GG. Giant cell arteritis with low erythrocyte sedimentation rate: frequency of occurence in a population-based study. Arthritis Rheum 2001:45:140–5.
64. Foroozan R, Danesh-Meyer H, Savino PJ, et al. Thrombocytosis in patients with biopsy-proven giant cell arteritis. Ophthalmology 2002;109:1267–71.
65. Hayreh SS, Podhajsky PA, Raman R, Zimmerman B. Giant cell arteritis: validity and reliability of various diagnostic criteria. Am J Ophthalmol 1997;123:285–96.
66. Guevara RA, Newman NJ, Grossniklaus HE. Positive temporal artery biopsy 6 months after prednisone treatment. Arch Ophthalmol 1998;116:1252–3.
67. Albert DM, Ruchman MC, Keltner JL. Skip areas in temporal arteritis. Arch Ophthalmol 1976;94:2072–7.
68. Chambers WABV. Specimen length in temporal artery biopsies. J Clin Neuroophthalmol 1988;8:121–5.
69. Sadda SR, Nee M, Miller NR, et al. Clinical spectrum of posterior ischemic optic neuropathy. Am J Ophthalmol 2001:132:743–50.
70. Hayreh SS. Anterior Ischemic optic neuropathy. Int Ophthalmol 1978;1:9–18.
71. Hollenhorst RW. Effect of posture on retinal ischemia from temporal arteritis. Arch Ophthalmol 1967;78:569–77.
72. Harrison EQ. Complications of herpes zoster ophthalmicus. Am J Ophthalmol 1965;60: 1111–4.
73. Miller N. Retrobulbar ischemic optic neuropathies. In: Miller NR, ed. Walsh and Hoyt's Clinical Neuro-Ophthalmology. Baltimore: Williams & Wilkins, 1982.
74. Buono LM, Foroozan R. Perioperative posterior ischemic optic neuropathy: review of the literature. Surv Ophthalmol 2005;50:15–26.

6

Compression of the Anterior Visual Pathways

ROD FOROOZAN AND LISA HINCKLEY

*U*nilateral or bilateral visual loss may occur from a *compressive* process affecting the intraorbital optic nerves, intracranial optic nerves, optic chiasm, or optic tracts. The term *compressive*, as used in this chapter, includes benign and malignant neoplasm, cyst, mucocele, and aneurysm. Also included is the orbital compression of the optic nerves by enlarged extraocular muscles in thyroid-associated orbitopathy.

The clinician should keep in mind the basic anatomy of the orbit, orbital apex (Fig. 6–1), and chiasm (Fig. 6–2) in forming an orderly differential diagnosis. Compressive processes of the visual pathways may be thought of as intrinsic, adjacent, remote, or infiltrative (Table 6–1).[1,2]

6-1 CAUSES OF COMPRESSIVE OPTIC NEUROPATHY

Many disease processes may cause compression of the optic nerve. This chapter discusses those conditions dealt with most frequently: glioma, craniopharyngioma, pituitary tumor, meningioma, aneurysm, and the optic neuropathy from thyroid associated orbitopathy.

6-2 SYMPTOMS OF COMPRESSIVE OPTIC NEUROPATHY

Most causes of visual pathway compression result in a slowly progressive decline in visual function over many months. Processes that may cause acute (hours to days) or acute-on-chronic visual loss (i.e., acute visual loss on a background of chronic

101

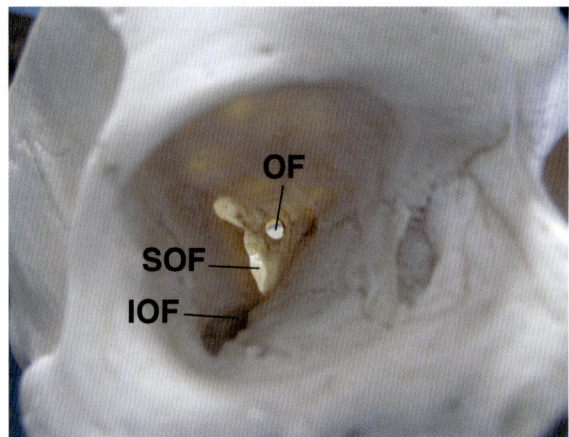

Figure 6–1. Bony anatomy of the right orbital apex. OF, optic foramen; SOF, superior orbital fissure; IOF, inferior orbital fissure.

visual disturbance) or acute visual loss in a patient discovered to have signs of a long-standing process (i.e., optic atrophy), include:

1. *Pituitary apoplexy.* Sudden intratumoral bleeding or infarction in a pituitary adenoma
2. *Mucocele.* Enlargement of a posterior ethmoidal or sphenoidal mucocele (Fig. 6–3)

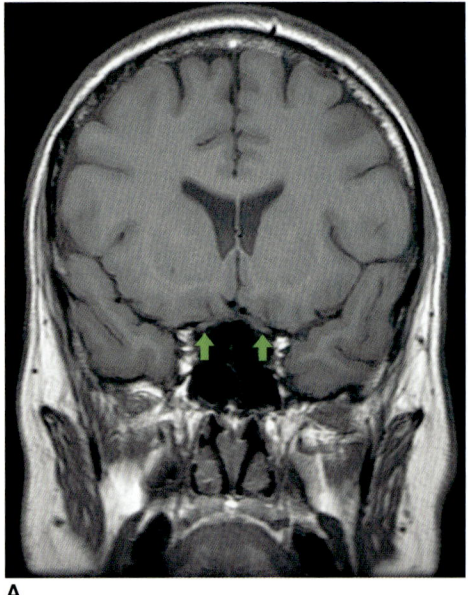
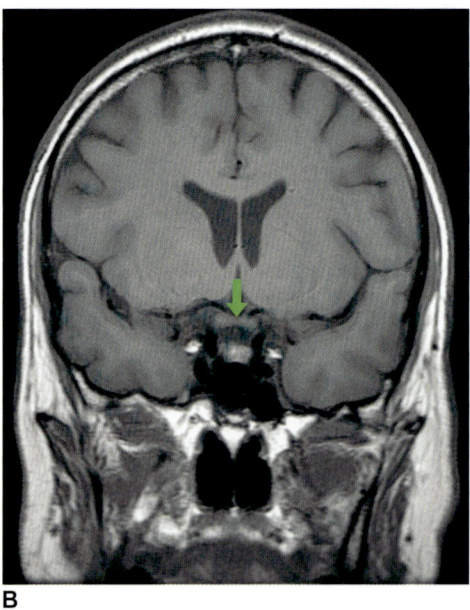

A   B

Figure 6–2. Magnetic resonance imaging (MRI) showing normal anatomy of the optic nerves, chiasm, sella, and optic tracts. (A) (above) Coronal T1-weighted MRI showing intracranial optic nerves (arrows). (B) Coronal T1-weighted MRI showing optic chiasm (arrow). (C) (opposite page) Sagittal T2-weighted MRI and (D) sagittal T1-weighted MRI with contrast showing pituitary gland (P), pituitary stalk (S), and optic chiasm (arrow). The average distance between the pituitary gland and optic chiasm is 10 mm. (E) Coronal and (F) axial T1-weighted MRI showing optic tracts (arrows).

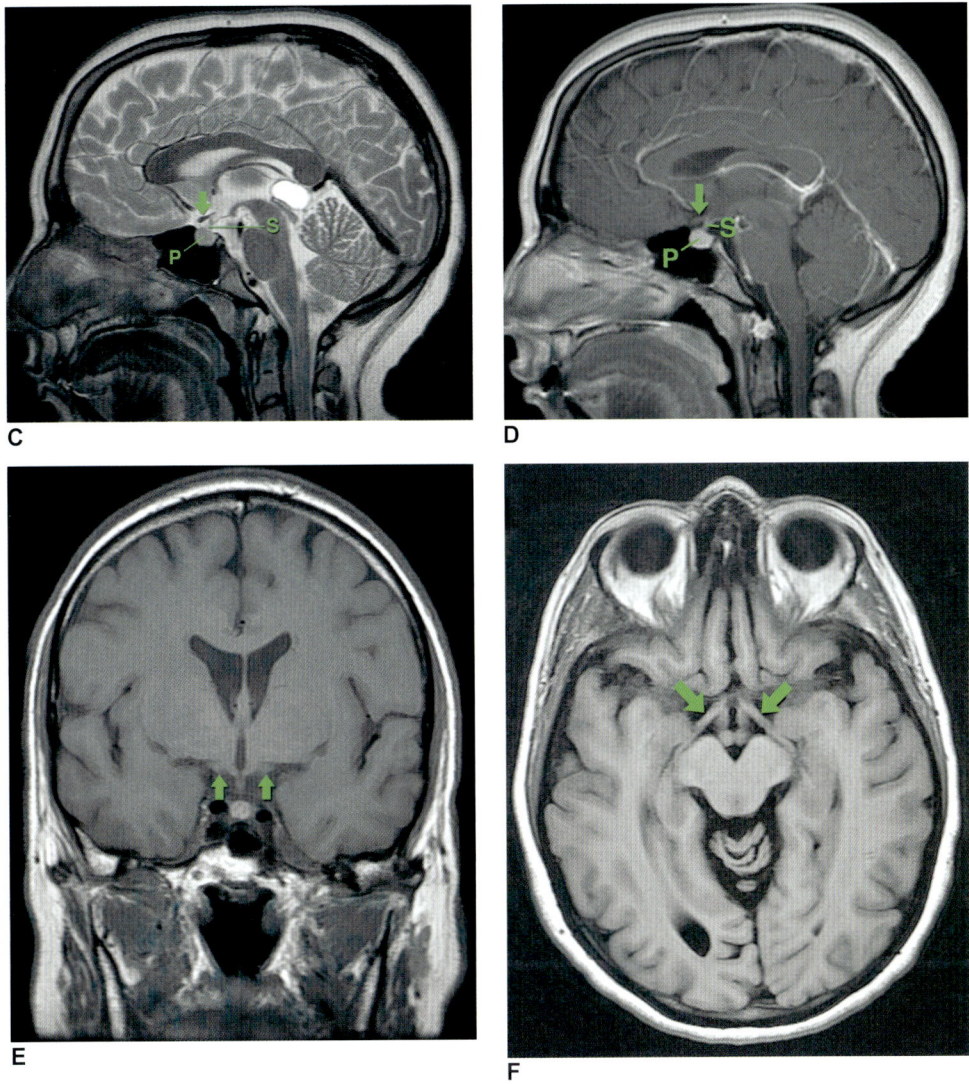

3. *Carotid–ophthalmic artery aneurysm.* Sudden expansion of a preexisting aneurysm
4. *Craniopharyngioma.* Enlargement of a cystic component or hemorrhage within the tumor

Processes that usually cause subacute (days to weeks) visual loss include:

1. *Infiltrative optic neuropathies.* Sarcoidosis, lymphoma, leukemia
2. *Leptomeningeal processes.* Inflammatory, neoplastic (Fig. 6–4)
3. *Malignant optic nerve glioma of adulthood.* Juvenile optic nerve glioma (discussed in section 6-5) is a low-grade astrocytoma. However, a glioma of adulthood involving the optic nerve most commonly represents a malignant glioblastoma multiforme. This begins in the chiasm or optic nerve,[3,4] with a mean age of onset is 50 years. Total blindness, which is invariably bilateral, ensues over a 2–4 month period, and death occurs within 6–12 months.[5]

Table 6–1 Compressive Lesions of the Anterior Visual Pathways

Intraorbital Process	Type of Lesion
Intrinsic	Optic nerve glioma
	Optic nerve sheath meningioma
	Optic nerve ganglioglioma[212]
	Optic nerve cavernous angioma[213]
	Optic nerve hemangioblastoma[214]
Adjacent	Cavernous hemangioma[215, 216]
	Other orbital tumors[217]
	Thyroid-associated orbitopathy
Remote	Metastases to optic nerve[217]
Infiltrative	Extension of intracranial process (see below)
Intracranial Process	
Intrinsic	Optic/chiasmal glioma[3–5]
Adjacent	Pituitary adenoma (pituitary apoplexy)
	Suprasellar meningioma
	Craniopharyngioma
	Germinoma[218]
	Carotid-paraophthalmic artery aneurysm and other vascular abnormalities[219]
	Mucocele (sphenoid sinus)[220]
	Sphenoid sinus tumor[221]
	Third ventricle tumor[222]
Remote	Metastases to optic nerve/chiasm[223]
	Leptomeningeal metastases[224, 225]
Infiltrative	Lymphoma[224, 226, 227]
	Leukemia[228]
	Myeloma[229]
	Sarcoidosis[230]

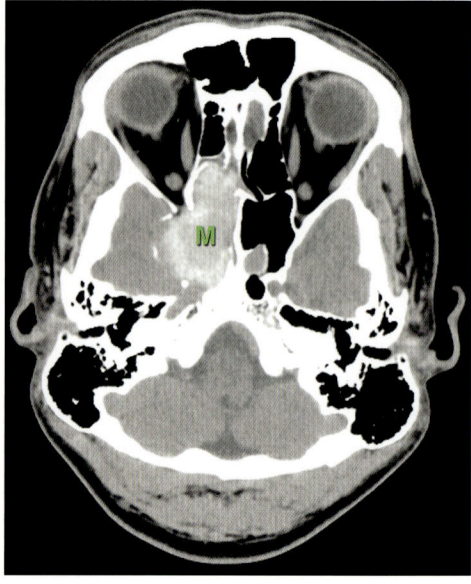

Figure 6–3. Axial computed tomography (CT) showing mucocele (M) of the right sphenoid sinus, which has become infected with fungus. Visual loss resulted from compression of the optic nerve in the orbital apex.

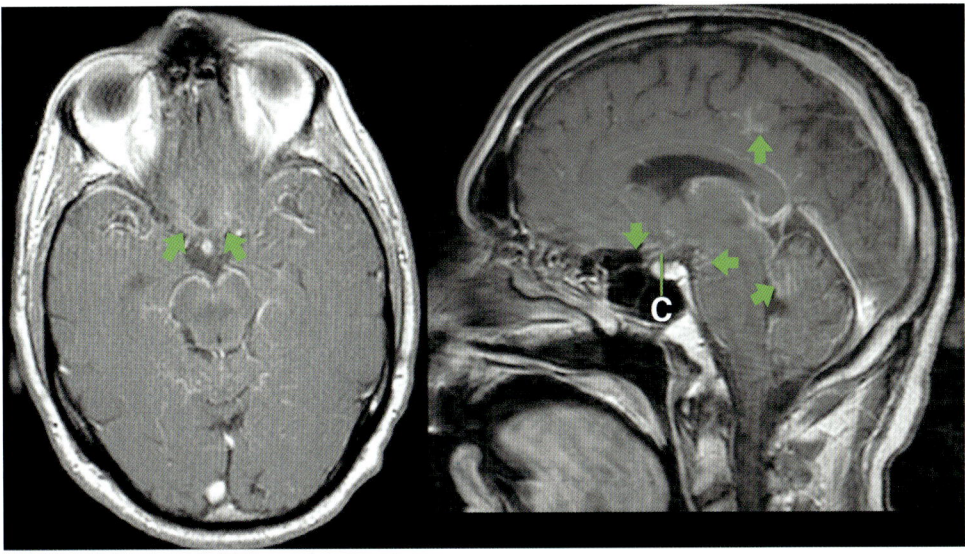

Figure 6–4. Axial (left) and sagittal (right) T1-weighted MRI with contrast showing leptomeningeal metastasis from cutaneous melanoma. Both optic nerves (left figure, arrows) and the optic chiasm (C) enhance. Multiple other areas involving the leptomeninges (right figure, arrows) also enhance.

Combined occlusion of the central retinal artery and vein often occurs as the tumor progresses.

Other findings that may accompany visual loss due to a compressive lesion include:

1. *Diplopia* due to a process affecting the extraocular muscles or due to an intracranial process affecting the ocular motor cranial nerves as they traverse the cerebrospinal fluid cisterns, cavernous sinuses, or superior orbital fissures
2. *Headache or eye pain*
3. *Pituitary dysfunction,* including amenorrhea, galactorrhea, decreased libido, acromegaly
4. *Skin changes compatible with neurofibromatosis,* such as café-au-lait spots, iris Lisch nodules, neurofibromas
5. *Decreased sense of smell,* as, for example, due to an olfactory groove meningioma
6. *Weight loss*—for example, due to a systemic malignancy
7. *Other neurologic symptoms,* such as multiple cranial nerve palsies due to leptomeningeal metastases

6-3 SIGNS OF COMPRESSIVE OPTIC NEUROPATHY

The signs accompanying compressive optic neuropathy include visual loss, dyschromatopsia, relative afferent pupillary defect, and various abnormalities of the orbit, eyelid, and extraocular movement.

1. *Visual loss.* Visual field defects of the optic nerve type (central, cecocentral, nerve fiber bundle defects), chiasmal type (bitemporal hemianopia, junctional defect), or optic tract involvement (incongruous homonymous hemianopia)

2. *Acquired dyschromatopsia.* Unilateral or bilateral color vision disturbance, especially when visual acuity is reduced

3. *Relative afferent pupillary defect.* May be subtle in cases of mild unilateral visual dysfunction; should also be seen in asymmetric bilateral optic neuropathy or chiasmal disease

4. *Orbital and eyelid signs.* Proptosis, retropulsion defect, enophthalmos (e.g., as may be seen with metastatic scirrhous carcinoma of the breast), eyelid abnormalities (ptosis, eyelid lag, eyelid retraction)

5. *Extraocular movement abnormalities.* No specific pattern if primarily a myopathic process or may follow the pattern of a specific ocular motor cranial nerve palsy

6-3-1 Optic Disc Findings. Among the numerous optic disc findings in compressive optic neuropathy are atrophy, edema, papilledema, shunt vessels, and Foster Kennedy syndrome.

1. *Optic atrophy.* This is the most common finding; early in the clinical course of optic nerve or chiasmal compression, the optic disc may appear normal. While some optic disc cupping may occur from causes of compressive optic neuropathy, optic disc pallor occurs out of proportion to the degree of cupping (see chapter 10).[6] Decreased thickness of the retinal nerve fiber layer occurs with the development of optic atrophy (Fig. 6–5).[7]

2. *Band or bowtie optic atrophy.* A type of atrophy (Fig. 6–6) seen with chiasmal or optic tract compression in an eye with a temporal hemianopic defect (loss of decussating nasal retinal fibers). Sparing of temporal retinal fibers (and the nasal field) results in relatively normal arcuate bundles, which are located in symmetric superior and inferior wedges on the disc. Temporal fibers of the papillomacular bundle and nasal peripheral fibers are atrophic, resulting in optic atrophy in a horizontal bowtie distribution (Fig. 6–7). This pattern of thinning of the retinal nerve fiber layer has been noted in vivo using scanning laser polarimetry and optical coherence tomography.[8]

3. *Optic disc edema* may be seen with compressive processes affecting the orbital or intracanalicular optic nerve; it is due to blockage of axoplasmic transport (e.g., meningioma of the optic nerve sheath) (Fig. 6–8). Intracranial compression of the optic nerve may result in optic atrophy but not swelling (see section 6–9).

4. *Papilledema* (see Chapter 3) is rarely caused by the tumors under consideration here; craniopharyngioma may occasionally cause papilledema by compressing the anterior third ventricle, causing hydrocephalus (see section 6–6).

5. *Optociliary shunt vessels* accompanied by optic disc edema or optic atrophy (Fig. 6–9) reflect impaired retinal venous outflow and often occur with meningiomas of the optic nerve sheath. However, they may be seen with other compressive lesions, especially those affecting the intraorbital optic nerve.

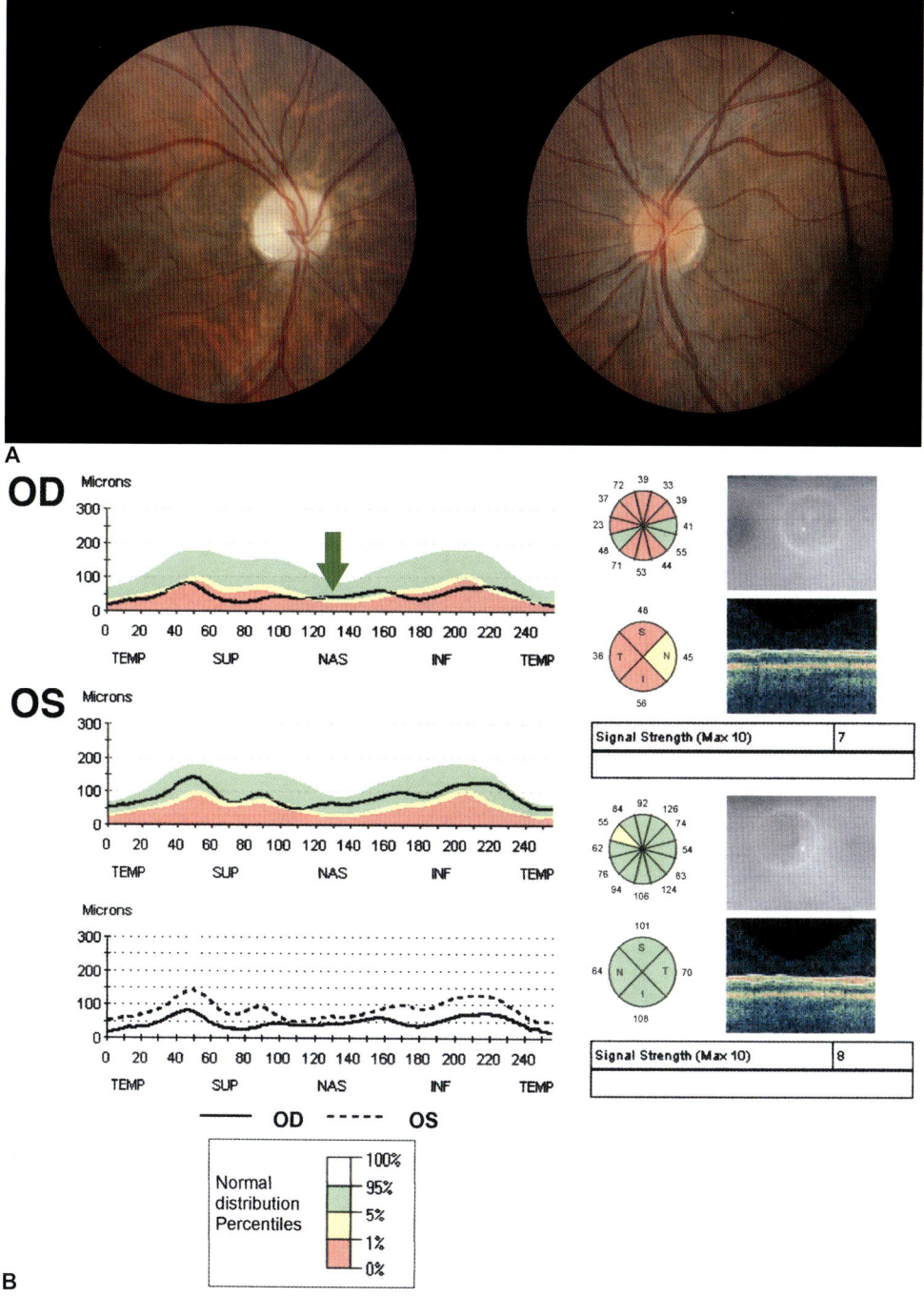

Figure 6–5. Decreased thickness of the retinal nerve fiber layer in a patient with optic atrophy due to a meningioma of the right optic nerve sheath. (A) Fundus photographs show optic atrophy on the right and a normal left optic nerve. (B) Optical coherence tomography (OCT) is a technique that measures reflected laser light within the eye. The measures of reflected light correlate with retinal thickness, including the thickness of the retinal nerve fiber layer, with the normal retinal nerve fiber layer thickest superiorly and inferiorly along the optic disc (see also Chapter 1, section 1–1). Normal retinal thickness for 95% of age-matched subjects is represented by the shaded green area. This OCT shows decreased thickness of the retinal nerve fiber layer of the right eye (arrow) due to the meningioma of the optic nerve sheath. The thickness of the retinal nerve fiber layer of the left eye is normal.

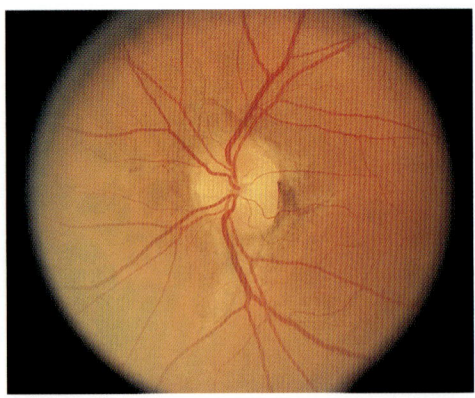

Figure 6–6. Bowtie atrophy of left optic disc. There is atrophy of the nasal and temporal horizontal quadrants with relative sparing of superior and inferior poles.

6. *Foster Kennedy syndrome*[9] is a rare finding, with large subfrontal tumors, usually meningiomas; optic atrophy, and decreased vision on one side (the side of optic nerve compression), while the fellow optic nerve demonstrates papilledema (see section 3-5). Pseudo–Foster Kennedy syndrome[10] is seen in anterior ischemic optic neuropathy when acute visual loss and disc swelling in one eye are evident, with optic atrophy and visual loss in the fellow eye from a previous episode.

A summary of the clinical characteristics and sites of lesions causing optic atrophy is shown in Table 6–2.[6]

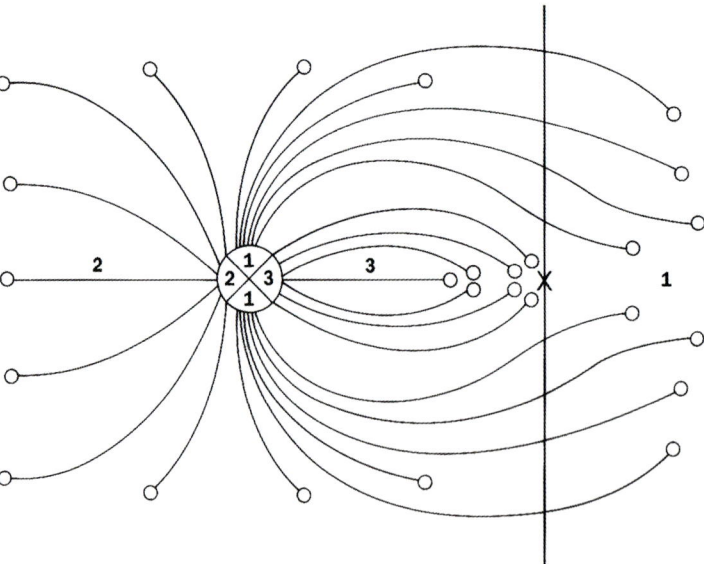

Figure 6–7. Left optic nerve and retinal axons. Those axons arising from the temporal retina (subserving the nasal visual field), which comprise superior and inferior areas of the optic disc (1), are spared in this patient with a left temporal hemianopia respecting the vertical meridian. Nasal retinal axons (those arising from 2) and the nasal aspect of the papillomacular bundle (3) (subserving the temporal visual field), however, will atrophy, resulting in bowtie or band optic atrophy. X, fovea.

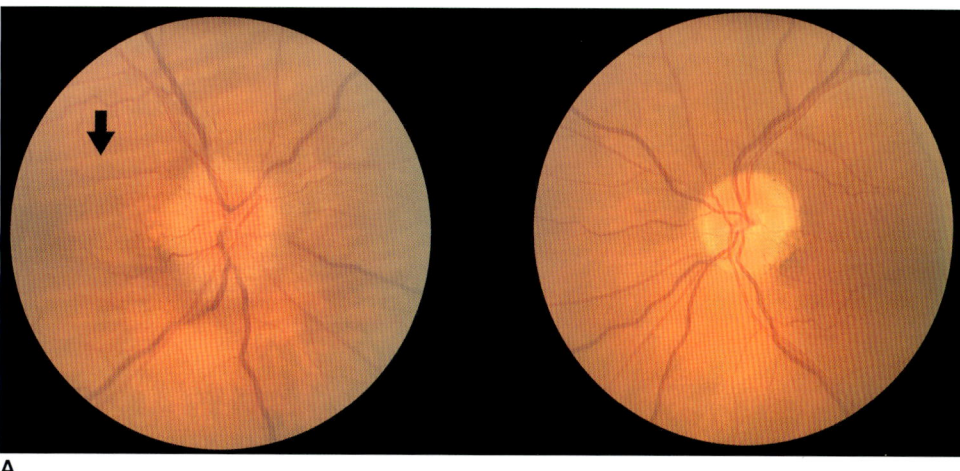

A

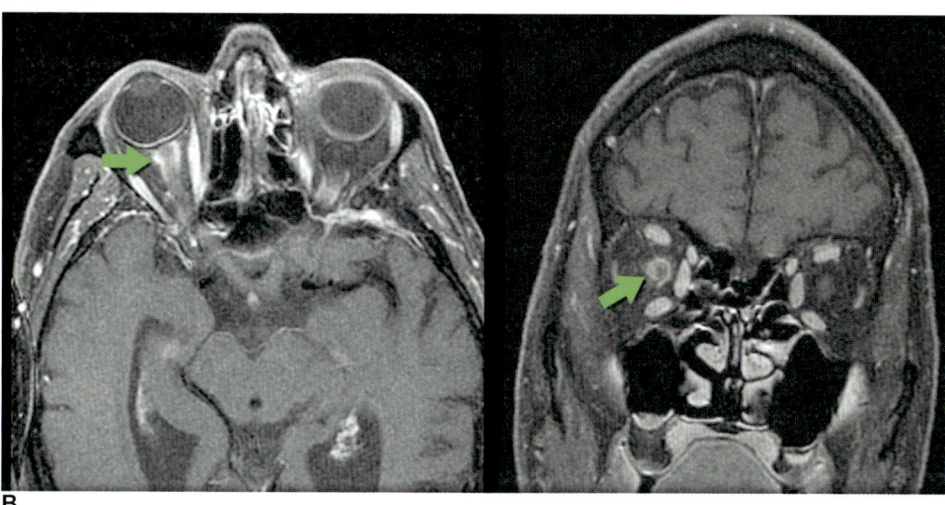

B

Figure 6–8. Optic disc edema from meningioma of the optic nerve sheath. (A) Fundus photographs show optic disc edema and choroidal folds (arrow) in the right eye; the left optic disc is normal. (B) T1-weighted MRI with fat supression demonstrates enhancement (arrows) of the right optic nerve sheath on axial (left) and coronal (right) scans.

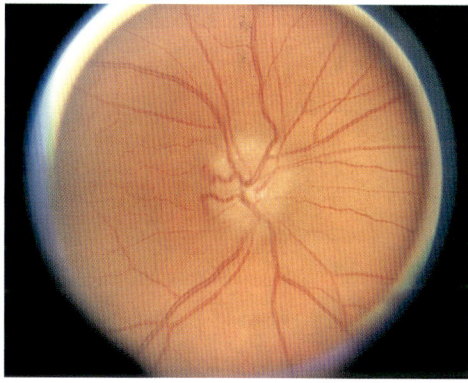

Figure 6–9. Two optociliary shunt vessels on the temporal aspect of the right optic disc in a patient with a meningioma of the optic nerve sheath. Visual acuity in the right eye was 20/80. The left optic nerve was normal.

Table 6-2 Clinical Characteristics and Sites of Lesions Causing Optic Atrophy

Site of Lesion	Visual Acuity	Visual Field Defect	Color Vision	Pupillary Response	Funduscopy
Optic nerve	Mildly to markedly reduced	Central or nerve fiber bundle	Mildly to markedly reduced	RAPD with unilateral/ asymmetric lesion, bilaterally sluggish pupils with symmetric optic neuropathy	Optic disc pallor
Optic chiasm	Normal to markedly reduced	Unilateral temporal, junctional, or bitemporal	Normal to markedly reduced	May be normal with subtle chiasmal lesion; with extensive lesion, may see RAPD or bilaterally sluggish pupils	Band atrophy
Optic tract	Normal unless optic chiasm and/ or optic nerves also affected	Homonymous hemianopia, typically incongruous	May be normal	RAPD contralateral to the side of the lesion unless the ipsilateral optic nerve is also affected	Band atrophy in eye with temporal visual field loss, diffuse atrophy in fellow eye

RAPD = relative afferent pupillary defect

Source: Modified from Foroozan R. The pale optic nerve. Contemp Ophthalmol 2003;2:1–10.

6-4 PATIENT EVALUATION

Additional components in evaluating a patient with compressive optic neuropathy include neuroimaging, a careful physical examination with selected laboratory tests, and a neurologic examination.

1. *Neuroimaging.* This requires computed tomography (CT) with intravenous contrast and/or magnetic resonance imaging (MRI) after gadolinium-DPTA administration. MRI can directly image the optic chiasm, intracranial optic nerves, and optic tracts (see Fig. 6–2) and is the procedure of choice in imaging anterior visual pathways. Orbital MRI with fat suppression and intravenous gadolinium allows for a detailed examination of intraorbital and intracanalicular optic nerves, while fat suppression is a key technique in the assessment of enhancement within the retrobulbar space (see Fig. 6–8). MRI may show thinning of the optic nerve in patients with optic atrophy (Fig. 6–10); it may also detect leptomeningeal metastases (see Fig. 6–4). CT is excellent for the evaluation of orbital processes because it allows for evaluation of surrounding bone; moreover, the presence of calcium in tumors can best be appreciated with CT.
2. *Physical examination* plus complete blood count, bone marrow biopsy, and oncologic examination as indicated.
3. *Neurologic examination* may include lumbar puncture to exclude conditions such as leptomeningeal metastases, lymphoma, and hemorrhage.

6-5 GLIOMA

Optic nerve or chiasmal glioma of childhood, a slowly progressive lesion, should be distinguished from the malignant lesion of adulthood (discussed in section 6–2), which is rare and is not discussed further in this chapter. The term *optic nerve glioma* denotes primarily an intraorbital astrocytoma, which may be associated with chiasmal extension, an optic nerve glioma of the fellow eye, or a distinct chiasmal lesion. Similarly, chiasmal glioma may extend anteriorly to either optic nerve, posteriorly along the optic tract, or posteriorly into the hypothalamus. Optic nerve and chiasmal gliomas are often associated with neurofibromatosis type 1 (NF-1).[11-13]

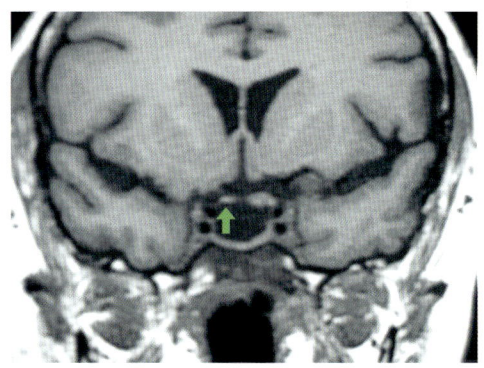

Figure 6–10. T1-weighted coronal MRI in a patient with right optic disc pallor demonstrates atrophy (arrow) of the right optic nerve.

Depending on the report, about 50% of gliomas affecting the anterior optic pathway are associated with NF, and 30% of patients with NF-1 will harbor such a glioma.[14] There is some controversy as to whether patients with NF-1 and gliomas of the anterior visual pathway may have a better prognosis than those who have sporadic gliomas.[15,16] However, it does appear that those gliomas that affect only the optic nerve have a better prognosis than those occurring more posteriorly and involving the hypothalamus, optic tracts, or optic chiasm.[17,18]

6-5-1 Optic Nerve Glioma

6-5-1-1 *Clinical Features.* Optic nerve glioma is usually detected in the first decade of life. Common signs include decreased visual acuity and color vision, an afferent pupillary defect, proptosis, strabismus, optic atrophy, and optic disc edema.[12,19] Visual loss, which is typically painless, may be stable or slowly progressive.

Neuroimaging shows fusiform enlargement of the optic nerve with discrete tumor margins (Fig. 6–11).

Typically the optic nerve does not enhance with contrast. MRI is preferred to CT for several reasons[20]:

1. A child found to have an optic nerve tumor will require multiple follow-up scans over the ensuing years. MRI spares the child the cumulative effect of radiation.
2. MRI images the orbital and intracranial contents in axial, coronal, and sagittal views without the need to reposition the child.
3. Intracanalicular and chiasmal extension of tumor is consistently imaged with MRI. These findings are critical for both diagnosis and therapy. Although CT, with bone window settings, can often show widening of the optic canal and intracranial extension when present, the proximity of tumor to bone in these cases leads to inferior soft tissue resolution. However, the intraorbital portion of the tumor is often seen equally well with CT.

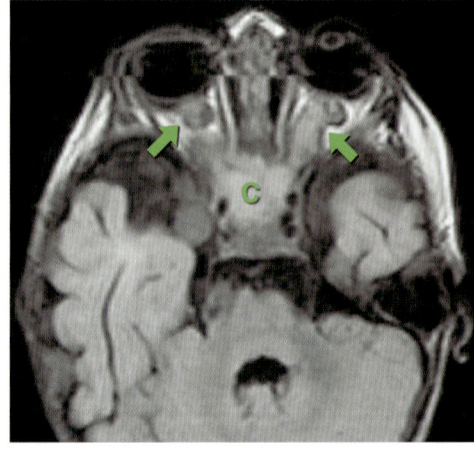

Figure 6–11. Bilateral optic nerve gliomas (arrows) extending to the optic chiasm (C) on axial T1-weighted MRI. Both optic nerves have fusiform thickening, which is characteristic of optic nerve gliomas. With tumorous involvement, the chiasm is enlarged as well.

Optic pathway gliomas may develop subsequent to initially normal neuro-imaging.[21] The diagnosis of optic nerve glioma is generally made by clinical as well as imaging criteria. A biopsy of the optic nerve or chiasmal mass may be hazardous and actually hasten visual morbidity.[13] One caveat, however, is in order: If the diagnosis is not clear-cut, biopsy and/or removal of the lesion may be imperative. An example is the optic nerve sheath meningioma of childhood, which has a much more aggressive clinical course than that of optic nerve glioma.

6-5-1-2 *Histopathology.* The histopathology of optic nerve and chiasmal gliomas is of a low-grade astrocytoma, mostly of the juvenile pilocytic type. Peritumoral arachnoid hyperplasia and tumoral enlargement caused by the accumulation of mucin may be seen.

6-5-1-3 *Natural History.* The clinical course is variable as some patients have a slow deterioration in visual function while others will remain stable.[20,22,23] Spontaneous visual improvement has been confirmed in some reports.[17,18]

6-5-1-4 *Management Options.* The treatment of optic nerve gliomas is controversial and there are no definitive studies to guide patient management. Furthermore, patients with spontaneous regression of optic nerve gliomas have been well documented.[24]

1. All patients should undergo cranial MRI if possible. Those patients with involvement of the chiasm or fellow optic nerve at presentation should be observed. Optic nerve or chiasmal biopsy in cases with clear-cut clinical and neuroradiologic features is not indicated and may result in further visual compromise.
2. Stable cases of presumed optic nerve glioma with intraorbital tumor should be followed up with serial MRI and clinical examinations.
3. Patients in whom visual progression occurs should be carefully evaluated for extension of tumor into the intracanalicular and intracranial space. Radiation therapy (including stereotactic radiation)[25] and chemotherapy have been used for patients with progressive tumors. Surgical excision of the glioma in total is typically reserved for patients with severe visual loss and proptosis. Surgical intervention may also be indicated when there is evidence of extension to the optic chiasm.
4. Patients with more modest levels of visual loss should be observed carefully. The low risk of intracranial extension must be weighed against the side effects of therapy.
5. Infectious, inflammatory, or neoplastic causes of optic neuropathy should be considered in atypical cases (Fig. 6–12).

6-5-2 *Chiasmal Glioma*

6-5-2-1 *Clinical Features.* Chiasmal glioma is more common than optic nerve glioma. It typically presents within the first few years of life.[16,26,27] Common ophthalmologic signs on presentation include visual loss, visual field defects, and optic

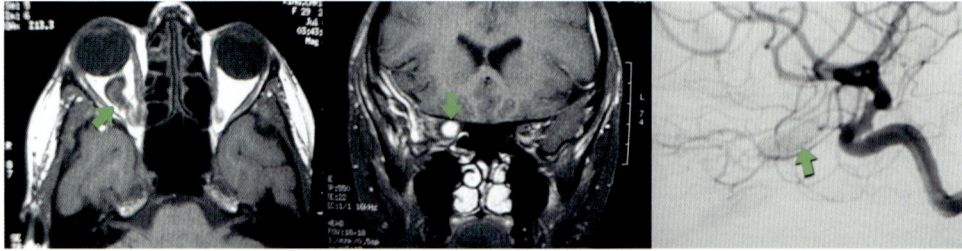

Figure 6–12. Optic nerve thickening (arrow) on T1-weighted MRI (left) without contrast. On coronal (center) T1-weighted MRI with contrast and fat suppression, the right optic nerve enhances markedly with contrast (arrow), a finding not typical of optic nerve glioma of childhood. The cerebral angiogram (right) shows early tumor blush (arrow) consistent with a hemangioblastoma of the optic nerve.

atrophy. The pattern of visual field defects in chiasmal glioma does not consistently correspond to the extent of the chiasmal tumor.[28]

1. Patients with nystagmus resembling that from spasmus nutans may harbor a chiasmal glioma.[29,30]
2. Hydrocephalus may occur from obstruction of the third ventricle.[30]
3. Patients with low-grade gliomas involving the hypothalamus may develop Russell's diencephalic syndrome, which is generally seen in children under 2 years of age who present with failure to thrive.[31–33] Presumably, after a normal period of growth, these children become emaciated despite adequate nutrition. Additional hypothalamic signs of chiasmal glioma include pendular rotary (see-saw) nystagmus and precocious sexual development.
4. More than half of patients with chiasmal glioma have neurofibromatosis.[34] Conversely, patients with neurofibromatosis have a 15% incidence of the entity.

Other features of chiasmal glioma, as determined by MRI, may include chiasmal enlargement (Fig. 6–13) and extension of tumor into intracranial optic nerves, optic tracts, hypothalamus, and less commonly the lateral geniculate body and optic radiations. The latter finding is highly suggestive but not pathognomonic of glioma.[35] Other presumed hamartomas of the basal ganglia, white matter, and cerebellum may be seen.[36]

6-5-2-2 *Natural History.* In patients with chiasmal gliomas, therapeutic decision-making is difficult.[34,37] Like optic nerve gliomas, chiasmal gliomas may regress spontaneously.[38]

6-5-2-3 *Management Options.* Chiasmal glioma may be managed by surgery, observation, radiation, or chemotherapy:

1. *Surgery.* For the most part, surgery is unwarranted. It does not improve vision, nor has total resection been shown to prolong life. Surgical biopsy may cause further visual loss and associated hypothalamic dysfunction. Biopsy

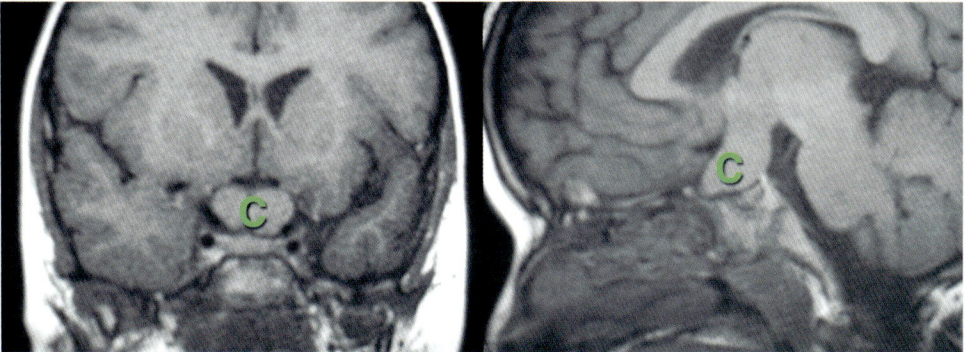

Figure 6–13. Optic chiasmal glioma on coronal (left) and sagittal (right) T1-weighted MRI. There is extension of the glioma into the hypothalamus.

should be recommended only when clinical or neuroradiologic features are atypical (Fig. 6–14). Occasionally, removal of an exophytic portion of tumor[39,40] or drainage of a cystic component[41] may result in improvement; however, these situations are rare. Hydrocephalus may require a cerebro-spinal diversion procedure.[40]

2. *Observation.* In patients who are stable visually and neurologically, observation seems warranted.[37,42]

3. *Radiotherapy.* In Russell's diencephalic syndrome, treatment with some combination of surgical excision, chemotherapy, and radiotherapy is generally indicated.[43,44] Otherwise, radiotherapy for chiasmal glioma is thought to stabilize the disease, at least temporarily, in many cases.[45–50] Radiation therapy of the young brain is not without major side effects and may include intellectual deterioration, vascular occlusion,[51] remote infarcts,[52]

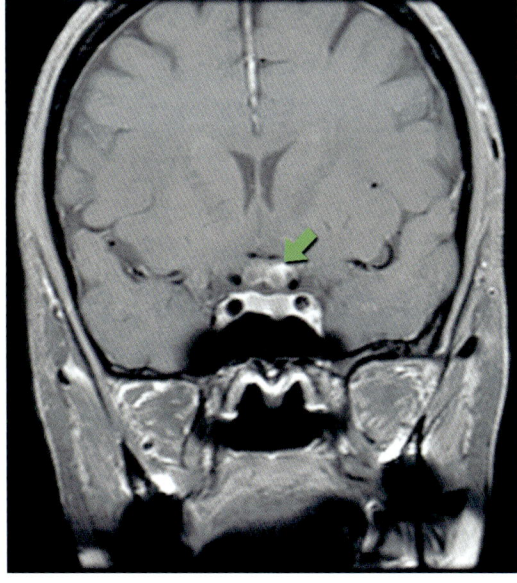

Figure 6–14. Thickening of the optic chiasm from sarcoidosis, with enhancement (arrow) on coronal T1-weighted MRI.

calcification of lenticular nuclei, and delayed radionecrosis of the optic chiasm and optic nerves.[53,54]

4. *Chemotherapy.* Progressive chiasmal glioma is typically treated. Because radiotherapy of immature brains, especially under the age of 6 years, may be hazardous, chemotherapy protocols have been developed.[55,56] Chemotherapy may be helpful alone or may delay the need for radiotherapy until an age when it is better tolerated.[44]

6-6 CRANIOPHARYNGIOMA

Although craniopharyngioma constitutes only 3% of intracranial neoplasms, it accounts for over 50% of suprasellar tumors in children and 20% in adults.[57] The mean age at diagnosis is 29 years (range 1–85 years), and the age incidence is bimodal, with one peak in the first two decades of life and the second in the years 50–70.[58] Craniopharyngioma has no gender predilection, is considered a congenital tumor, and may be present in the neonate.

Review of the embryology of the pituitary gland may clarify how and when craniopharyngiomas are formed (Fig. 6–15). Most authorities believe that craniopharyngiomas arise from vestigial squamous epithelial cells that are remnants of Rathke's pouch, while others think the tumor is derived from squamous metaplasia of cells in the anterior pituitary gland.[59,60]

6-6-1 *Clinical Features.* Clinical findings in patients with craniopharyngioma include growth failure, impotence, galactorrhea, amenorrhea, and visual loss.[61–63] The diagnosis may be delayed in some patients. Typically the visual loss is gradual and progressive, but in some patients rapid growth or enlargement of the cyst may cause sudden visual loss.[62] Endocrinopathy may include hypothyroidism, hypoadrenalism, and diabetes insipidus.[63] Headache may occur in 50% of patients with craniopharyngioma.[64]

Craniopharyngioma may be suggested by three neuroradiologic criteria: (1) the tumor primarily extends into the suprasellar cistern, (2) the tumor usually has both cystic and solid components and often exhibits hemorrhagic products, and (3) intratumoral calcification is often present, especially in childhood. Edema within the optic tracts is a fourth characteristic that has been described as suggestive of craniopharyngioma.[65] Although CT remains the best way to detect calcification, MRI will optimally demonstrate the extent of tumor and its relationship to neighboring structures, such as the chiasm, hypothalamus, and third ventricle (Fig. 6–16).

6-6-2 *Histopathology.* Craniopharyngiomas are benign tumors: 60% are exclusively cystic, and half of the cysts contain viscous fluid while in the others the fluid is clear.[64,66]

Two distinct patterns are evident on microscopic examination: (1) a solid nest of squamous cells, forming squamous "pearls," and (2) a loose collection of "stellate cells" surrounded by a single layer of pseudostratified columnar cells resting on a thin basement membrane (adamantinomatous pattern). In one-third of cases,

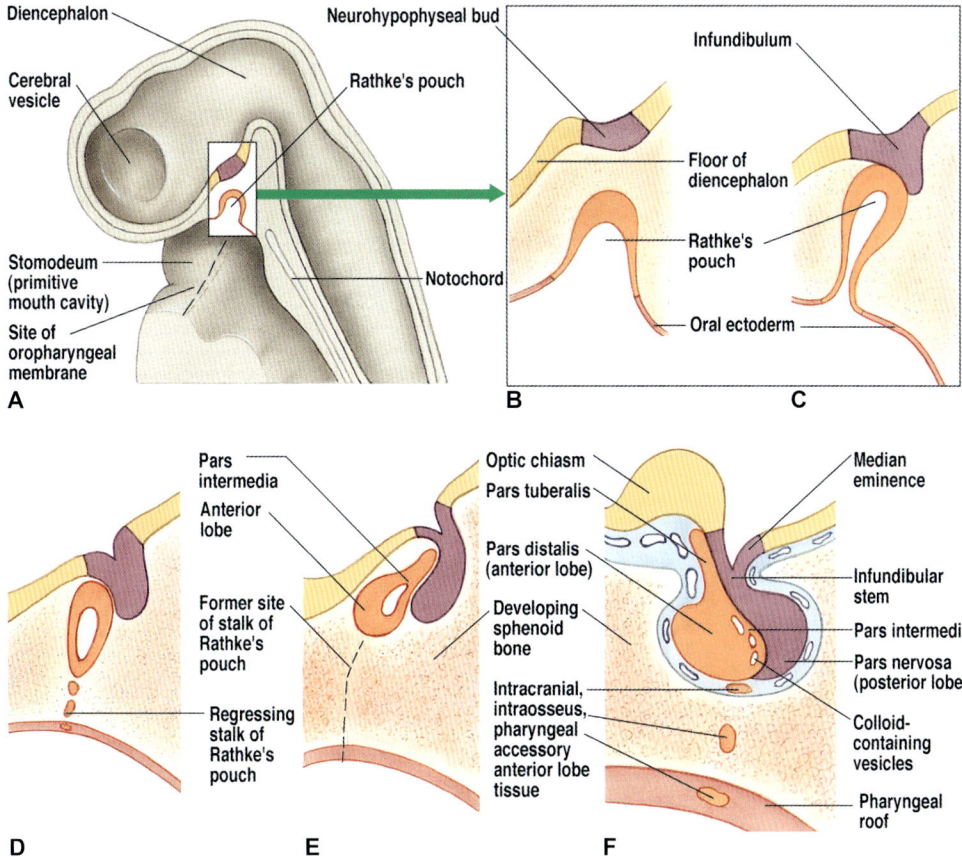

Figure 6–15. Development of pituitary gland (hypophysis). (A) Sagittal section of cranial end of embryo at 4 weeks, showing Rathke's pouch as upgrowth from roof of primitive mouth cavity and neurohypophyseal bud from forebrain. (B,C,D) Successive stages of developing pituitary gland. By 8 weeks, Rathke's pouch loses its connection with the oral cavity. (E,F) Later stages, showing proliferation of the anterior wall of Rathke's pouch and obliteration of its lumen. Orange, Rathke's pouch of stomodeum (upgrowth from roof of primitive mouth). Purple, infundibulum of diencephalon (downgrowth from floor of forebrain). (Redrawn with permission from Moore KL, Hay JC: The Developing Human: Clinically Oriented Embryology. Philadelphia: Saunders, 1973.)

the adamantinomatous forms predominate, in another third, the squamous type; and in the final third, a mixture of both. Tumoral calcification is present in 75% of patients.

6-6-3 *Management Options.* Optimal management of craniopharyngioma is controversial.[67] Some neurosurgeons contend that complete removal of tumor is required,[68] while others believe that judicious subtotal removal followed by radiotherapy is acceptable.[61,69–71]

Total removal of a craniopharyngioma can be accomplished in only a small proportion of patients. Incomplete removal of tumor followed by radiotherapy, either external beam or interstitial brachytherapy,[69] seems to afford an excellent

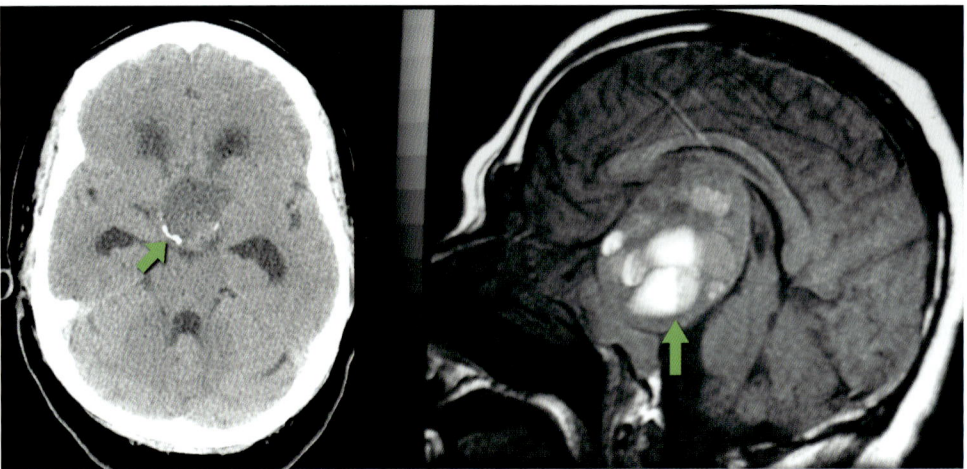

Figure 6–16. Craniopharyngioma with obstructive hydrocephalus on axial CT (left), demonstrating rim calcification (arrow). Noncontrast sagittal T1-weighted MRI (right) showing multiple tumoral cysts and hemorrhagic sediment levels (arrow).

survival rate as well as a low recurrence rate. A radical attempt at removal of a tenacious tumor may lead to morbidity, death, or late psychosocial deficits from damage to nearby structures such as the hypothalamus and carotid artery. However, radiotherapy for craniopharyngioma in young children may be fraught with the same complications as described earlier for chiasmal glioma. Postoperative endocrine defects must also be managed.[63] Intracystic chemotherapy has been used successfully in some patients with craniopharyngioma.[72,73]

Depending on the duration of optic nerve compression and the degree of preoperative visual deficit, decompression of the cyst may lead to marked visual improvement.[62,74–76]

6-7 PITUITARY ADENOMA

Pituitary tumors, mostly benign adenomas, are clinically common, representing 10% of symptomatic intracranial neoplasms. Moreover, asymptomatic pituitary adenomas must be quite prevalent, as judged by the high incidence detected at routine postmortem examination. In one study, approximately one-quarter harbored microadenomas.[77] Most pituitary adenomas (75%) are secretory, with the majority secreting prolactin (PL), while others produce growth hormone (GH), adrenocorticotrophic hormone (ACTH), thyroid-stimulating hormone (TSH), and follicle-stimulating hormone (FSH). Histologically, two types of tumors, the oncocytoma and the null-cell tumor, are thought to be nonsecretory (in the older literature referred to as *chromophobe adenomas*).[78–81]

6-7-1 Clinical Features. Pituitary adenomas may present in two important ways. First, those tumors that are hormonally active may give rise to symptoms and signs while they are still small.[82–84] Second, when tumors grow larger and show mass effect, they may encroach on the suprasellar cistern and cause visual dysfunction or grow laterally into the cavernous sinus and cause diplopia. These patients may also have associated endocrine symptoms, but they usually present initially to ophthalmologists. Many cases in which headaches predominate are initially evaluated by internists or neurologists.

6-7-1-1 *Visual Signs.* Pituitary adenoma is the most common tumor known to cause optic nerve or chiasmal compression. A pituitary adenoma must typically grow approximately 10 mm above the diaphragma sellae before it compresses the visual apparatus (see Fig. 6–2).[85] A pituitary adenoma that is larger than 10 mm is designated a macroadenoma and is easily seen on neuroimaging studies (Fig. 6–17).

Visual loss is slowly progressive, with symptoms over many months. It may be bilateral but is often asymmetric. Loss of visual acuity and color vision is often evident in one or both eyes. Loss of stereopsis[86] and photophobia[87] may occur. The hallmark visual field disturbance due to chiasmal disease is temporal field loss with respect of the vertical meridian.[88] The most common patterns are bitemporal hemianopia and junctional syndrome.[89] In the latter, central field loss in one eye is combined with a temporal field defect in the fellow eye. Pituitary adenomas cause chiasmal syndromes that result in preferential loss of the superior temporal visual field (inferior retinal ganglion cell fibers) in each eye. Preferential loss of the inferior temporal visual field in each eye should raise the suspicion for a different cause of a chiasmal syndrome.[90] A relative afferent pupillary defect is likely unless visual loss is symmetric, and optic atrophy is typical. Motility defects, often in the form of unilateral third or sixth nerve palsy, are due to parasellar extension of the tumor

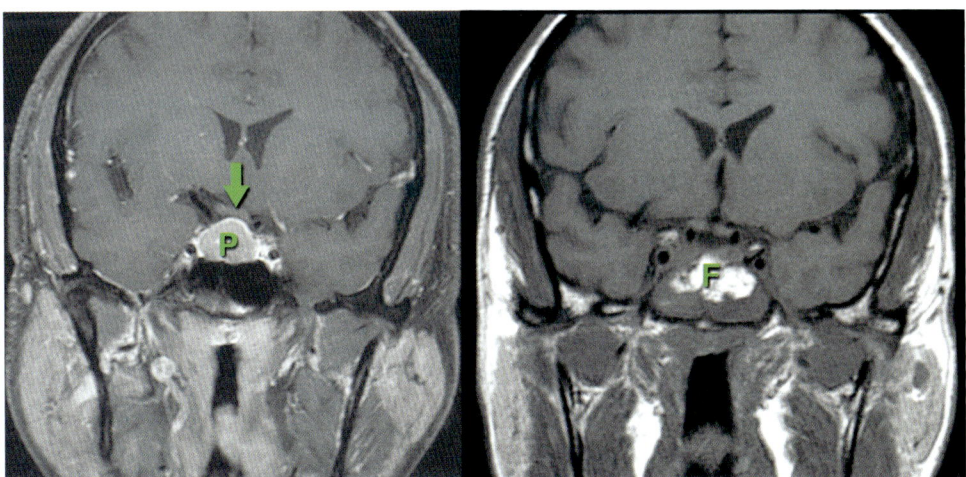

Figure 6–17. Pituitary macroadenoma (P) preoperatively (coronal T1–weighted MRI with contrast, left) and postoperatively (coronal T1-weighted MRI, right) after transsphenoidal resection. The tumor abuts the inferior portion of the optic chiasm (arrow). Fat has been used (F) to pack the sella after resection of the adenoma.

affecting the ocular motor cranial nerves within the cavernous sinus. Nystagmus may occur with extension of the tumor outside the sella.[91]

Sudden expansion of an existing adenoma due to intratumoral hemorrhage (Fig. 6–18) or infarction gives rise to the syndrome of pituitary apoplexy.[92,93] The typical triad of findings is (1) headache with or without meningeal irritation or signs of subarachnoid hemorrhage, (2) visual loss, and (3) diplopia from cavernous sinus extension. Frequently, the full triad is not seen. Less frequently, death from acute hypothalamic compression may occur.[94] Precipitating factors for pituitary apoplexy include radiotherapy, treatment with bromocriptine, dialysis, anticoagulation, recent surgery, trauma, and pregnancy.[95] Rapid neurosurgical decompression is warranted, and hormonal replacement, including corticosteroids, for hypopituitarism may be critical.[96]

6-7-1-2 *Endocrine Signs.* Prolactin-secreting tumors present differently in women than in men. In women, amenorrhea and galactorrhea are more commonly reported.[97] Symptoms of impotence frequently are not reported by male patients, so that the diagnosis is often delayed. Gynecomastia and galactorrhea are rare presenting signs in men. Additional manifestations of the hyperprolactinemic state may include emotional lability, unexplained weight gain, and osteoporosis.

Growth hormone–secreting tumors cause acromegaly. Bone and soft tissue enlargement of the face, feet, and hands may be detected. In addition, severe arthritic disease has been reported in 40% of cases, while other manifestations include heart disease, carpal tunnel syndrome, hypertension, diabetes mellitus, menstrual dysfunction, impotence, and sterility.[98] Early detection of endocrine dysfunction probably results in tumor detection before extrasellar spread can occur. Because the metabolic effects of growth hormone cause significant morbidity and mortality, aggressive treatment of such tumors is warranted.

As with GH-secreting tumors, ACTH-secreting adenomas cause a plethora of mostly nonocular clinical signs, encompassing Cushing's syndrome including obe-

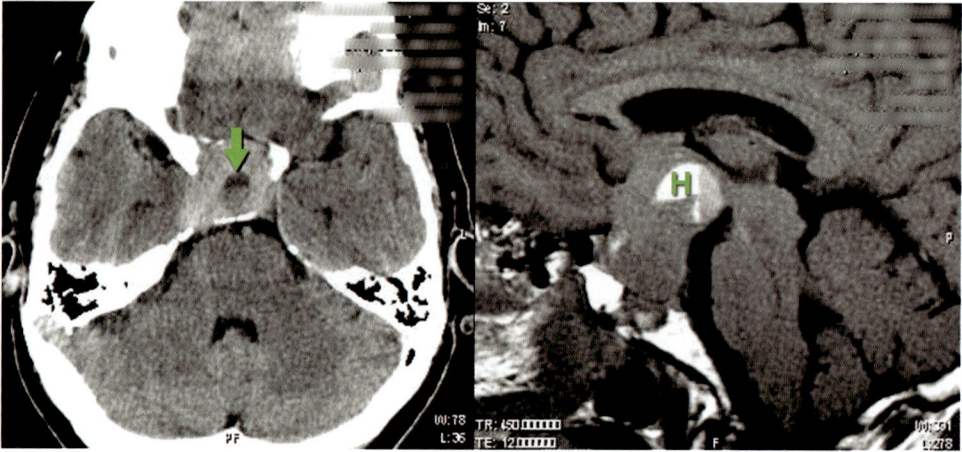

Figure 6–18. Pituitary apoplexy on axial CT (left) and sagittal T1-weighted MRI (right). There are areas of hypodensity (arrow) and hyperintensity (H) consistent with recent hemorrhage.

sity, hypertension, diabetes mellitus, and ketoacidosis.[99] In addition, primary tumors secreting TSH and secondary tumors secreting TSH and FSH due to target-organ failure are rarely reported.

6-7-2 *Neuroimaging.* MRI with gadolinium enhancement is currently the best method for detecting a pituitary adenoma. MRI affords a direct view of the anterior visual pathways in relationship to the tumor. Intratumoral hemorrhage and cysts are well seen (see Fig. 6–18). Invasion of the cavernous sinuses and displacement of parasellar vasculature are also well imaged with MRI. Other suprasellar masses, such as meningioma and aneurysm, can usually be differentiated with MRI.

After resection of a pituitary adenoma, MRI is superior to CT for patients who require postoperative neuroimaging (see Fig. 6–17).

6-7-3 *Management Options.* The goal of therapy for pituitary adenoma is two-fold: to eliminate the effects of the endocrine imbalance and to eliminate the mass effect of the tumor and its compression on neural structures, including the visual pathways. Pharmacologic treatment and neurosurgical intervention are discussed.

6-7-3-1 *Therapy of Prolactinoma.* The dopamine agonists bromocriptine and cabergoline have been shown to inhibit prolactin secretion and shrink pituitary tumors.[97,100] These agents appear to decrease the intracellular synthesis of prolactin and to impair lactotroph cell processes such as exocytosis. Dopamine agonists thus decrease the mass effect of the tumor and reverse amenorrhea, galactorrhea, and impotence while also inhibiting the progression of osteoporosis. Bromocriptine is usually tolerated orally, and often only low doses (7.5 mg daily) are necessary to be effective. There is no evidence of teratogenesis.

Several reports document the efficacy of dopamine agonists for both micro-adenomas and macroadenomas,[101] including impressive endocrinologic and visual improvement.[102]

For microadenoma patients not tolerating dopamine agonists, transsphenoidal resection has a high cure rate, with minimal morbidity and mortality.[103] For those maintained on medical therapy, two points should be considered: (1) dopamine agonists may have to be taken indefinitely, as discontinuing the medication may lead to tumor recurrence and secretory activity, and (2) dopamine agonists have been reported to cause fibrotic changes in the pituitary adenoma, which may make subsequent surgical removal difficult.[104]

In cases of macroadenoma with chiasmal compression or endocrine symptoms, dopamine agonists should be offered. If endocrine and visual symptoms abate, patients may be maintained on this therapy. Those who fail to respond fully or who cannot tolerate medical therapy should be offered surgery. Radiotherapy may be used adjunctively in those patients who are poor surgical risks.

In tumors that erode the sellar floor, the use of dopamine agonists with subsequent tumor shrinkage may rarely result in "unplugging" a connection between the intracranial and extracranial space, leading to cerebrospinal fluid leak and its attendant risk of infection.

6-7-3-2 Therapy of Other Secreting Tumors. The therapy of GH- and ACTH-secreting tumors is beyond the scope of this chapter; the reader may consult suitable references.[105–108] Most but not all secreting tumors may be discovered prior to visual pathway compression. For example, primary hypothyroidism may lead to secondary pituitary enlargement.[109] Thus, a complete endocrinologic evaluation should be considered in all patients with pituitary adenoma.

6-7-3-3 Therapy of Nonsecreting Tumors. In general, visual improvement after transsphenoidal decompression of the chiasm should be rapid and noticed by the patient within days of the surgery.[110] A later, more mild phase of improvement may take weeks to months. Dramatic visual improvement may even occur after surgery in patients with marked visual loss from pituitary apoplexy.[111]

6-7-3-4 Adverse Outcomes. Lack of visual improvement may result from long-standing compression of the optic chiasm. Failure of typical visual improvement or new visual loss may necessitate neuroimaging of the sellar area to exclude treatment outcomes that require surgical intervention. These include postoperative hematoma, chiasmal compression from overpacking of the operative bed (Fig. 6–19),[112] cerebrospinal fluid leak related to a transsphenoidal approach to the sellar floor, and inadequate resection of the tumor. Treatment of a pituitary adenoma, which has previously caused remodeling and expansion of the sella, may result in an "empty sella," which may predispose to chiasmal herniation into the sella and visual loss (Fig. 6–20).[113]

6-8 MENINGIOMA

6-8-1 Suprasellar Meningioma. Meningiomas comprise about 15% of all brain tumors. They occur far more commonly in adults than in children and with twice the

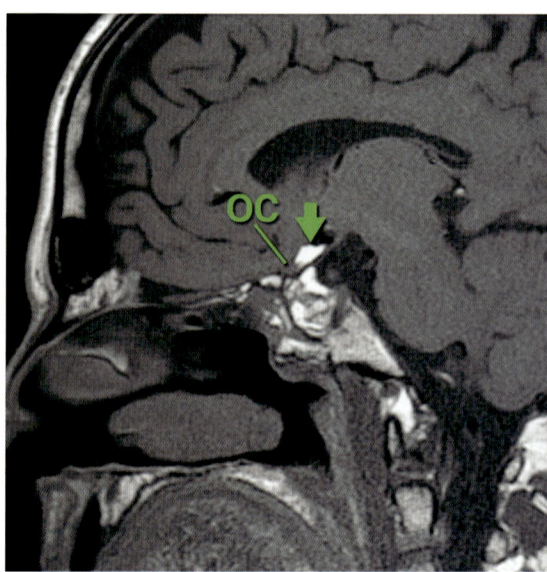

Figure 6–19. Postoperative sagittal T1-weighted MRI after transsphenoidal resection of a pituitary adenoma shows fat graft (arrow), which migrated to the suprasellar region and compressed the optic chiasm (OC).

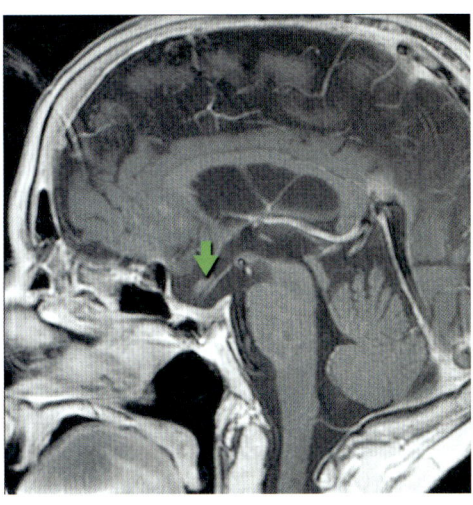

Figure 6–20. Postoperative sagittal T1-weighted MRI after transsphenoidal resection of a pituitary adenoma shows herniation of the optic chiasm (arrow) into an "empty sella."

frequency in women than in men.[114] Convexity meningiomas (parasagittal, falcine, and lateral cerebral convexity) are most prevalent, accounting for half of all tumors. Basal meningiomas (olfactory groove, sphenoid wing, suprasellar) account for 40%, while posterior fossa tumors comprise 10% of all cases.[115]

Meningiomas arise from meningothelial arachnoid cells and usually compress rather than invade adjacent brain. An osteoblastic reaction of adjacent bone, termed *hyperostosis*, may occur. Another well-described phenomenon characteristic of meningiomas is *pneumosinus dilatans*, a reactive pneumotization of bone underlying the meningioma.[116] A meningioma most often has well-circumscribed borders and appears as a sessile or pedunculated mass. Infrequently, a tumor may grow flat along the dural surface, making its soft tissue component difficult to identify radiographically; this is termed an *en plaque meningioma*.

In general, meningiomas are benign tumors, both histologically and clinically. The onset of neurologic symptoms is typically insidious and progressive, but rapid clinical deterioration has been reported. One such example is the accelerated growth of meningiomas during pregnancy.[117,118]

At least five histologic patterns of meningioma have been described: meningothelial, fibrous, transitional, papillary, and angioblastic.[119] The meningothelial type, the most common, consists of large epithelial-like cells with indistinct borders in a lobulated pattern. A whorl pattern of the cells is characteristic, and the psammoma body, a centrally located area of calcification, is characteristic. The incidence of malignancy in meningioma ranges from 2% to 10%, but distant metastases are rare.[119–122]

6-8-1-1 *Clinical Features.* Patients with suprasellar meningiomas are typically women, with a mean age of 50 years.[123] Progressive visual loss is the most common and often the only complaint; the visual loss may be unilateral or bilateral.[124,125] Less frequently, headache, personality change, proptosis, diplopia, and endocrinologic symptoms may be present. The specific location of the suprasellar meningioma accounts for the symptoms and signs seen and is also important regarding therapy and prognosis.[124] Typical locations are described below; the boldface numbers correspond to those in Fig. 6–21.

1. *Tuberculum sellae* (1). Tumors that originate and do not extend beyond here lead to visual dysfunction in one or both eyes. Posterior growth of such tumors results in chiasmal compression.
2. *Planum sphenoidale and olfactory groove* (3,9). Tumors that affect only the

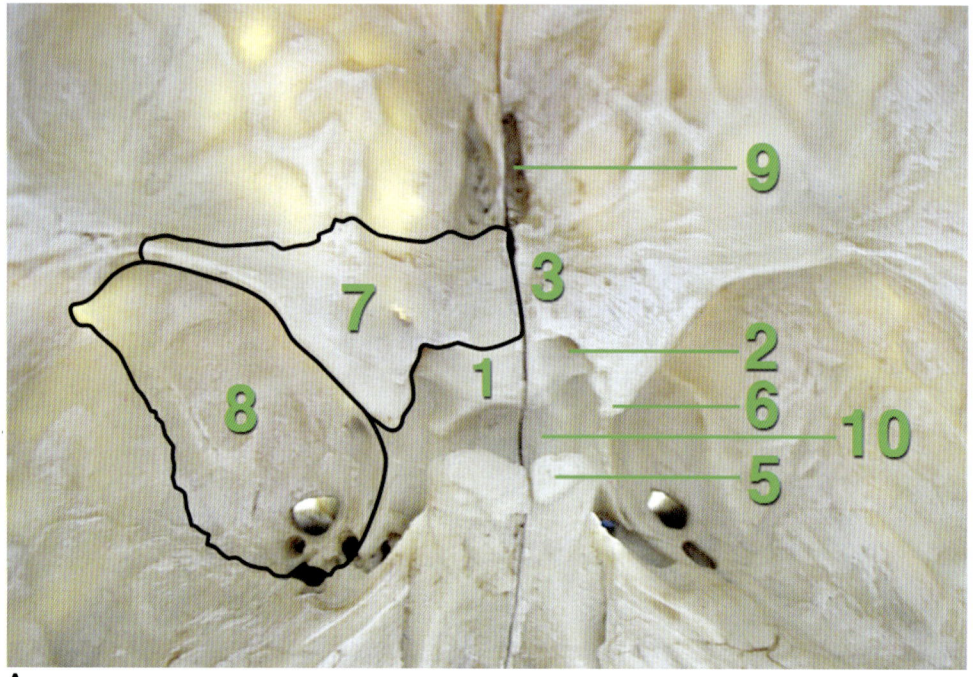

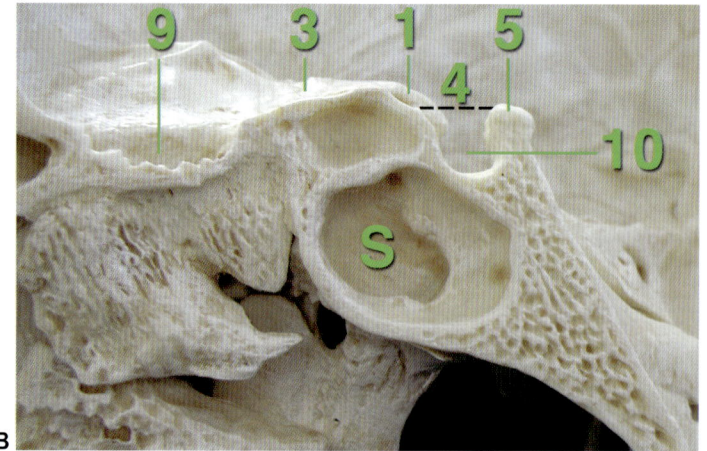

Figure 6–21. Bony anatomy of sella turcica and neighboring structures. (A) Top view. (B) Midsagittal view. 1, tuberculum sellae; 2, optic canal; 3, planum sphenoidale; 4, diaphragma sella (dotted line); 5, dorsum sellae; 6, anterior clinoid process; 7, lesser wing of sphenoid; 8, greater wing of sphenoid; 9, olfactory groove; 10, sella turcica; S, sphenoid sinus.

olfactory groove do not result in visual loss. These tumors must first grow posteriorly over the planum sphenoidale before contacting the superior aspect of the intracranial optic nerves and then the chiasm. These tumors are therefore large before visual dysfunction occurs. Other symptoms may include anosmia and personality change due to compression of the overlying frontal lobes.[123]

3. *Optic canal and anterior clinoid process* (2,6). Tumors isolated to this location cause unilateral optic neuropathy. Extension into the orbit may occur. Tumors that originate in other locations (e.g., tuberculum sellae) and extend to the optic foramen seem to have an overall worse prognosis for total removal and visual recovery (see below).

4. *Lesser and greater wings of the sphenoid* (7,8). Tumors of the lesser wing of the sphenoid may cause a unilateral optic neuropathy in addition to unilateral ophthalmoplegia. The latter is due to involvement of cranial nerves in the area of the superior orbital fissure and cavernous sinus. Tumors limited to the greater wing of the sphenoid cause proptosis but not optic nerve dysfunction.

5. *Diaphragma sellae* (4). Tumors that originate here compress the optic nerves and chiasm. In addition, they may grow into the sella, making it difficult to distinguish them from pituitary adenomas.

6. *Intrasellar meningioma* (10). Very rare and may be confused with other intrasellar tumors, especially pituitary adenoma.[123,126,127]

6-8-1-2 *Neuroimaging*. In the evaluation of patients harboring a meningioma, cranial CT and MRI are complementary. CT accurately shows a suprasellar tumor that is well circumscribed and homogeneously enhancing after intravenous contrast. Appropriate window settings may show hyperostosis or pneumosinus dilatans of adjacent bones, which is highly suggestive of meningioma. Intratumoral calcification may also be noted (Fig. 6–22). Gadolinium-enhanced MRI accurately depicts the extent of meningioma and its relationship to the anterior visual pathways (Fig. 6–23) and may show enhancement of the adjacent dura ("dural tail"). MRI may be helpful in those unusual cases in which suprasellar meningioma with intrasellar extension masquerades as pituitary adenoma (Fig. 6–24). Such distinction is

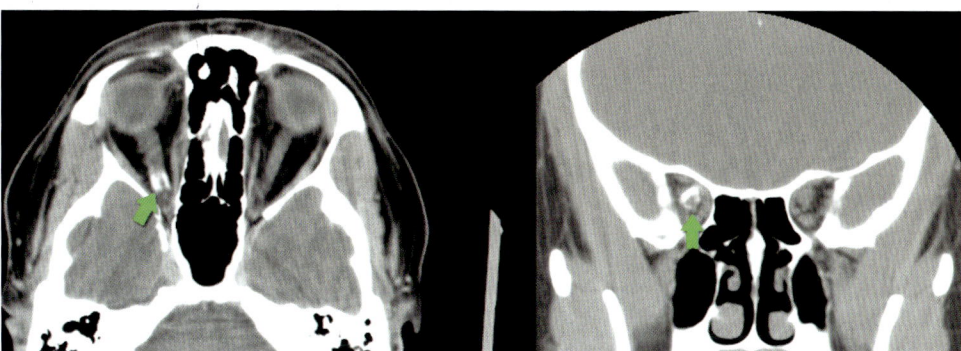

Figure 6–22. Meningioma of the right optic nerve sheath on axial (left) and coronal (right) CT shows calcification (arrows).

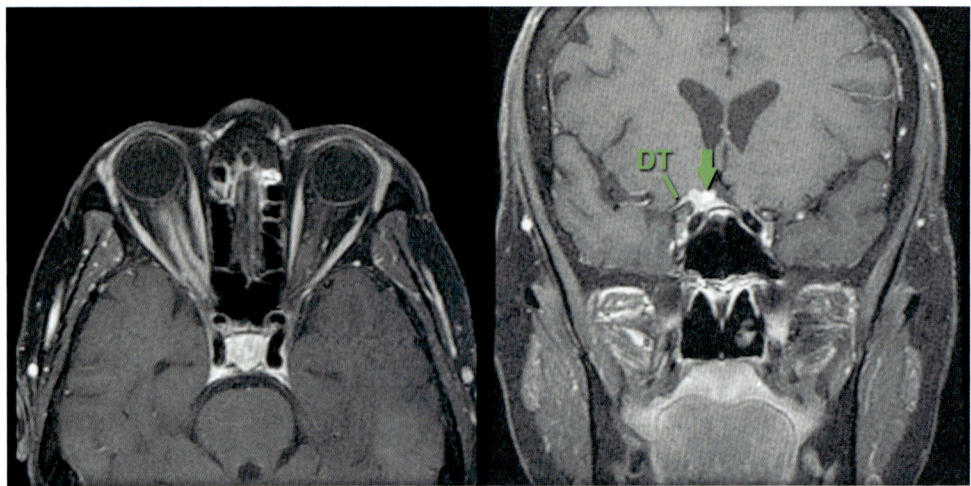

Figure 6–23. Right anterior paraclinoid meningioma. Left, axial T1-weighted MRI reveals meningioma resulting in a characteristic tram-track appearance. Right, coronal view demonstrates meningioma (arrow) with dural tail (DT).

critical, because a pituitary adenoma is often treated by transsphenoidal resection, while an intrasellar meningioma often requires craniotomy. Large aneurysms with intrasellar extension may occasionally be misdiagnosed by CT. Ordering both standard MRI and MRA avoids this potential pitfall. Cerebral angiography is generally not necessary for routine evaluation of meningioma but is helpful in preoperative planning.[128]

6-8-1-3 *Management Options.* The treatment of meningioma must be tailored to the individual patient.

1. *Observation.* In patients with minimal visual loss over a long period of time, observation may be appropriate. Since meningioma is in most cases a slow-growing tumor, observation may also be a reasonable alternative to surgery in patients who are poor surgical risks.
2. *Chemotherapy.* Chemotherapy has largely been disappointing for patients with meningiomas, but further investigation is ongoing.[129–131] Research into these agents was prompted by the fact that progesterone receptors have been

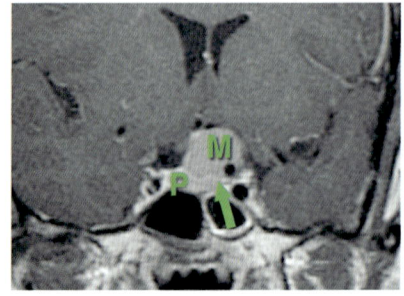

Figure 6–24. Meningioma (M) on T1-weighted MRI with contrast compresses the adjacent pituitary gland (P) and elevates the optic chiasm. There is a tissue plane (arrow) between the tumor and the normal pituitary gland.

found in the majority of meningiomas,[132] as well as by clinical studies suggesting that meningiomas grow during pregnancy.

3. *Surgery.* Microsurgical resection of tumor is the treatment of choice for some meningiomas affecting the visual system.[124,125] Patients with visual symptoms for less than a year have an excellent prognosis for visual recovery.[127] Tumors restricted to the tuberculum sellae have a better outcome than those that extend to other locations. Attempts at total removal of tumor without causing further damage to visual structures should be made. Growth of residual tumor and recurrence of symptoms are not uncommon.

4. *Radiotherapy.* Radiation therapy has played an increasingly important role in the treatment of meningiomas involving the visual pathways.[133] Radiation may be given alone or as an adjunct to surgery. This form of treatment seems prudent in those patients with progressive visual loss from meningioma who are considered poor surgical risks because of age or other medical problems. Radiation may halt further growth of tumor and may decrease the incidence of recurrence following subtotal resection. One serious complication of radiotherapy is late radionecrosis of the optic nerves and chiasm, which may result in devastating visual loss (Fig. 6–25). Most investigators agree that radionecrosis is a rare event when daily doses of radiation are less than 200 cGy and the total dose is less than 4500 cGy (see Chapter 10); however visual loss may still develop with stereotactic fractionated radiation.[53,54,134,135]

6-8-2 *Optic Nerve Sheath Meningioma.* Primary meningioma of the optic nerve sheath should be distinguished from other meningiomas. Examples of the latter include sphenoid wing meningioma, which involves the orbit and orbital apex with secondary optic nerve compression, and intracranial meningioma, which may extend into the orbit through the optic canal (see Fig. 6–23).[1]

6-8-2-1 *Clinical Features.* Optic nerve sheath meningioma (ONSM) is most commonly found in women, with an average age of 45 years. This form of meningioma is well reported in children (less than 18 years) and may be more aggressive than in adults.[1,136]

Slowly progressive unilateral visual loss is the most common presenting symptom. Other complaints include transient visual obscurations (occurring spontaneously or associated with eye movement), headache, and proptosis. In all cases,

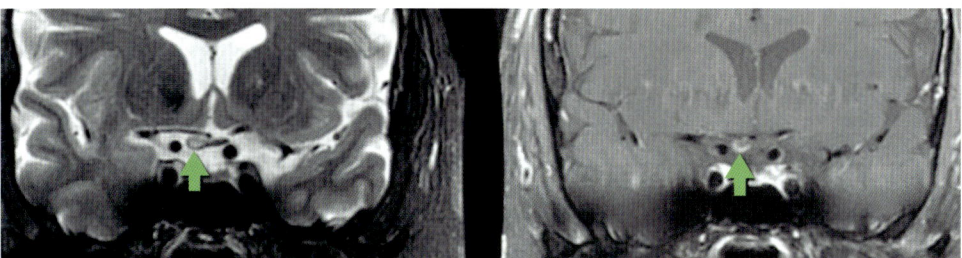

Figure 6–25. Radiation-induced injury to the optic chiasm on coronal T2-weighted (left) and T1-weighted MRI with contrast (right). The right side of the optic chiasm (arrows) is thickened and enhances.

neuro-ophthalmologic examination demonstrates findings compatible with unilateral or, infrequently, bilateral optic neuropathy. Signs of visual dysfunction include decreased acuity, visual field defects, color vision impairment, and contrast sensitivity disturbance. An afferent pupillary defect is noted in almost all cases. The appearance of the optic disc is almost always abnormal, with either optic disc swelling (in tumors involving the more proximal optic nerve) or optic disc pallor. Intrapapillary refractile bodies may be evident in a minority of cases with swollen discs. Optociliary shunt vessels (see Fig. 6–9) may be present in 15%–30% of patients.

6-8-2-2 *Neuroimaging.* The diagnosis of ONSM is most often established with neuroimaging studies. On CT scanning the optic nerve sheath is often in a tubular pattern and frequently contains areas of calcification (see Fig. 6–22).[137,138] The posterior apical aspect of the optic nerve is the most common site of involvement among all subtypes. The pattern of radiographic enlargement may not correlate with the degree of visual dysfunction. At times, axial CT scanning may reveal the "tram-track sign"—a central lucency representing the optic nerve surrounded by tumorous calcification. Despite the enlargement of the nerve sheath, the optic nerve can typically still be distinguished.

Currently, the imaging procedure of choice for diagnosis of ONSM is MRI of the brain and orbits with fat suppression and contrast.[138–140] Meningioma on T1- and T2-weighted images is often isointense to gray matter but enhances markedly after administration of contrast. Intracanalicular and intracranial extension of tumor is well demonstrated.[139] MRI increases the likelihood of detecting intracanalicular involvement because artifact from the surrounding bone is minimized. In addition, the fat-suppression technique eliminates the bright signal from intraorbital fat and allows the peripheral margins of a meningioma to be well demonstrated with contrast (see Figs. 6–8 and 6–23).

The combination of typical clinical symptoms and signs and radiographic appearance with involvement of the optic nerve sheath on fat-suppressed MRI with contrast makes an initial tissue biopsy unnecessary in most patients. As opposed to ONSM, intrinsic optic nerve enlargement is characteristic of optic nerve glioma, sarcoidosis (Fig. 6–26), and lymphoproliferative disease. In these three entities, subacute rather than slowly progressive visual loss would be expected. If pain is present and the condition is thought to be idiopathic inflammatory optic perineuritis, a trial of systemic corticosteroids may be cautiously instituted. If a diagnosis cannot be firmly established or an atypical clinical course occurs, a biopsy of the optic nerve may be necessary.[141] However, this diagnostic procedure may further compromise vision and, rarely, opening the dura can result in further expansion of the tumor into the orbit.

6-8-2-3 *Management Options.* Surgery appears to be unwarranted in the management of most ONSMs.[142–144] General guidelines for the treatment of ONSM include the following:

1. In patients with good visual function (including visual acuity equal to or better than 20/40), observation seems prudent. In some patients, ONSM may spontaneously regress with a concordant improvement in visual function.[145] In those

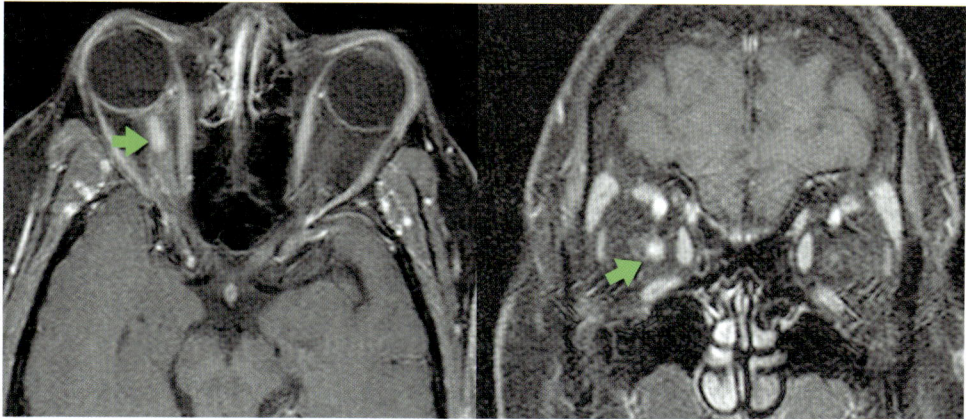

Figure 6–26. Optic nerve enhancement from sarcoidosis on axial (left) and coronal (right) fat-suppressed T1-weighted MRI with contrast. As compared with nerve sheath enhancement from a meningioma (Figs. 6–8 and 6–23), the enhancement from an inflammatory process involves the optic nerve itself.

with vision worse than 20/40 who have shown progression of symptoms, radiotherapy (stereotactic fractionated radiotherapy)[146–148] should be considered. In cases of meningioma involving the optic nerve sheath, radiotherapy has been shown to slow the rate of visual deterioration.[149] Accumulating evidence supports the use of a specific technique, stereotactic fractionated radiotherapy, for ONSM.[146–148,150,151] Stereotactic fractionated radiotherapy stabilizes or may improve vision in patients with this condition.

2. In patients with progressive visual loss despite radiotherapy in whom vision is no longer useful and the tumor is growing, complete removal of the intraorbital tumor with the optic nerve may be performed. These patients should be studied carefully with MRI following intravenous gadolinium to exclude intracranial spread.

3. In eyes already blind from ONSM without intracranial spread, close observation with serial neuroimaging is possible. However, removal of the intraorbital tumor and optic nerve will result in a cure.

4. Management of patients with intracranial extension remains a difficult question.[136,152] Treatment of the intracranial component should be considered when there is progressive growth with compression of the chiasm or fellow optic nerve resulting in visual loss.

6-9 INTRACRANIAL ANEURYSM

Intracranial aneurysms can be divided into three categories[153]:

1. Saccular, discussed below
2. Mycotic, involving weakening and dilation of an artery from a septic process (e.g., subacute bacterial endocarditis)
3. Fusiform, resulting in diffuse enlargement of an artery rather than a localized outpouching, and associated with atherosclerotic vascular disease[154]

Saccular aneurysms are localized outpouchings, typically arising at the bifurcation of the arteries of the circle of Willis or its branches. They are presumably developmental defects in the media and elastica of arteries, although it appears probable that aneurysms develop in later life and are unusual in childhood. Aneurysms occur more frequently in women, with no racial predilection. On the basis of arteriographic studies, the prevalence of cerebral aneurysms has been calculated to be 0.65%, with an estimated annual rate of rupture of 1%–2%.[155] About 25% of the patients have multiple aneurysms. The most common location is the anterior portion of the circle of Willis: internal carotid, middle cerebral, anterior cerebral, and anterior communicating arteries (Fig. 6–27).[153,156] Aneurysms may vary in size, ranging from 2 mm to greater than 25 mm in "giant aneurysms." [157,158] Aneurysms that cause neuroophthalmic symptoms[159–161] are typically larger than 3 mm.

Most intracranial aneurysms are asymptomatic; with rupture, however, the most common findings are those of subarachnoid hemorrhage, including severe headache, stiff neck, mental status changes, coma, and delayed cerebral infarction due to vasospasm.[153,157] The mortality from aneurysmal bleed and early rebleeding within days to weeks is approximately 50%.[153] Emergent treatment with obliteration of the aneurysm and preservation of the parent artery should be performed as soon as feasible. A second symptomatic presentation of aneurysms is compression

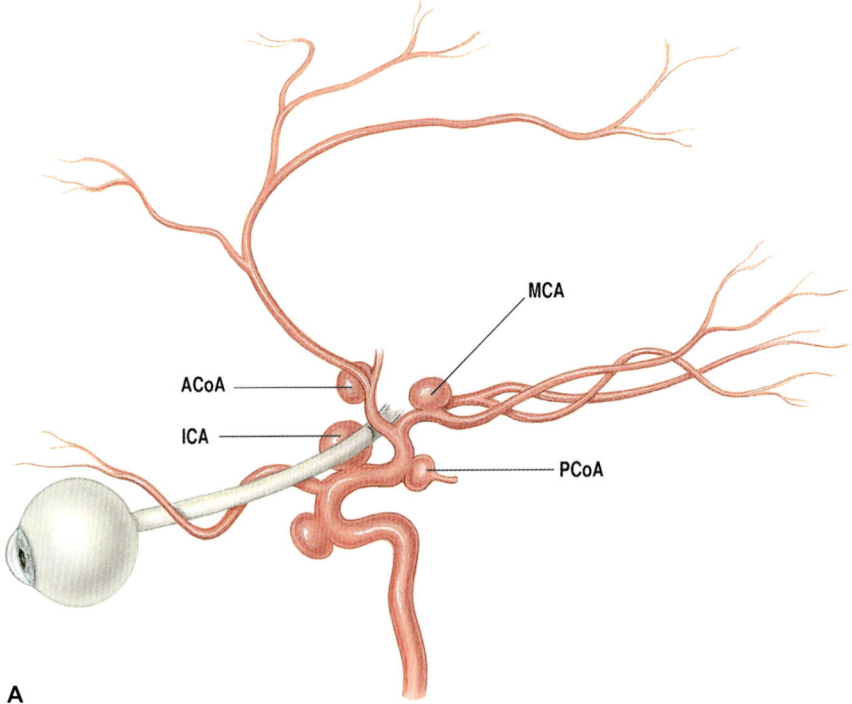

A

Figure 6–27. Location of aneurysms of the circle of Willis in (A) lateral and (B) (opposite page) inferior views. ACoA, anterior communicating artery; MCA, middle cerebral artery; ICA, internal carotid artery; PCoA, posterior communicating artery; PCA, posterior cerebral artery; VA, vertebral artery; BA, basilar artery. (Redrawn with permission of S. Karger AG, Basel, from Krayenbuhl H. Klassifikation und klinische Symptomatologie der zerebralen Aneurysmen. Ophthalmologica 1973;167:122.)

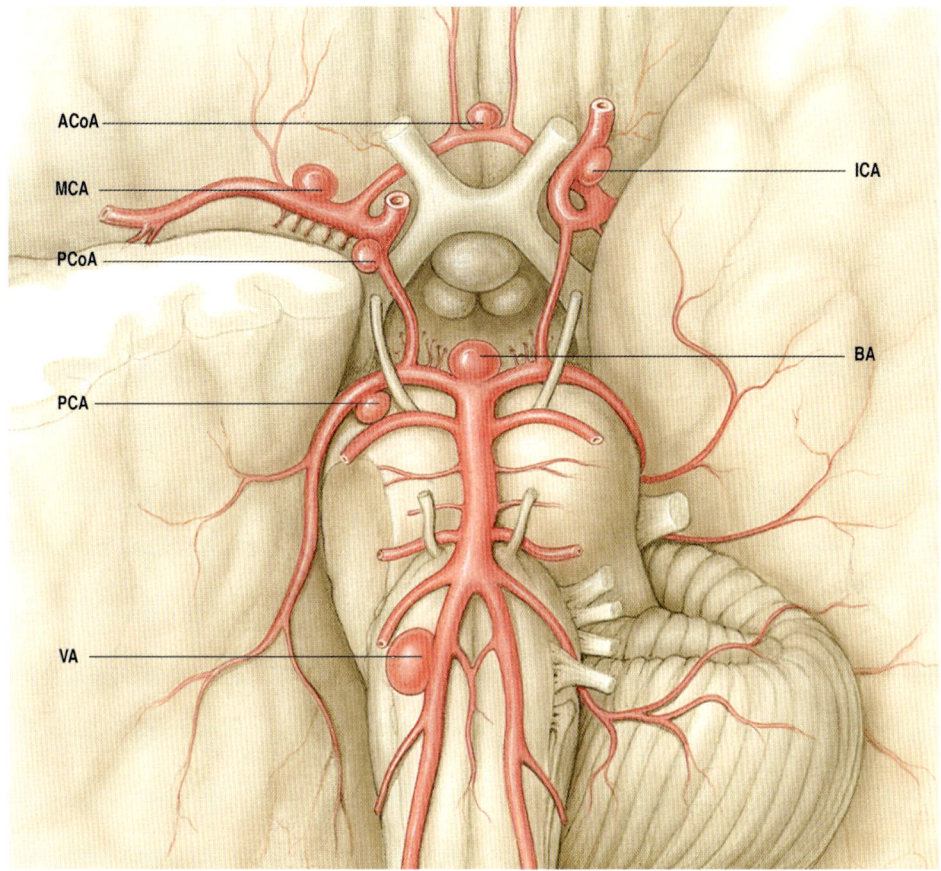

B

Figure 6–27 (continued)

of adjacent structures, such as cranial nerves or the anterior visual pathway (Fig. 6–28).[162] Aneurysms may infrequently present with transient neurologic signs or ischemic infarction due to emboli within the aneurysmal sac.[163]

6-9-1 Clinical Features. Aneurysms affecting the anterior visual system may be categorized according to their origin. However, in many instances, the aneurysmal neck may be so wide that such a classification may be difficult.

1. *Ophthalmic artery,* Aneurysms involving only the ophthalmic artery, either intraorbital or intracranial, are extremely rare. Most cases present with progressive monocular visual acuity and field loss, optic atrophy, or optic disc edema.[164] Rarely, acute monocular blindness and proptosis may occur due to orbital hemorrhage.[165]
2. *Carotid–paraophthalmic artery.* These aneurysms arise from the internal carotid artery above the cavernous sinus, at the origin of the ophthalmic artery. The frequency of this particular aneurysm ranges from 1.5%–8%. In reported series, the most frequent clinical presentation is subarachnoid hemorrhage.[165] Unilateral visual acuity and field loss may occur, depending on the varying projection of the aneurysm.

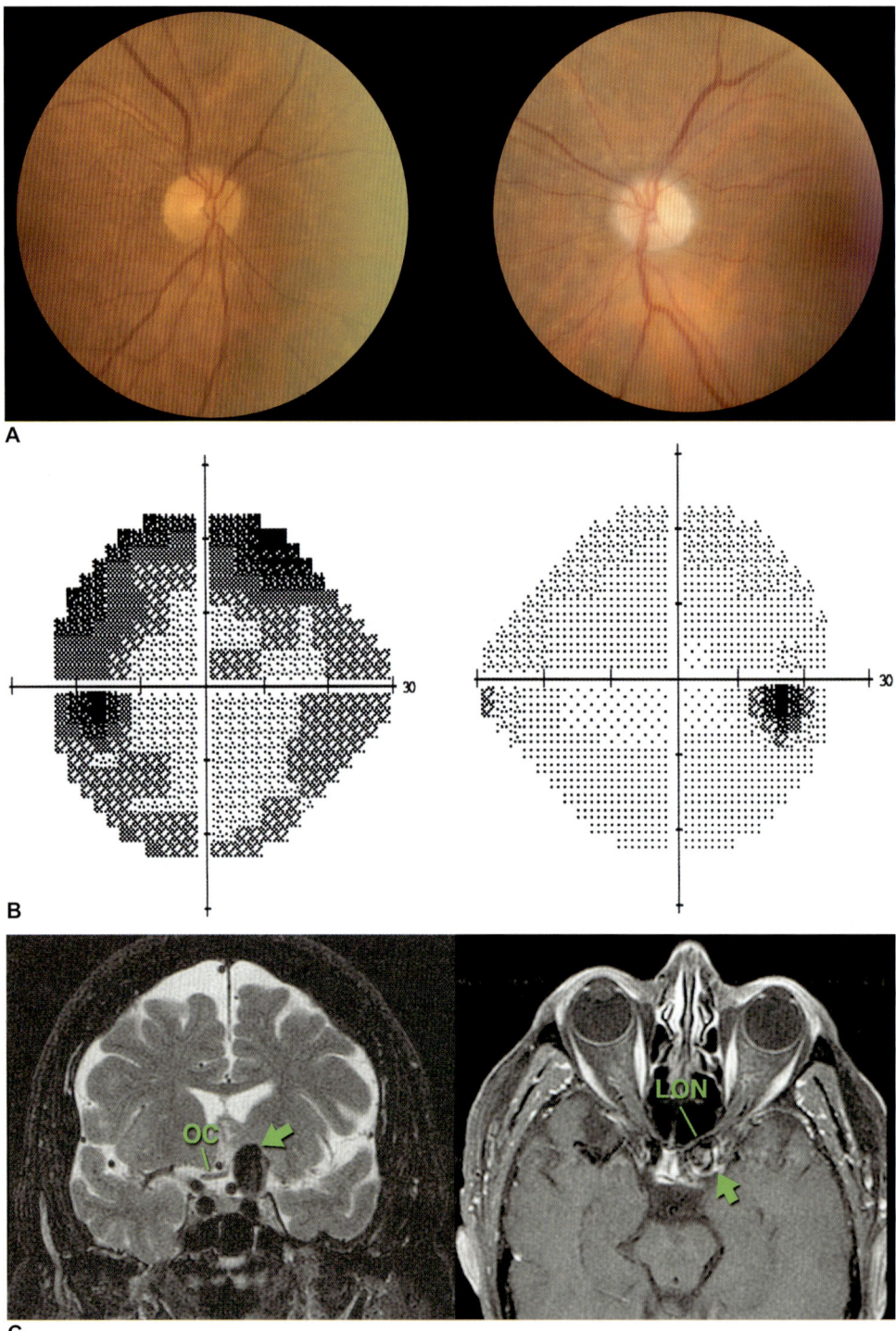

Figure 6–28. Optic neuropathy from a left carotid–paraophthalmic artery aneurysm. (A) Fundus photographs show a normal optic disc on the right and optic atrophy on the left. (B) Automated perimetry shows a normal visual field on the right and nerve fiber bundle defects on the left. (C) Coronal T2-weighted MRI (left) and axial T1-weighted MRI with fat suppression and contrast (right) show a carotid-paraophthalmic aneurysm (arrows) displacing the optic chiasm (OC) and compressing the left intracranial optic nerve (LON).

3. *Supraclinoid carotid artery.* These aneurysms arise from the internal carotid artery distal to the origin of the ophthalmic artery and may slowly enlarge to compress the anterior visual pathways. Proximal supraclinoid aneurysms produce asymmetric visual loss, with greater involvement of the ipsilateral optic nerve. Distal aneurysms of the carotid terminus (at the bifurcation of anterior and middle cerebral arteries) may mimic suprasellar tumors, causing bitemporal hemianopia. Posterior extension of a supraclinoid aneurysm may compress the optic tract.[166]

4. *Anterior communicating artery* Most of these aneurysms present with subarachnoid hemorrhage. Local compression of the optic nerves occurs infrequently.[167]

Visual loss from aneurysmal compression may have no predictable pattern and may be gradual or acute. Abrupt loss of vision may be related to a sudden change in the size of the aneurysm, variation in intracranial pressure, and arterial spasm with subarachnoid hemorrhage. Subarachnoid hemorrhage may cause characteristic intraocular hemorrhages (Terson syndrome) (Fig. 6–29). These hemorrhages may occur in multiple intraocular structures including the vitreous, subhyaloid space, and subretinal space.[168] Macular hemorrhages may cause persistent visual loss.

6-9-2 *Neuroimaging.* Neuroimaging is mandatory in the evaluation of patients suspected of harboring an aneurysm. Evidence of subarachnoid hemorrhage may be apparent with CT or, less commonly, MRI. However, if neuroimaging is negative and subarachnoid hemorrhage is still suspected, a lumbar puncture is required.[153] CT will reveal a well-circumscribed mass lesion, and enhancement may be diffusely homogeneous or inhomogeneous or show rim enhancement only with thrombosed aneurysms. However, MRI is the scanning procedure of choice. The changes in signal intensity may include flow void in all pulsing sequences due to rapidly flowing blood, intermediate or increased heterogeneous signal due to thrombosis, and peripheral areas of low intensity due to hemosiderin or intramural calcium. Cerebral angiog-

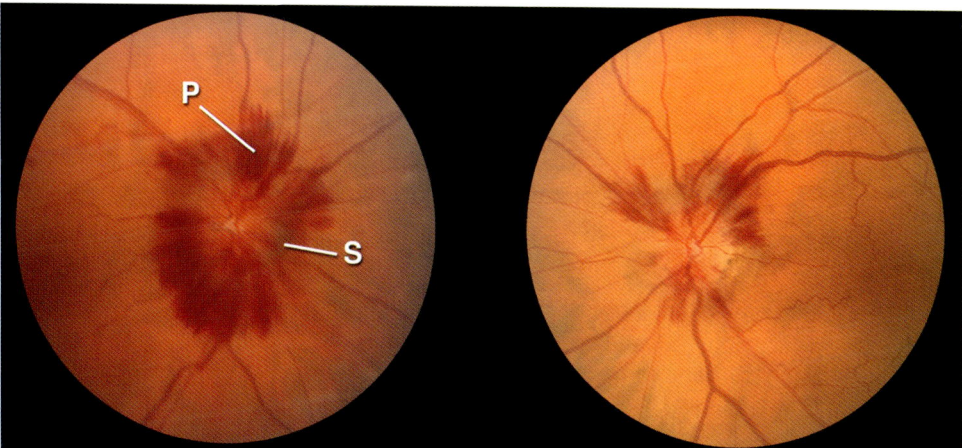

Figure 6–29. Fundus photographs showing preretinal (P) and subretinal (S) hemorrhages from Terson syndrome after subarachnoid hemorrhage. Bilateral vitreous hemorrhages (not noted photographically) were also present.

raphy is often performed to confirm the diagnosis and plan treatment. This modality also detects the presence of other aneurysms. Magnetic resonance angiography (MRA) and computed tomographic angiography (CTA) are noninvasive techniques for visualizing the intracranial vasculature (Fig. 6–30).[169–174] Both MRI/MRA and

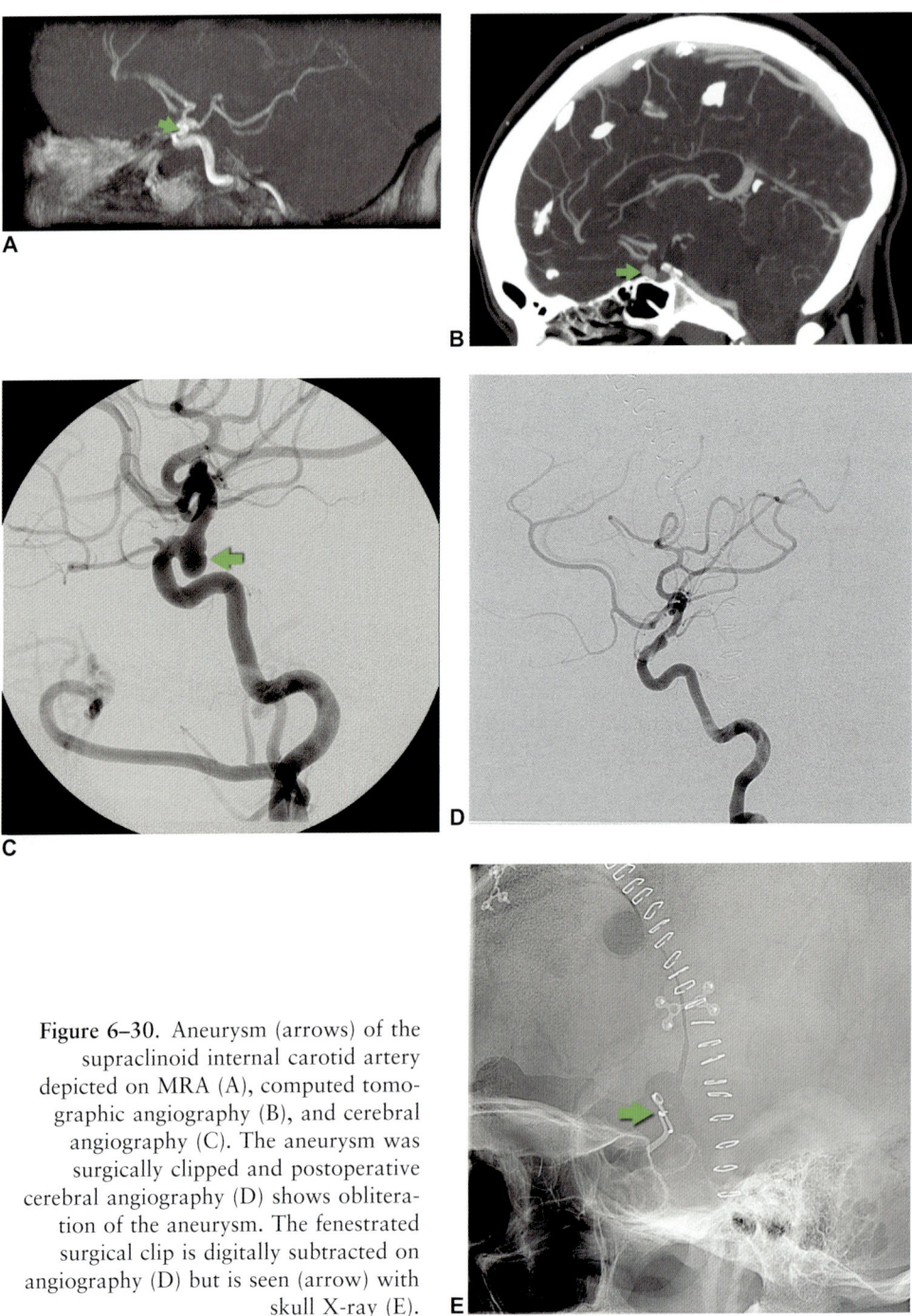

Figure 6–30. Aneurysm (arrows) of the supraclinoid internal carotid artery depicted on MRA (A), computed tomographic angiography (B), and cerebral angiography (C). The aneurysm was surgically clipped and postoperative cerebral angiography (D) shows obliteration of the aneurysm. The fenestrated surgical clip is digitally subtracted on angiography (D) but is seen (arrow) with skull X-ray (E).

CTA are sensitive in the detection of cerebral aneurysms to a resolution of 2 mm, including those that cause visual pathway compression. However, cerebral angiography remains the standard in the diagnosis of aneurysms and other vascular disorders of the central nervous system that may cause compressive optic neuropathy (Fig. 6–31).[171,175]

6-9-3 *Management Options.* Aneurysms causing compressive optic neuropathy are typically treated both to prevent rupture and reverse progressive optic neuropathy.[169,176]

The decision to treat an unruptured aneurysm depends on several factors, and in some cases remains controversial.[169,176] Therapy of aneurysms includes surgical and endovascular techniques (Fig. 6–32). The use of a particular treatment modality depends on several factors, including the size and location of the aneurysm and the configuration of the aneurysmal neck.

1. *Surgical*
   A. *Direct surgery.* Direct ligation of the aneurysmal neck or the base of the aneurysm ("clipping") historically has been the therapy of choice (see Fig. 6–30). With this method, the aneurysmal dome may be opened and extirpated, relieving compression of the visual system.[165,177,178]
   B. *Surgical trapping.* Surgically occluding the parent vessel proximal and distal to the aneurysm is uncommonly done. However, cerebral ischemia cannot necessarily be predicted beforehand. If cross-circulation is deemed poor, a primary extracranial-intracranial bypass procedure must first be performed.

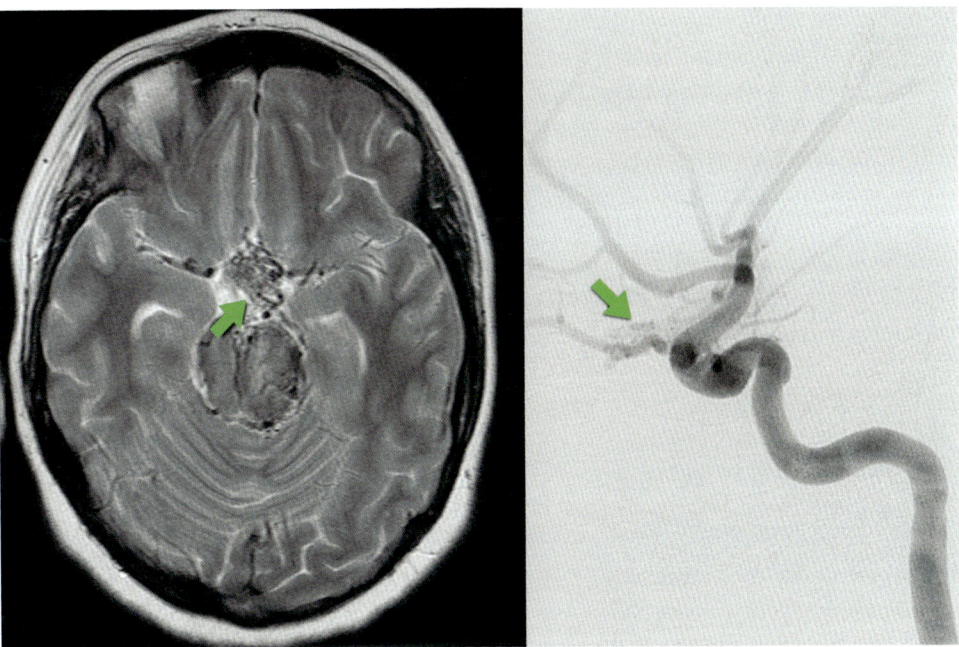

Figure 6–31. Paraclinoid arteriovenous malformation (arrows) on axial T2-weighted MRI (left), primarily fed by the ophthalmic artery on cerebral angiography (right).

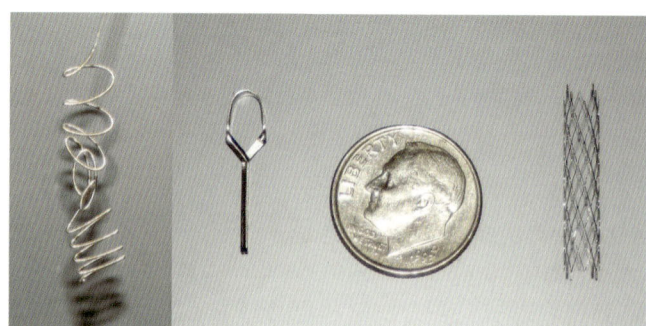

Figure 6–32. Platinum coil (left), neurosurgical clip (center), and intravascular stent (right) used to treat intracerebral aneurysms.

C. *Wrapping.* The aneurysmal dome may be reinforced by wrapping in gauze or plastic coating.

2. *Endovascular.* Endovascular embolization using platinum coils and remodeling of a wide aneurysmal neck with intraluminal stents are now routinely used as primary therapeutic options (Fig. 6–33).[169,178–180] The use of platinum coils has gained favor in part because they are MRI-compatible.

6-10 OPTIC NEUROPATHY FROM THYROID-ASSOCIATED ORBITOPATHY

Thyroid-associated orbitopathy (TAO) is an immune-mediated inflammatory disorder of the orbit. Involvement of the extraocular muscles has been extensively studied with orbital imaging techniques[181–184] and pathologic examination.[185–188] Many of the clinical manifestations, including proptosis, periorbital edema, and limited ocular motility, can be explained by increased extraocular muscle volume.[184] Common eyelid signs such as eyelid retraction and eyelid lag cannot be explained on a similar basis. Visual loss from TAO has two major causes: corneal exposure and optic neuropathy.[189] The former is due to severe proptosis from the underlying inflammatory process, while the latter is due to compression of the apical portion of the optic nerve by enlarged extraocular muscles.

The incidence of optic neuropathy from TAO is around 5% among patients with typical thyroid disease.[190] This unusual manifestation, however, may result in devastating visual loss if untreated.

6-10-1 *Clinical Features.* The optic neuropathy from TAO is similar to other types of compressive neuropathies. Symptoms consist of unilateral or bilateral progressive visual loss, typically over several months, although some patients may report more abrupt visual failure. Transient visual obscurations, as seen with optic nerve sheath meningioma, are not typically described, and fluctuation in vision over a short period of time is unusual.[191] Although the optic neuropathy is often bilateral, it may be markedly asymmetric and may occur in the absence of clinical signs of overt orbitopathy. The optic disc is normal in appearance in 50% of patients, swollen in 35%, and pale in 15%; choroidal folds may be present. Although visual loss from TAO has been reported to result from proptosis and stretching of the optic

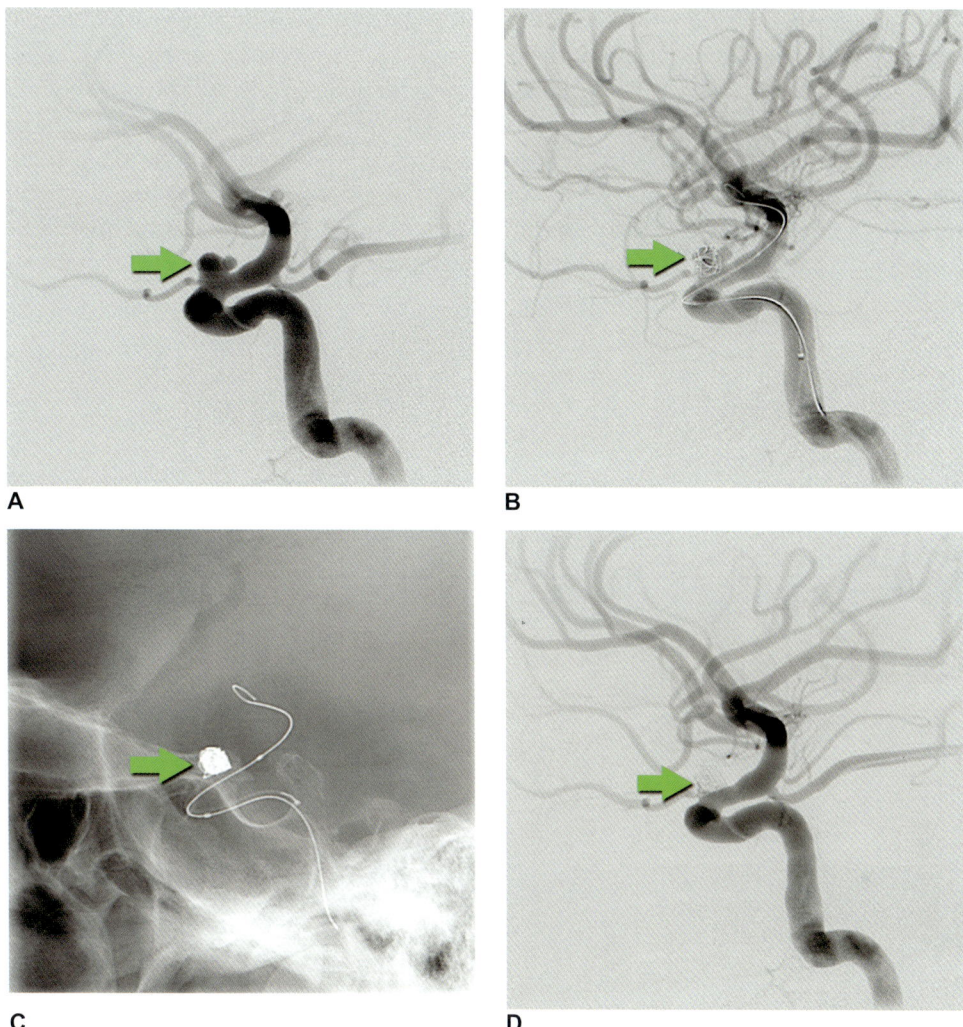

A

B

C

D

Figure 6–33. Paraophthalmic aneurysm (arrow) of the internal carotid artery on cerebral angiography (A). (B) During treatment, an intravascular catheter places platinum coils within the aneurysm (arrow). Skull X-ray demonstrates coil cast (arrow) after placement of the coils has been completed (C). (D) Postembolization cerebral angiography shows obliteration of the aneurysm (arrow).

nerve,[192] most patients who develop visual loss have crowding of the orbital apex from thickened extraocular muscles, often best noted using axial orbital imaging (Fig. 6–34).

There is a correlation between extraocular muscle limitation and periorbital swelling and the development of optic neuropathy.[193] The degree of proptosis correlates less well with optic neuropathy; eyelid retraction and eyelid lag have shown no correlation.

6-10-2 *Management Options.* Patients with suspected optic neuropathy from TAO should undergo orbital imaging before treatment options are considered. Occasionally, other entities may masquerade as thyroid eye disease, including idiopathic orbital inflammation, lymphoma, and carcinomatous enlargement of the extraocular muscles. Enlargement of the belly of the extraocular muscle with relative sparing of the tendon is fairly characteristic although not completely specific for thyroid disease. The proclivity for rectus muscle involvement is in the following order: inferior, medial, superior, and lateral (see Fig. 6–34). When the pattern of extraocular muscle thickening does not follow this order, conditions other than thyroid eye disease should be considered (Table 6–3). The following management options are available:

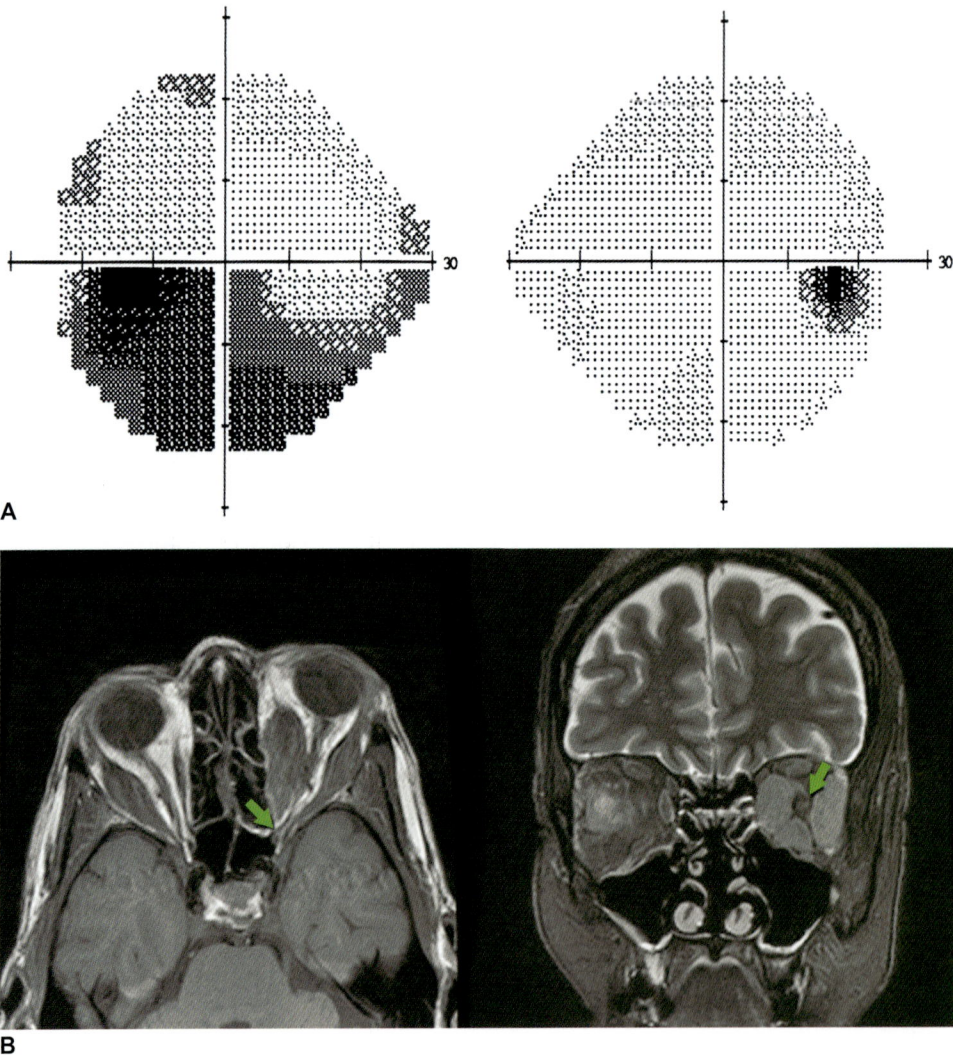

Figure 6–34. TAO causing left optic neuropathy. (A) Automated perimetry is normal on the right and shows an inferior altitudinal defect on the left. (B) There is enlargement of the extraocular muscles within the right orbit with sparing of the tendons. More significantly, axial (left) and coronal (right) T2-weighted MRI shows marked thickening of the inferior, medial, and lateral rectus muscles within the left orbit with crowding of the orbital apex and compression of the left optic nerve (arrows). (C) (opposite page) Automated perimetry after left orbital decompression shows marked improvement of the left visual field.

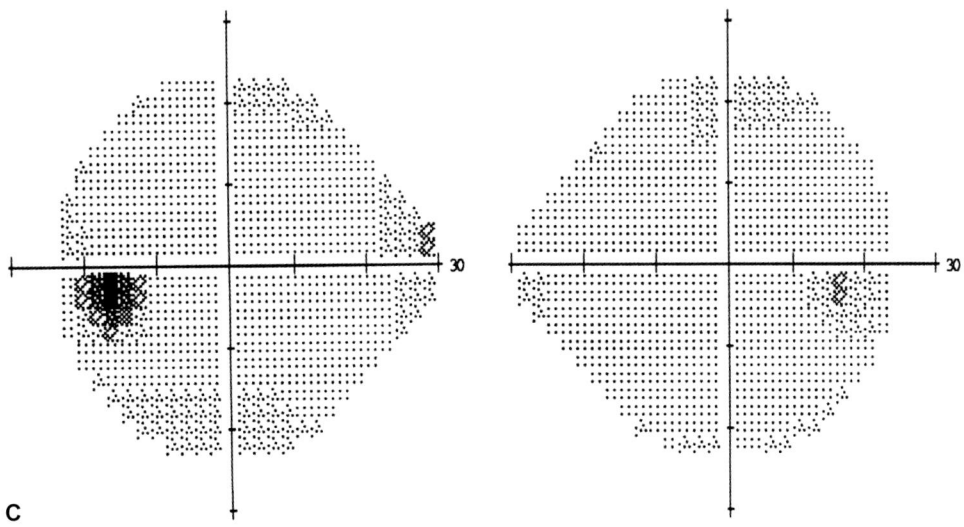

C

Figure 6–34 (continued)

Table 6-3 Nonthyroid Causes of Extraocular Muscle Enlargement

1. *Inflammation*

   Specific: Sarcoidosis, Wegener's granulomatosis, Crohn's disease, Whipple's disease, systemic lupus erythematosus, rheumatoid arthritis
   Nonspecific: Idiopathic orbital inflammation

2. *Vascular*

   Carotid-cavernous fistula
   Arteriovenous malformation

3. *Neoplastic*

   Local invasion
   Metastasis

4. *Infectious*

   Primary: viral, bacterial, fungal, parasitic
   Secondary: orbital cellulitis

5. *Deposition*

   Amyloid

6. *Traumatic*

7. *Iatrogenic*

   Following orbital/ sinus surgery
   Drug-induced: lithium, chloroquine

8. *Congenital*

   Fibrosis syndromes
   Neurofibromatosis

9. *Miscellaneous*

   Acromegaly
   Vitamin E deficiency

Source: Modified from Lacey,[231] with permission.

1. *Observation* It seems reasonable to observe closely those patients with minimal visual dysfunction.[191,194–196]
2. *Oral corticosteroids.* A number of reports have documented visual improvement using systemic corticosteroids.[191,197] Improvement typically begins within 72 hours and is maximal by 6 to 8 weeks, such that if a response to therapy is not seen within 3–4 weeks, prolonged corticosteroid therapy is less likely to be effective.
3. *Orbital decompression surgery.* Surgical decompression of the orbit for patients with optic neuropathy from TAO has been shown to be highly effective in restoring visual function (see Fig. 6–34).[198–201] Most investigators suggest at least a two-wall decompression procedure (orbital floor and medial wall) and, in more severe cases, a three-wall procedure (orbital floor, medial wall, and lateral wall).[201] Surgery limited to either the lateral wall or the orbital roof is infrequently performed as a primary procedure.[202] Complications include transient or permanent infraorbital anesthesia and diplopia, often requiring strabismus surgery.[203–206]
4. *Radiotherapy.* Radiotherapy for TAO remains controversial.[207] In most reports, radiotherapy is reserved as a second line of treatment, usually in those patients who have not responded to corticosteroids.[208] Some clinicians have used radiation therapy as a primary treatment modality for optic neuropathy from TAO.[209,210] Most investigators suggest a total dose in the range of 2000 cGy, because complications in this range are unusual. Nevertheless, radiation retinopathy may still occur with these doses.[207,211] Radiotherapy should be administered by radiotherapists experienced in treating orbital disease.

References

1. Miller NR. Primary tumours of the optic nerve and its sheath. Eye 2004;18(11):1026–37.
2. Foroozan R. Chiasmal syndromes. Curr Opin Ophthalmol 2003;14(6):325–31.
3. Hoyt WF, Meshel LG, Lessell S, et al. Malignant optic glioma of adulthood. Brain 1973;96(1):121–32.
4. Spoor TC, Kennerdell JS, Martinez AJ, Zorub D. Malignant gliomas of the optic nerve pathways. Am J Ophthalmol 1980;89(2):284–92.
5. Wabbels B, Demmler A, Seitz J, et al. Unilateral adult malignant optic nerve glioma. Graefes Arch Clin Exp Ophthalmol 2004;242(9):741–8.
6. Foroozan R. The pale optic nerve. Contemporary Ophthalmology 2003;2(26):1–10.
7. Jonas JB, Dichtl A. Evaluation of the retinal nerve fiber layer. Surv Ophthalmol 1996; 40(5):369–78.
8. Kanamori A, Nakamura M, Matsui N, et al. Optical coherence tomography detects characteristic retinal nerve fiber layer thickness corresponding to band atrophy of the optic discs. Ophthalmology 2004;111(12):2278–83.
9. Kennedy F. Retrobulbar neuritis as an exact diagnostic sign of certain tumors and abscesses in the frontal lobes. Am J Med Sci 1911;142:355–68.
10. Schatz NJ, Smith JL. Non-tumor causes of the Foster Kennedy syndrome. J Neurosurg 1967;27(1):37–44.
11. Thiagalingam S, Flaherty M, Billson F, North K. Neurofibromatosis type 1 and optic pathway gliomas: follow-up of 54 patients. Ophthalmology 2004;111(3):568–77.
12. Suharwardy J, Elston J. The clinical presentation of children with tumours affecting the anterior visual pathways. Eye 1997;11(Pt 6):838–44.

13. Jacobson DM. Gliomas of the anterior visual pathways. Neurosurg Clin North Am 1999;10(4):683–98.
14. Gayre GS, Scott IU, Feuer W, et al. Long-term visual outcome in patients with anterior visual pathway gliomas. J Neuroophthalmol 2001;21(1):1–7.
15. Astrup J. Natural history and clinical management of optic pathway glioma. Br J Neurosurg 2003;17(4):327–35.
16. Czyzyk E, Jozwiak S, Roszkowski M, Schwartz RA. Optic pathway gliomas in children with and without neurofibromatosis 1. J Child Neurol 2003;18(7):471–8.
17. Liu GT, Brodsky MC, Phillips PC, et al. Optic radiation involvement in optic pathway gliomas in neurofibromatosis. Am J Ophthalmol 2004;137(3):407–14.
18. Balcer LJ, Liu GT, Heller G, et al. Visual loss in children with neurofibromatosis type 1 and optic pathway gliomas: relation to tumor location by magnetic resonance imaging. Am J Ophthalmol 2001;131(4):442–5.
19. Wright JE, McNab AA, McDonald WI. Optic nerve glioma and the management of optic nerve tumours in the young. Br J Ophthalmol 1989;73(12):967–74.
20. Haik BG, Saint Louis L, Bierly J, et al. Magnetic resonance imaging in the evaluation of optic nerve gliomas. Ophthalmology 1987;94(6):709–17.
21. Massry GG, Morgan CF, Chung SM. Evidence of optic pathway gliomas after previously negative neuroimaging. Ophthalmology 1997;104(6):930–5.
22. Frohman LP, Epstein F, Kupersmith MJ. Atypical visual prognosis with an optic nerve glioma. J Clin Neuroophthalmol 1985;5(2):90–4.
23. McDonnell P, Miller NR. Chiasmatic and hypothalamic extension of optic nerve glioma. Arch Ophthalmol 1983;101(9):1412–5.
24. Parsa CF, Hoyt CS, Lesser RL, et al. Spontaneous regression of optic gliomas: thirteen cases documented by serial neuroimaging. Arch Ophthalmol 2001;119(4):516–29.
25. Combs SE, Schulz-Ertner D, Moschos D, et al. Fractionated stereotactic radiotherapy of optic pathway gliomas: tolerance and long-term outcome. Int J Radiat Oncol Biol Phys 2005;62(3):814–9.
26. Alvord EC, Jr., Lofton S. Gliomas of the optic nerve or chiasm. Outcome by patients' age, tumor site, and treatment. J Neurosurg 1988;68(1):85–98.
27. Khafaga Y, Hassounah M, Kandil A, et al. Optic gliomas: a retrospective analysis of 50 cases. Int J Radiat Oncol Biol Phys 2003;56(3):807–12.
28. Glaser JS, Hoyt WF, Corbett J. Visual morbidity with chiasmal glioma. Long-term studies of visual fields in untreated and irradiated cases. Arch Ophthalmol 1971;85(1):3–12.
29. Koenig SB, Naidich TP, Zaparackas Z. Optic glioma masquerading as spasmus nutans. J Pediatr Ophthalmol Strabismus 1982;19(1):20–4.
30. Lavery MA, O'Neill JF, Chu FC, Martyn LJ. Acquired nystagmus in early childhood: a presenting sign of intracranial tumor. Ophthalmology 1984;91(5):425–53.
31. Russell A. A diencephalic syndrome of emaciation in infancy and childhood. Arch Dis Child 1951;26:274.
32. Layden WE, Edwards WC. Ocular manifestations of the diencephalic syndrome. Am J Ophthalmol 1972;73(1):78–82.
33. Poussaint TY, Barnes PD, Nichols K, et al. Diencephalic syndrome: clinical features and imaging findings. AJNR Am J Neuroradiol 1997;18(8):1499–505.
34. Imes RK, Hoyt WF. Childhood chiasmal gliomas: update on the fate of patients in the 1969 San Francisco Study. Br J Ophthalmol 1986;70(3):179–82.
35. Lourie GL, Osborne DR, Kirks DR. Involvement of posterior visual pathways by optic nerve gliomas. Pediatr Radiol 1986;16(4):271–4.
36. Patronas NJ, Dwyer AJ, Papathanasiou M, et al. Contributions of magnetic resonance imaging in the evaluation of optic gliomas. Surg Neurol 1987;28(5):367–71.

37. Grill J, Laithier V, Rodriguez D, et al. When do children with optic pathway tumours need treatment? An oncological perspective in 106 patients treated in a single centre. Eur J Pediatr 2000;159(9):692–6.

38. Liu GT, Lessell S. Spontaneous visual improvement in chiasmal gliomas. Am J Ophthalmol 1992;114(2):193–201.

39. Coppeto JR, Monteiro ML, Uphoff DF. Exophytic suprasellar glioma: a rare cause of chiasmatic compression. Case report. Arch Ophthalmol 1987;105(1):28.

40. Medlock MD, Scott RM. Optic chiasm astrocytomas of childhood. 2. Surgical management. Pediatr Neurosurg 1997;27(3):129–36.

41. Albright AL, Sclabassi RJ. Cavitron ultrasonic surgical aspirator and visual evoked potential monitoring for chiasmal gliomas in children. Report of two cases. J Neurosurg 1985;63(1):138–40.

42. Medlock MD, Madsen JR, Barnes PD, et al. Optic chiasm astrocytomas of childhood. 1. Long-term follow-up. Pediatr Neurosurg 1997;27(3):121–8.

43. DeSousa AL, Kalsbeck JE, Mealey J Jr, Fitzgerald J. Diencephalic syndrome and its relation to opticochiasmatic glioma: review of twelve cases. Neurosurgery 1979;4(3): 207–9.

44. Silva MM, Goldman S, Keating G, et al. Optic pathway hypothalamic gliomas in children under three years of age: the role of chemotherapy. Pediatr Neurosurg 2000;33(3): 151–8.

45. Chutorian AM, Schwartz JF, Evans RA, Carter S. Optic Gliomas in Children. Neurology 1964;14:83–95.

46. Danoff BF, Kramer S, Thompson N. The radiotherapeutic management of optic nerve gliomas in children. Int J Radiat Oncol Biol Phys 1980;6(1):45–50.

47. Taveras JM, Mount LA, Wood EH. The value of radiation therapy in the management of glioma of the optic nerves and chiasm. Radiology 1956;66(4):518–28.

48. Packer RJ, Savino PJ, Bilaniuk LT, et al. Chiasmatic gliomas of childhood. A reappraisal of natural history and effectiveness of cranial irradiation. Childs Brain 1983;10(6):393–403.

49. Flickinger JC, Torres C, Deutsch M. Management of low-grade gliomas of the optic nerve and chiasm. Cancer 1988;61(4):635–42.

50. Tao ML, Barnes PD, Billett AL, et al. Childhood optic chiasm gliomas: radiographic response following radiotherapy and long-term clinical outcome. Int J Radiat Oncol Biol Phys 1997;39(3):579–87.

51. Beyer RA, Paden P, Sobel DF, Flynn FG. Moyamoya pattern of vascular occlusion after radiotherapy for glioma of the optic chiasm. Neurology 1986;36(9):1173–8.

52. Fletcher WA, Imes RK, Hoyt WF. Chiasmal gliomas: appearance and long-term changes demonstrated by computerized tomography. J Neurosurg 1986;65(2):154–9.

53. Crompton MR, Layton DD. Delayed radionecrosis of the brain following therapeutic x-radiation of the pituitary. Brain 1961;84:85–101.

54. Kline LB, Kim JY, Ceballos R. Radiation optic neuropathy. Ophthalmology 1985;92(8): 1118–26.

55. Packer RJ, Sutton LN, Bilaniuk LT, et al. Treatment of chiasmatic/hypothalamic gliomas of childhood with chemotherapy: an update. Ann Neurol 1988;23(1):79–85.

56. Mitchell AE, Elder JE, Mackey DA, et al. Visual improvement despite radiologically stable disease after treatment with carboplatin in children with progressive low-grade optic/thalamic gliomas. J Pediatr Hematol Oncol 2001;23(9):572–7.

57. Koos WT, Miller MH. Intracranial tumors of infants and children. St Louis: Mosby, 1971; 188.

58. Bartlett JR. Craniopharyngiomas. An analysis of some aspects of symptomatology, radiology and histology. Brain 1971;94(4):725–32.

59. Arseni C, Maretsis M. Craniopharyngioma. Neurochirurgia (Stuttg) 1972;15(1):25–32.

60. Wang KC, Hong SH, Kim SK, Cho BK. Origin of craniopharyngiomas: implication on the growth pattern. Childs Nerv Syst 2005;21(8–9):628–34.

61. Baskin DS, Wilson CB. Surgical management of craniopharyngiomas. A review of 74 cases. J Neurosurg 1986;65(1):22–7.

62. Chen C, Okera S, Davies PE, et al. Craniopharyngioma: a review of long-term visual outcome. Clin Exp Ophthalmol 2003;31(3):220–8.

63. Ullrich NJ, Scott RM, Pomeroy SL. Craniopharyngioma therapy: long-term effects on hypothalamic function. Neurologist 2005;11(1):55–60.

64. Petito CK, DeGirolami U, Earle KM. Craniopharyngiomas: a clinical and pathological review. Cancer 1976;37(4):1944–52.

65. Hirunpat S, Tanomkiat W, Sriprung H, Chetpaophan J. Optic tract edema: a highly specific magnetic resonance imaging finding for the diagnosis of craniopharyngiomas. Acta Radiol 2005;46(4):419–23.

66. Miller DC. Pathology of craniopharyngiomas: clinical import of pathological findings. Pediatr Neurosurg 1994;21 Suppl 1:11–7.

67. Isaac MA, Hahn SS, Kim JA, et al. Management of craniopharyngioma. Cancer J 2001; 7(6):516–20.

68. Katz EL. Late results of radical excision of craniopharyngiomas in children. J Neurosurg 1975;42(1):86–93.

69. Kalapurakal JA. Radiation therapy in the management of pediatric craniopharyngiomas: a review. Childs Nerv Syst 2005;21(8–9):808–16.

70. Carmel PW, Antunes JL, Chang CH. Craniopharyngiomas in children. Neurosurgery 1982;11(3):382–9.

71. Fischer EG, Welch K, Belli JA, et al. Treatment of craniopharyngiomas in children: 1972–1981. J Neurosurg 1985;62(4):496–501.

72. Anderson DR, Trobe JD, Taren JA, Gebarski SS. Visual outcome in cystic craniopharyngiomas treated with intracavitary phosphorus-32. Ophthalmology 1989;96(12):1786–92.

73. Mottolese C, Stan H, Hermier M, et al. Intracystic chemotherapy with bleomycin in the treatment of craniopharyngiomas. Childs Nerv Syst 2001;17(12):724–30.

74. Repka MX, Miller NR, Miller M. Visual outcome after surgical removal of craniopharyngiomas. Ophthalmology 1989;96(2):195–9.

75. Merchant TE, Kiehna EN, Sanford RA, et al. Craniopharyngioma: the St. Jude Children's Research Hospital experience 1984–2001. Int J Radiat Oncol Biol Phys 2002;53(3):533–42.

76. Kalapurakal JA, Goldman S, Hsieh YC, et al. Clinical outcome in children with recurrent craniopharyngioma after primary surgery. Cancer J 2000;6(6):388–93.

77. Burrow GN, Wortzman G, Rewcastle NB, et al. Microadenomas of the pituitary and abnormal sellar tomograms in an unselected autopsy series. N Engl J Med 1981;304(3): 156–8.

78. McCormick WF, Halmi NS. Absence of chromophobe adenomas from a large series of pituitary tumors. Arch Pathol 1971;92(4):231–8.

79. Kovacs K, Horvath E, Ryan N, Ezrin C. Null cell adenoma of the human pituitary. Virchows Arch A Pathol Anat Histol 1980;387(2):165–74.

80. Wilson CB. A decade of pituitary microsurgery. The Herbert Olivecrona lecture. J Neurosurg 1984;61(5):814–33.

81. Ironside JW. Best Practice No 172: pituitary gland pathology. J Clin Pathol 2003; 56(8):561–8.

82. Hollenhorst R, Younge B. Ocular manifestations produced by adenomas of the pituitary gland: analysis of 1000 cases. In: Kohler PO, Ross GT, eds. Diagnosis and Treatment of Pituitary Tumors. New York,: American Elsevier, 1973.

83. Wray SH. Neuro-ophthalmologic manifestations of pituitary and parasellar lesions. Clin Neurosurg 1977;24:86–117.

84. Anderson D, Faber P, Marcovitz S, et al. Pituitary tumors and the ophthalmologist. Ophthalmology 1983;90(11):1265–70.

85. Gnjidic Z, Ivekovic R, Rumboldt Z, et al. Chiasma syndrome in acromegalic patients: correlation of neuroradiologic and neuroophthalmologic findings. Coll Antropol 2002;26(2):601–8.

86. Hirai T, Ito Y, Arai M, et al. Loss of stereopsis with optic chiasmal lesions and stereoscopic tests as a differential test. Ophthalmology 2002;109(9):1692–702.

87. Kawasaki A, Purvin VA. Photophobia as the presenting visual symptom of chiasmal compression. J Neuroophthalmol 2002;22(1):3–8.

88. Fujimoto N, Saeki N, Miyauchi O, Adachi-Usami E. Criteria for early detection of temporal hemianopia in asymptomatic pituitary tumor. Eye 2002;16(6):731–8.

89. Karanjia N, Jacobson DM. Compression of the prechiasmatic optic nerve produces a junctional scotoma. Am J Ophthalmol 1999;128(2):256–8.

90. Mejico LJ, Miller NR, Dong LM. Clinical features associated with lesions other than pituitary adenoma in patients with an optic chiasmal syndrome. Am J Ophthalmol 2004;137(5):908–13.

91. Unsold R, Ostertag C. Nystagmus in suprasellar tumors: recent advances in diagnosis and therapy. Strabismus 2002;10(2):173–7.

92. Rovit RL, Fein JM. Pituitary apoplexy: a review and reappraisal. J Neurosurg 1972; 37(3):280–8.

93. Sibal L, Ball SG, Connolly V, et al. Pituitary apoplexy: a review of clinical presentation, management and outcome in 45 cases. Pituitary 2004;7(3):157–63.

94. Wakai S, Fukushima T, Teramoto A, Sano K. Pituitary apoplexy: its incidence and clinical significance. J Neurosurg 1981;55(2):187–93.

95. Biousse V, Newman NJ, Oyesiku NM. Precipitating factors in pituitary apoplexy. J Neurol Neurosurg Psychiatry 2001;71(4):542–5.

96. Randeva HS, Schoebel J, Byrne J, et al. Classical pituitary apoplexy: clinical features, management and outcome. Clin Endocrinol (Oxf) 1999;51(2):181–8.

97. Schlechte JA. Clinical practice. Prolactinoma. N Engl J Med 2003;349(21):2035–41.

98. Baskin DS, Boggan JE, Wilson CB. Transsphenoidal microsurgical removal of growth hormone–secreting pituitary adenomas. A review of 137 cases. J Neurosurg 1982; 56(5):634–41.

99. Boggan JE, Tyrrell JB, Wilson CB. Transsphenoidal microsurgical management of Cushing's disease. Report of 100 cases. J Neurosurg 1983;59(2):195–200.

100. Spark RF, Baker R, Bienfang DC, Bergland R. Bromocriptine reduces pituitary tumor size and hypersection. Requiem for pituitary surgery? JAMA 1982;247(3):311–6.

101. Corenblum B. The medical treatment of the hypersecreting pituitary gland. Can J Neurol Sci 1985;12(3):243–50.

102. Moster ML, Savino PJ, Schatz NJ, et al. Visual function in prolactinoma patients treated with bromocriptine. Ophthalmology 1985;92(10):1332–41.

103. Barker FG II, Klibanski A, Swearingen B. Transsphenoidal surgery for pituitary tumors in the United States, 1996–2000: mortality, morbidity, and the effects of hospital and surgeon volume. J Clin Endocrinol Metab 2003;88(10):4709–19.

104. Landolt AM, Keller PJ, Froesch ER, Mueller J. Bromocriptine: Does it jeopardise the result of later surgery for prolactinomas? Lancet 1982;2(8299):657–8.

105. Besser GM, Wass JA, Thorner MO. Acromegaly: results of long term treatment with bromocriptine. Acta Endocrinol Suppl (Copenh) 1978;216:187–98.

106. Wass JA, Thorner MO, Morris DV, et al. Long-term treatment of acromegaly with bromocriptine. Br Med J 1977;1(6065):875–8.

107. Ross DA, Wilson CB. Results of transsphenoidal microsurgery for growth hormone–secreting pituitary adenoma in a series of 214 patients. J Neurosurg 1988;68(6):854–67.

108. Lindholm J, Riishede J, Vestergaard S, et al. No effect of bromocriptine in acromegaly: a controlled trial. N Engl J Med 1981;304(24):1450–4.

109. Yamamoto K, Saito K, Takai T, et al. Visual field defects and pituitary enlargement in primary hypothyroidism. J Clin Endocrinol Metab 1983;57(2):283–7.

110. Ebersold MJ, Quast LM, Laws ER Jr, et al. Long-term results in transsphenoidal removal of nonfunctioning pituitary adenomas. J Neurosurg 1986;64(5):713–9.

111. Agrawal D, Mahapatra AK. Visual outcome of blind eyes in pituitary apoplexy after transsphenoidal surgery: a series of 14 eyes. Surg Neurol 2005;63(1):42–6.

112. Slavin ML, Lam BL, Decker RE, et al. Chiasmal compression from fat packing after transsphenoidal resection of intrasellar tumor in two patients. Am J Ophthalmol 1993;115(3):368–71.

113. Jones SE, James RA, Hall K, Kendall-Taylor P. Optic chiasmal herniation: an under recognized complication of dopamine agonist therapy for macroprolactinoma. Clin Endocrinol (Oxf) 2000;53(4):529–34.

114. Kuratsu J, Kochi M, Ushio Y. Incidence and clinical features of asymptomatic meningiomas. J Neurosurg 2000;92(5):766–70.

115. Escourolle R, Poirier J. Manual of basic neuropathology. Philadelphia,: Saunders, 1973; 51–4.

116. Hirst LW, Miller NR, Hodges FJ III, et al. Sphenoid pneumosinus dilatans. A sign of meningioma originating in the optic canal. Neuroradiology 1982;22(4):207–10.

117. Slavin ML. Acute, severe, symmetric visual loss with cecocentral scotomas due to olfactory groove meningioma. J Clin Neuroophthalmol 1986;6(4):224–7.

118. Bickerstaff ER, Small JM, Guest IA. The relapsing course of certain meningiomas in relation to pregnancy and menstruation. J Neurol Neurosurg Psychiatry 1958;21(2): 89–91.

119. Kumar V, Abbas AK, Fausto N, et al. The central nervous system. In: Robbins and Cotran Pathologic Basis of Disease, 7th / ed. Philadelphia: Saunders, 2005.

120. Jaaskelainen J, Haltia M, Laasonen E, et al. The growth rate of intracranial meningiomas and its relation to histology. An analysis of 43 patients. Surg Neurol 1985;24(2): 165–72.

121. Jaaskelainen J, Haltia M, Servo A. Atypical and anaplastic meningiomas: radiology, surgery, radiotherapy, and outcome. Surg Neurol 1986;25(3):233–42.

122. Slavin ML. Metastatic malignant meningioma. J Clin Neuroophthalmol 1989;9(1): 55–9.

123. Andrews BT, Wilson CB. Suprasellar meningiomas: the effect of tumor location on postoperative visual outcome. J Neurosurg 1988;69(4):523–8.

124. Ciric I, Rosenblatt S. Suprasellar meningiomas. Neurosurgery 2001;49(6):1372–7.

125. Chicani CF, Miller NR. Visual outcome in surgically treated suprasellar meningiomas. J Neuroophthalmol 2003;23(1):3–10.

126. Grisoli F, Vincentelli F, Raybaud C, et al. Intrasellar meningioma. Surg Neurol 1983; 20(1):36–41.

127. Rosenberg LF, Miller NR. Visual results after microsurgical removal of meningiomas involving the anterior visual system. Arch Ophthalmol 1984;102(7):1019–23.

128. Bendszus M, Rao G, Burger R, et al. Is there a benefit of preoperative meningioma embolization? Neurosurgery 2000;47(6):1306–11.

129. Lamberts SW, Tanghe HL, Avezaat CJ, et al. Mifepristone (RU 486) treatment of meningiomas. J Neurol Neurosurg Psychiatry 1992;55(6):486–90.

130. Lesch KP, Engl HG, Gross S. Androgen receptor binding activity in meningiomas. Surg Neurol 1987;28(3):176–80.

131. Hahn BM, Schrell UM, Sauer R, et al. Prolonged oral hydroxyurea and concurrent 3d-conformal radiation in patients with progressive or recurrent meningioma: results of a pilot study. J Neurooncol 2005;74(2):157–65.

132. Thom M, Martinian L. Progesterone receptors are expressed with higher frequency by optic nerve sheath meningiomas. Clin Neuropathol 2002;21(1):5–8.

133. Stafford SL, Pollock BE, Foote RL, et al. Meningioma radiosurgery: tumor control, outcomes, and complications among 190 consecutive patients. Neurosurgery 2001; 49(5):1029–37.

134. Harris JR, Levene MB. Visual complications following irradiation for pituitary adenomas and craniopharyngiomas. Radiology 1976;120(1):167–71.

135. Subramanian PS, Bressler NM, Miller NR. Radiation retinopathy after fractionated stereotactic radiotherapy for optic nerve sheath meningioma. Ophthalmology 2004; 111(3):565–7.

136. Saeed P, Rootman J, Nugent RA, et al. Optic nerve sheath meningiomas. Ophthalmology 2003;110(10):2019–30.

137. Sibony PA, Krauss HR, Kennerdell JS, et al. Optic nerve sheath meningiomas. Clinical manifestations. Ophthalmology 1984;91(11):1313–26.

138. Mafee MF, Goodwin J, Dorodi S. Optic nerve sheath meningiomas. Role of MR imaging. Radiol Clin North Am 1999;37(1):37–58.

139. Zimmerman CF, Schatz NJ, Glaser JS. Magnetic resonance imaging of optic nerve meningiomas. Enhancement with gadolinium-DTPA. Ophthalmology 1990;97(5):585–91.

140. Lindblom B, Truwit CL, Hoyt WF. Optic nerve sheath meningioma. Definition of intraorbital, intracanalicular, and intracranial components with magnetic resonance imaging. Ophthalmology 1992;99(4):560–6.

141. Behbehani RS, Vacarezza N, Sergott RC, et al. Isolated optic nerve lymphoma diagnosed by optic nerve biopsy. Am J Ophthalmol 2005;139(6):1128–30.

142. Wright JE, Call NB, Liaricos S. Primary optic nerve meningioma. Br J Ophthalmol 1980;64(8):553–8.

143. Kennerdell JS, Maroon JC, Malton M, Warren FA. The management of optic nerve sheath meningiomas. Am J Ophthalmol 1988;106(4):450–7.

144. Smith JL, Vuksanovic MM, Yates BM, Bienfang DC. Radiation therapy for primary optic nerve meningiomas. J Clin Neuroophthalmol 1981;1(2):85–99.

145. Egan RA, Lessell S. A contribution to the natural history of optic nerve sheath meningiomas. Arch Ophthalmol 2002;120(11):1505–8.

146. Miller NR. The evolving management of optic nerve sheath meningiomas. Br J Ophthalmol 2002;86(11):1198.

147. Andrews DW, Foroozan R, Yang BP, et al. Fractionated stereotactic radiotherapy for the treatment of optic nerve sheath meningiomas: preliminary observations of 33 optic nerves in 30 patients with historical comparison to observation with or without prior surgery. Neurosurgery 2002;51(4):890–902.

148. Turbin RE, Thompson CR, Kennerdell JS, et al. A long-term visual outcome compari-

son in patients with optic nerve sheath meningioma managed with observation, surgery, radiotherapy, or surgery and radiotherapy. Ophthalmology 2002;109(5):890–9.

149. Kupersmith MJ, Warren FA, Newall J, Ransohoff J. Irradiation of meningiomas of the intracranial anterior visual pathway. Ann Neurol 1987;21(2):131–7.

150. Carrasco JR, Penne RB. Optic nerve sheath meningiomas and advanced treatment options. Curr Opin Ophthalmol 2004;15(5):406–10.

151. Landert M, Baumert BG, Bosch MM, et al. The visual impact of fractionated stereotactic conformal radiotherapy on seven eyes with optic nerve sheath meningiomas. J Neuroophthalmol 2005;25(2):86–91.

152. Sarkies NJ. Optic nerve sheath meningioma: diagnostic features and therapeutic alternatives. Eye 1987;1 (Pt 5):597–602.

153. Schievink WI. Intracranial aneurysms. N Engl J Med 1997;336(1):28–40.

154. Guirgis MF, Lam BL, Falcone SF. Optic tract compression from dolichoectatic basilar artery. Am J Ophthalmol 2001;132(2):283–6.

155. Winn HR, Jane JA Sr, Taylor J, et al. Prevalence of asymptomatic incidental aneurysms: review of 4568 arteriograms. J Neurosurg 2002;96(1):43–9.

156. Krayenbuhl H. [Proceedings: Classification and clinical symptomatology of cerebral aneurysms]. Ophthalmologica 1973;167(2):122–64.

157. Ropper AH, Adams RD, Victor M, Brown RH. Cerebrovascular diseases. In: Adams and Victor's Principles of Neurology, 8th ed. New York: McGraw-Hill, 2005.

158. Unruptured intracranial aneurysms: risk of rupture and risks of surgical intervention. International Study of Unruptured Intracranial Aneurysms Investigators. N Engl J Med 1998;339(24):1725–33.

159. Kasner SE, Liu GT, Galetta SL. Neuro-ophthalmologic aspects of aneurysms. Neuroimaging Clin N Am 1997;7(4):679–92.

160. Biousse V, Mendicino ME, Simon DJ, Newman NJ. The ophthalmology of intracranial vascular abnormalities. Am J Ophthalmol 1998;125(4):527–44.

161. Cestari DM, Rizzo JF, 3rd. The neuroophthalmic manifestations and treatment options of unruptured intracranial aneurysms. Int Ophthalmol Clin 2004;44(1):169–87.

162. Bakker SL, Hasan D, Bijvoet HW. Compression of the visual pathway by anterior cerebral artery aneurysm. Acta Neurol Scand 1999;99(3):204–7.

163. Stewart RM, Samson D, Diehl J, et al. Unruptured cerebral aneurysms presenting as recurrent transient neurologic deficits. Neurology 1980;30(1):47–51.

164. Jea A, Baskaya MK, Morcos JJ. Penetration of the optic nerve by an internal carotid artery–ophthalmic artery aneurysm: case report and literature review. Neurosurgery 2003;53(4):996–9.

165. Huber A, Yasargil M. Ophthalmic artery aneurysms. In: Smith JL, ed. Neuro-ophthalmology Now! Chicago: Year Book Medical Publishers, 1986.

166. Farris BK, Smith JL, David NJ. The nasal junction scotoma in giant aneurysms. Ophthalmology 1986;93(7):895–905.

167. Hoeoek O, Norlen G. Aneurysms of the Internal Carotid Artery. Acta Neurol Scand 1964;40:200–18.

168. Schultz PN, Sobol WM, Weingeist TA. Long-term visual outcome in Terson syndrome. Ophthalmology 1991;98(12):1814–9.

169. Vargas ME, Kupersmith MJ, Setton A, et al. Endovascular treatment of giant aneurysms which cause visual loss. Ophthalmology 1994;101(6):1091–8.

170. Harrison MJ, Johnson BA, Gardner GM, Welling BG. Preliminary results on the management of unruptured intracranial aneurysms with magnetic resonance angiography and computed tomographic angiography. Neurosurgery 1997;40(5):947–55.

171. White PM, Teadsale E, Wardlaw JM, Easton V. What is the most sensitive non-invasive imaging strategy for the diagnosis of intracranial aneurysms? J Neurol Neurosurg Psychiatry 2001;71(3):322–8.

172. White PM, Teasdale EM, Wardlaw JM, Easton V. Intracranial aneurysms: CT angiography and MR angiography for detection prospective blinded comparison in a large patient cohort. Radiology 2001;219(3):739–49.

173. Suzuki IM, Matsui, Ueda F, et al. Contrast-enhanced MR angiography (enhanced 3-D fast gradient echo) for diagnosis of cerebral aneurysms. Neuroradiology 2002;44(1): 17–20.

174. Gibbs GF, Huston J III, Bernstein MA, et al. 3.0-Tesla MR angiography of intracranial aneurysms: comparison of time-of-flight and contrast-enhanced techniques. J Magn Reson Imaging 2005;21(2):97–102.

175. Jacobson DM, Trobe JD. The emerging role of magnetic resonance angiography in the management of patients with third cranial nerve palsy. Am J Ophthalmol 1999; 128(1):94–6.

176. Bederson JB, Awad IA, Wiebers DO, et al. Recommendations for the management of patients with unruptured intracranial aneurysms: A Statement for healthcare professionals from the Stroke Council of the American Heart Association. Stroke 2000; 31(11):2742–50.

177. Ferguson GG, Drake CG. Carotid-ophthalmic aneurysms: the surgical management of those cases presenting with compression of the optic nerves and chiasm alone. Clin Neurosurg 1980;27:263–307.

178. Britz GW. Clipping or coiling of cerebral aneurysms. Neurosurg Clin North Am 2005;16(3):475–85.

179. Kupersmith MJ, Berenstein A, Choi IS, et al. Percutaneous transvascular treatment of giant carotid aneurysms: neuro-ophthalmologic findings. Neurology 1984;34(3):328–35.

180. Molyneux AJ. Indications for treatment of cerebral aneurysms from an endovascular perspective: the creation of an evidence base for interventional techniques. Neurosurg Clin N Am 2005;16(2):313–6.

181. Trokel SL, Hilal SK. Recognition and differential diagnosis of enlarged extraocular muscles in computed tomography. Am J Ophthalmol 1979;87(4):503–12.

182. Trokel SL, Hilal SK. Submillimeter resolution CT scanning of orbital diseases. Ophthalmology 1980;87(5):412–7.

183. Enzmann D, Marshal WH Jr, Rosenthal AR, Kriss JP. Computed tomography in Graves' ophthalmopathy. Radiology 1976;118(3):615–20.

184. Boulos PR, Hardy I. Thyroid-associated orbitopathy: a clinicopathologic and therapeutic review. Curr Opin Ophthalmol 2004;15(5):389–400.

185. Trokel SL, Jakobiec FA. Correlation of CT scanning and pathologic features of ophthalmic Graves' disease. Ophthalmology 1981;88(6):553–64.

186. Tengroth B. Histological studies of orbital tissues in a case of endocrine exophthalmos before and after remission. Acta Ophthalmol (Copenh) 1964;42:588–91.

187. Kroll AJ, Kuwabara T. Dysthyroid ocular myopathy. Anatomy, histology, and electron microscopy. Arch Ophthalmol 1966;76(2):244–7.

188. Riley FC. Orbital pathology in Graves' disease. Mayo Clin Proc 1972;47:975–9.

189. Yeatts RP. Graves' ophthalmopathy. Med Clin North Am 1995;79(1):195–209.

190. Bartley GB, Fatourechi V, Kadrmas EF, et al. Clinical features of Graves' ophthalmopathy in an incidence cohort. Am J Ophthalmol 1996;121(3):284–90.

191. Trobe JD, Glaser JS, Laflamme P. Dysthyroid optic neuropathy. Clinical profile and rationale for management. Arch Ophthalmol 1978;96(7):1199–209.

192. Anderson RL, Tweeten JP, Patrinely JR, et al. Dysthyroid optic neuropathy without extraocular muscle involvement. Ophthalmic Surg 1989;20(8):568–74.

193. Feldon SE, Muramatsu S, Weiner JM. Clinical classification of Graves' ophthalmopathy. Identification of risk factors for optic neuropathy. Arch Ophthalmol 1984;102(10): 1469–72.

194. Igersheimer J. Visual changes in progressive exophthalmos. AMA Arch Ophthalmol 1955;53(1):94–104.

195. Hedges TR Jr, Scheie HG. Visual field defects in exophthalmos associated with thyroid disease. AMA Arch Ophthalmol 1955;54(6):885–92.

196. Henderson JW. Optic neuropathy of exophthalmic goiter (Graves' disease). AMA Arch Ophthalmol 1958;59(4):471–80.

197. Day RM, Carroll FD. Corticosteroids in the treatment of optic nerve involvement associated with thyroid dysfunction. Arch Ophthalmol 1968;79(3):279–82.

198. Carter KD, Frueh BR, Hessburg TP, Musch DC. Long-term efficacy of orbital decompression for compressive optic neuropathy of Graves' eye disease. Ophthalmology 1991;98(9):1435–42.

199. Chang EL, Bernardino CR, Rubin PA. Transcaruncular orbital decompression for management of compressive optic neuropathy in thyroid-related orbitopathy. Plast Reconstr Surg 2003;112(3):739–47.

200. Bartalena L, Marcocci C, Pinchera A. Treating severe Graves' ophthalmopathy. Baillieres Clin Endocrinol Metab 1997;11(3):521–36.

201. Goldberg RA, Weinberg DA, Shorr N, Wirta D. Maximal, three-wall, orbital decompression through a coronal approach. Ophthalmic Surg Lasers 1997;28(10):832–43.

202. Hallin ES, Feldon SE, Luttrell J. Graves' ophthalmopathy: III. Effect of transantral orbital decompression on optic neuropathy. Br J Ophthalmol 1988;72(9):683–7.

203. McNab AA. Orbital decompression for thyroid orbitopathy. Aust N Z J Ophthalmol 1997;25(1):55–61.

204. Shorr N, Neuhaus RW, Baylis HI. Ocular motility problems after orbital decompression for dysthyroid ophthalmopathy. Ophthalmology 1982;89(4):323–8.

205. Young JD. Ocular complications of transantral decompression for thyrotrophic exophthalmos. Proc R Soc Med 1971;64(9):929–31.

206. DeSanto LW. The total rehabilitation of Graves' ophthalmopathy. Laryngoscope 1980;90(10 Pt 1):1652–78.

207. Gorman CA, Garrity JA, Fatourechi V, et al. The aftermath of orbital radiotherapy for Graves' ophthalmopathy. Ophthalmology 2002;109(11):2100–7.

208. Ravin JG, Sisson JC, Knapp WT. Orbital radiation for the ocular changes of Graves' disease. Am J Ophthalmol 1975;79(2):285–8.

209. Rush S, Winterkorn JM, Zak R. Objective evaluation of improvement in optic neuropathy following radiation therapy for thyroid eye disease. Int J Radiat Oncol Biol Phys 2000;47(1):191–4.

210. Hurbli T, Char DH, Harris J, et al. Radiation therapy for thyroid eye diseases. Am J Ophthalmol 1985;99(6):633–7.

211. Miller ML, Goldberg SH, Bullock JD. Radiation retinopathy after standard radiotherapy for thyroid-related ophthalmopathy. Am J Ophthalmol 1991;112(5):600–1.

212. Sadun F, Hinton DR, Sadun AA. Rapid growth of an optic nerve ganglioglioma in a patient with neurofibromatosis 1. Ophthalmology 1996;103(5):794–9.

213. Glastonbury CM, Warner JE, MacDonald JD. Optochiasmal apoplexy from a cavernoma. Neurology 2003;61(2):266.

214. Kerr DJ, Scheithauer BW, Miller GM, et al. Hemangioblastoma of the optic nerve: case report. Neurosurgery 1995;36(3):573–80; discussion 80–1.

215. Harris GJ, Jakobiec FA. Cavernous hemangioma of the orbit. J Neurosurg 1979; 51(2):219–28.
216. Wright JE. Orbital vascular anomalies. Trans Am Acad Ophthalmol Otolaryngol 1974;78(4):OP606–16.
217. Rootman J. Diseases of the Orbit, 2nd ed. Philadelphia, Pa. London: Lippincott Williams & Wilkins, 2003.
218. Rutka JT, Hoffman HJ, Drake JM, Humphreys RP. Suprasellar and sellar tumors in childhood and adolescence. Neurosurg Clin N Am 1992;3(4):803–20.
219. Norwood EG, Kline LB, Chandra-Sekar B, Harsh GR III. Aneurysmal compression of the anterior visual pathways. Neurology 1986;36(8):1035–41.
220. Hejazi N, Witzmann A, Hassler W. Ocular manifestations of sphenoid mucoceles: clinical features and neurosurgical management of three cases and review of the literature. Surg Neurol 2001;56(5):338–43.
221. Harbison JW, Lessell S, Selhorst JB. Neuro-ophthalmology of sphenoid sinus carcinoma. Brain 1984;107 (Pt 3):855–70.
222. Rutka JD, Sharpe JA, Resch L, Fleming JF. Compressive optic neuropathy and ependymoma of the third ventricle. J Clin Neuroophthalmol 1985;5(3):194–8.
223. Lau JJ, Trobe JD, Ruiz RE, et al. Metastatic neuroblastoma presenting with binocular blindness from intracranial compression of the optic nerves. J Neuroophthalmol 2004;24(2):119–24.
224. Olson ME, Chernik NL, Posner JB. Infiltration of the leptomeninges by systemic cancer. A clinical and pathologic study. Arch Neurol 1974;30(2):122–37.
225. Susac JO, Smith JL, Powell JO. Carcinomatous optic neuropathy. Am J Ophthalmol 1973;76(5):672–9.
226. Bullock JD, Yanes B, Kelly M, McDonald LW. Non-Hodgkins lymphoma involving the optic nerve. Ann Ophthalmol 1979;11(10):1477–80.
227. Miller NR, Iliff WJ. Visual loss as the initial symptom in Hodgkin disease. Arch Ophthalmol 1975;93(11):1158–61.
228. Allen RA, Straatsma BR. Ocular involvement in leukemia and allied disorders. Arch Ophthalmol 1961;66:490–508.
229. Gudas PP Jr. Optic nerve myeloma. Am J Ophthalmol 1971;71(5):1085–9.
230. Frohman LP, Guirgis M, Turbin RE, Bielory L. Sarcoidosis of the anterior visual pathway: 24 new cases. J Neuroophthalmol 2003;23(3):190–7.
231. Lacey B, Chang W, Rootman J. Nonthyroid causes of extraocular muscle disease. Surv Ophthalmol 1999;44(3):187–213.

Developmental and Hereditary Optic Nerve Disorders

LANNING B. KLINE, EUGENE H. ENG,
AND R. MICHAEL SIATKOWSKI

*A*lthough a large body of literature deals with developmental anomalies of the optic nerve, the ophthalmologist encounters only a few in routine clinical practice.[1] This chapter discusses these developmental disorders and the more common forms of hereditary optic nerve disease. At times, optic disc anomalies may mimic an acquired optic neuropathy. Prompt recognition of developmental and hereditary disorders of the optic nerve eliminates unnecessary patient evaluation.

7-1 DEVELOPMENTAL OPTIC NERVE DISORDERS

7-1-1 *Anomalous Elevation of the Optic Nerve, or* Pseudopapilledema. Anomalous elevation of the optic nerve head (pseudopapilledema) is a major cause of unnecessary alarm, as it frequently leads to the diagnosis of papilledema. The distinction between acquired and congenital disc elevation can often be made on the basis of ophthalmoscopic findings.

Congenitally full optic discs may occur alone or in association with hyaloid remnants, myelinated retinal nerve fibers, hyperopia, and, most often, hyaline bodies (drusen):

1. *Congenitally full optic disc.* A variety of factors contribute to the full or crowded appearance of the nerve head in pseudopapilledema (Fig. 7–1). These include a small scleral canal, the relatively late embryologic consolidation of the lamina cribrosa, and regression of the hyaloid system. The ophthalmoscopic features

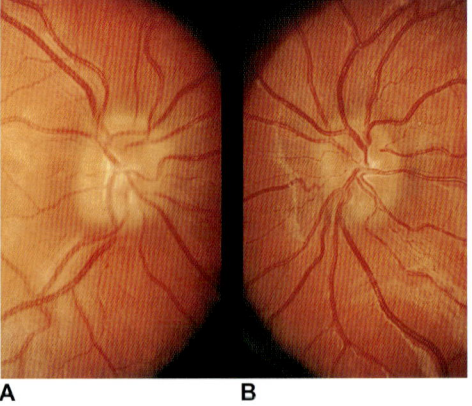

Figure 7–1. Congenitally full optic discs. Central physiologic cup is absent and blood vessels on surface of each disc have an anomalous pattern. (A) Right eye. (B) Left eye.

A   B

of congenitally full discs are summarized in Table 7–1. Although the disc appears elevated and at times the margins are indistinct, the nerve head is not hyperemic, the surface arteries are not obscured, and—importantly—the peripapillary nerve fiber layer is not opacified. The central cup is absent, and often glial remnants overlie the central disc. A frequent association is an anomalous branching of the retinal vessels as they course over the surface of the disc. At times, a single examination may be inadequate for a definitive diagnosis of pseudopapilledema; serial observations may be required to confirm the clinical diagnosis. Subsequent examinations may reveal progression of anomalous optic dics to visible optic disc drusen (see below).[2] The presence of spontaneous venous pulsations is strongly suggestive of pseudopapilledema.

2. *Hyaloid remnants.* During embryonic development, the hyaloid vascular system traverses the vitreous cavity and then atrophies. If a portion of the hyaloid system persists, it may overlie the disc and cause apparent blurring of the nerve head (Fig. 7–2). Careful ophthalmoscopy reveals that this anomaly is actually anterior to a normal optic disc.

3. *Myelinated retinal nerve fibers.* The nerve fiber layer is transparent, as myelination terminates at the lamina cribrosa. Myelination may extend onto the retina, resulting in opacified white areas. If the myelinated patches surround the optic disc, the margins may appear blurred (Fig. 7–3). Recent his-

Table 7–1 Ophthalmoscopic Features
of Pseudopapilledema

1. Elevated disc; margins obscured
2. Absence of central cup
3. Vascular anomalies with increased branching
4. Normal nerve fiber layer; disc transilluminates
5. ± Spontaneous venous pulse
6. ± Hyaline bodies
7. Hemorrhages absent
8. No exudates
9. No nerve fiber (cotton-wool) infarcts

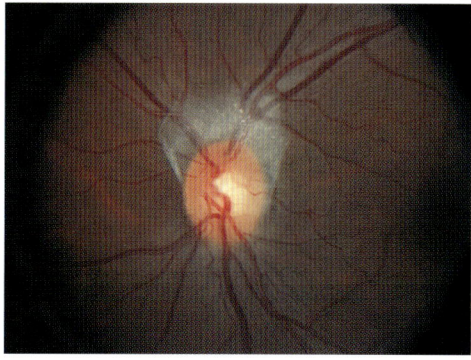

Figure 7–2. Hyaloid remnant. Glial veil overlies superior portion of optic disc.

topathologic evidence suggests that the abnormal myelination is due to ectopic oligodendrocytes within the retina.[3]

4. *Hyperopia.* Hyperopic eyes are smaller than average yet contain a full complement of retinal nerve fibers. These fibers must traverse a relatively small scleral canal, imparting an elevated and crowded appearance to the optic disc.

5. *Hyaline bodies (drusen).* Hyaline bodies, or optic disc drusen, are the most frequent cause of pseudopapilledema and often pose the most difficulty in distinguishing between acquired and congenital disc elevation (Table 7–2). They occur in 3.4 to 24 per 1000 people and are bilateral in 75%. Hyaline bodies are crystalline structures located anterior to the lamina cribrosa. Their origin is due to the presence of a crowded, small scleral canal leading to disruption of axonal metabolism resulting in continual calcium deposition.[4,5]

Optic discs containing intrapapillary hyaline bodies tend to have a characteristic appearance (Figs. 7–4 and 7–5).[6,7] They generally give the disc a yellow-white appearance, in contrast to the hyperemic, congested appearance of acquired disc swelling. At times, hemorrhages are associated with optic disc drusen, either on the surface of the disc, extending into the peripapillary nerve fiber layer, or under the retina or retinal pigment epithelium. Subretinal neovascularization may occur in the macula or adjacent to the disc (Fig. 7–6). Alterations in the peripapillary retinal pigment epithelium, a frequent ophthalmoscopic finding with disc drusen, are thought to result from resolved subretinal pigment epithelial hemor-

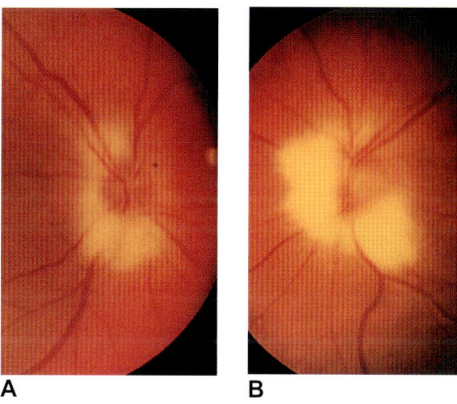

A   B

Figure 7–3. Myelinated retinal nerve fibers obscure borders of each optic disc. (A) Right eye. (B) Left eye.

Table 7–2 Comparison of Optic Disc Drusen and Early Papilledema

Feature	Drusen	Early Papilledema
Symptomatology	Incidental findings: visual disturbances due to (1) vitreous hemorrhages, (2) field loss, or (3) macular dysfunction from subretinal hemorrhage or serous detachment; occasional transient visual obscurations	Headache and transient visual obscurations; visual acuity unaffected
Family history	Irregular dominant inheritance May be sporadic	Rare familial occurrence of pseudotumor cerebri
Associated conditions	Retinitis pigmentosa from any cause	Increased intracranial pressure
Race	Caucasians overwhelmingly	Any
Age at onset	Definite age-related progression from buried to exposed	Any
Optic cup	Small or absent	Preserved
Elevation	Obviously elevated with tendency for center of disc to be highest point of elevation	Minimally elevated
Margins	Irregular or "lump-bumpy" appearance	Obscured by opacification of nerve fiber layer; superior and inferior margins affected first
Color	Pink to yellowish pink with variable bright lemon-yellow excrescence	Hyperemic
Nerve fiber layer	Normal or decreased	Dulling and opacification of peripapillary nerve fiber layer light reflexes
Vessels	Situated in center of disc; frequently anomalous with trifurcations; spontaneous venous pulsations often present	Normal distribution of vessels; absent venous pulsations with full veins; telangiectasia of preexisting capillary network on disc
Hemorrhages	Types: (1) peripapillary nerve fiber splinter hemorrhage, (2) subretinal or subpigment epithelial, (3) subretinal neovascularization removed from disc, (4) vitreous hemorrhage	Multiple splinter hemorrhages in nerve fiber layer most common

Source: Adapted from Hitchings RA, Corbett JJ, Winkleman J, et al: Hemorrhages with optic nerve drusen. *Arch Neurol* 1976;33:675–677.

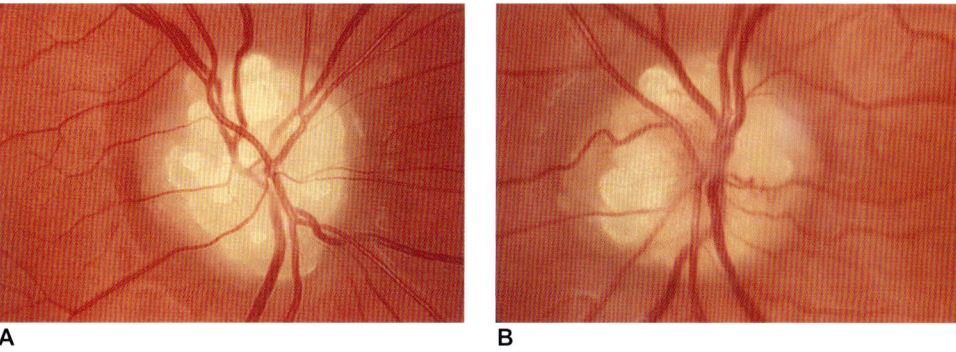

A   **B**

Figure 7–4. Optic disc drusen. (A) Right eye. (B) Left eye.

rhages (Fig. 7–7). Rarely with these hemorrhagic phenomena, the optic nerve head may become edematous (Fig. 7–8).

Hyaline bodies are usually not visible at birth or during infancy, but they tend to become more prominent with age. Often familial, they are inherited as an autosomal dominant trait with irregular penetrance. This fact makes examination of family members mandatory when the distinction between true papilledema and pseudopapilledema is in doubt.

Up to 73% of patients with visible disc drusen and 36% with buried disc drusen have associated visual field loss, although the field defect is usually asymptomatic.[6,8,9] Over a 3-year period, the rate of visual field loss is estimated to be around 1.6% per year.[10] Most defects are nerve-fiber-bundle in type, with loss nasally being the most common. Only rarely is central fixation affected; thus a patient with disc drusen

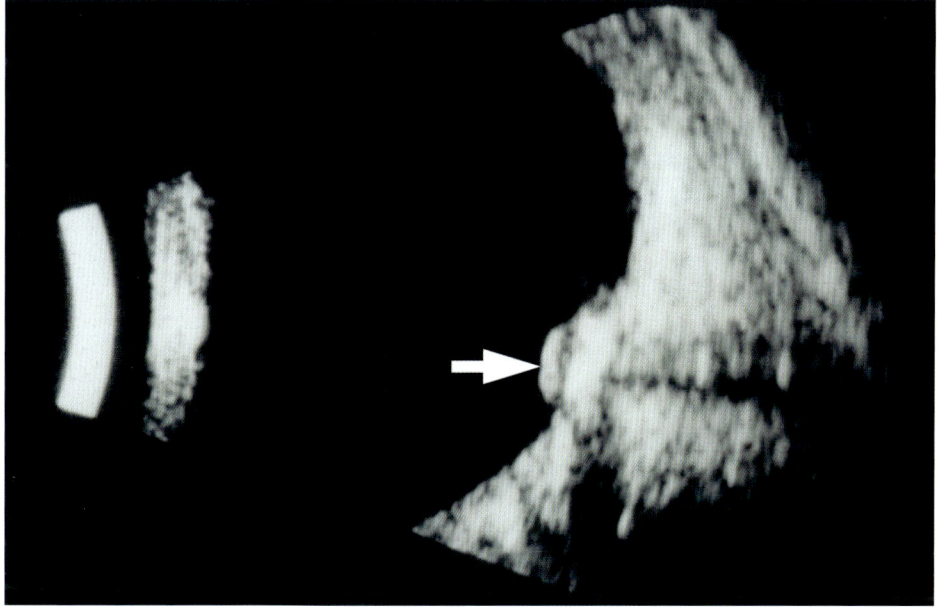

Figure 7–5. B Scan of optic disc drusen (arrow). Courtesy Bradley K Farris, MD.

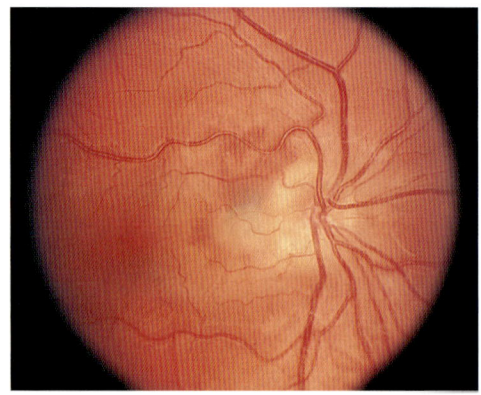

Figure 7–6. Subretinal and intraretinal hemorrhages with optic disc drusen. Fluorescein angiography revealed peripapillary choroidal neovascularization.

and decreased visual acuity must first be evaluated with a cranial neuroimaging study for another cause of the visual loss.[11] Due to the potential vascular complications and visual field changes, patients with drusen should undergo periodic visual field testing and detailed examinations of the nerve fiber layer.[5]

There is very little evidence of other associations with optic disc drusen. However, there does appear to be a definite relationship of optic disc drusen with tapetoretinal degeneration, particularly retinitis pigmentosa (RP).[6] Approximately 10% of patients with RP have optic disc or peripapillary drusen.[12]

7-1-2 Optic Nerve Hypoplasia. Optic nerve hypoplasia is a variable condition that may be unilateral or bilateral, marked or minimal, associated with good or poor visual function, and may occur in isolation or in association with other ocular or neurologic abnormalities.[13] Once considered a rare finding, optic nerve hypoplasia is now the most common congenital optic disc anomaly encountered in pediatric ophthalmic practice and a common cause of congenital blindness.

The optic disc appears smaller than normal on ophthalmoscopy, although this finding may be subtle (Fig. 7–9).[14] At times, the hypoplastic disc is surrounded by a ring of sclera and a ring of hyperpigmentation: the "double-ring sign" (Fig. 7–10).

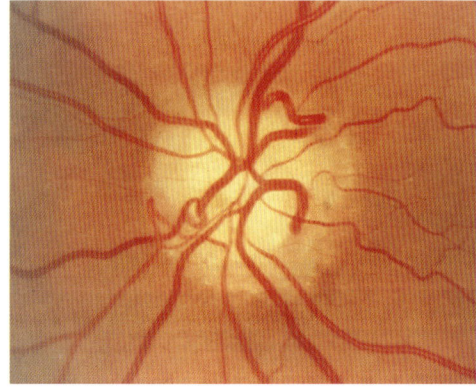

Figure 7–7. Optic disc drusen with alteration in peripapillary retinal pigment epithelium.

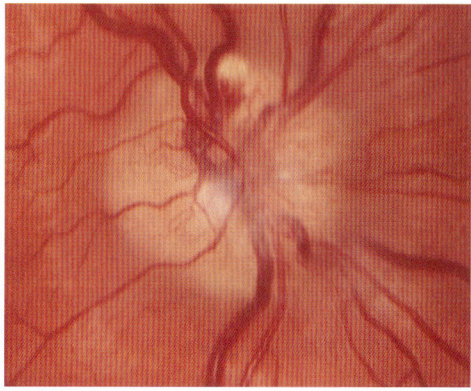

Figure 7–8. Acute edema and hemorrhages of optic disc associated with disc drusen.

Recognition of this abnormality is important, since potential correction of endocrinologic, neurologic, and other ocular deficits may allow normal growth and development.[15] If optic nerve hypoplasia occurs in isolation, it may be accompanied by strabismus and/or nystagmus. It is unusual for unilateral optic nerve hypoplasia to be associated with the systemic abnormalities mentioned above. Because it may be difficult to assess growth and development during the first 2 years of life, children in this age group should undergo neurologic and endocrinologic evaluation. If overall development appears normal by 2 years of age in a child with unilateral optic nerve hypoplasia, a more conservative approach may be taken.

Neurologic abnormalities accompanying bilateral optic nerve hypoplasia (BONH) include forebrain malformations and endocrinologic defects.[16] Nearly half of patients with BONH will show absence of the corpus callosum or septum pellucidum on neuroimaging.[17]

Careful magnetic resonance imaging (MRI) of the neurohypophysis revealing posterior pituitary ectopia or absence of the posterior pituitary infundibulum may help to predict the presence and type of endocrinologic deficiencies (Fig. 7–11).[18–20] One-fourth of patients will display some endocrinologic abnormality.[17] Growth-hormone deficiency is the most prevalent endocrinologic abnormality, but multiple abnormalities reported include hypothyroidism, sexual infantilism or precocity, neonatal hypoglycemia, hypoadrenalism, hyperprolactinemia, and diabetes insipidus.[21]

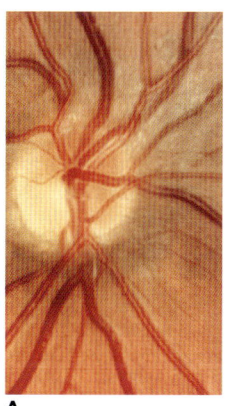
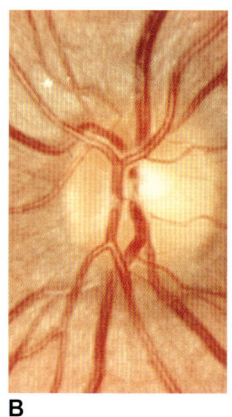

A   **B**

Figure 7–9. Mild optic nerve hypoplasia of (A) right optic disc when compared to (B) left disc.

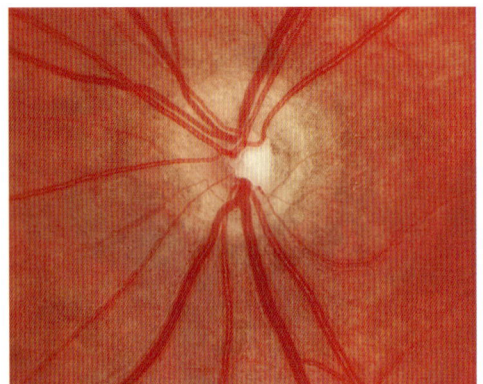

Figure 7–10. Hypoplastic optic disc surrounded by rings of increased and decreased pigmentation: the "double-ring sign."

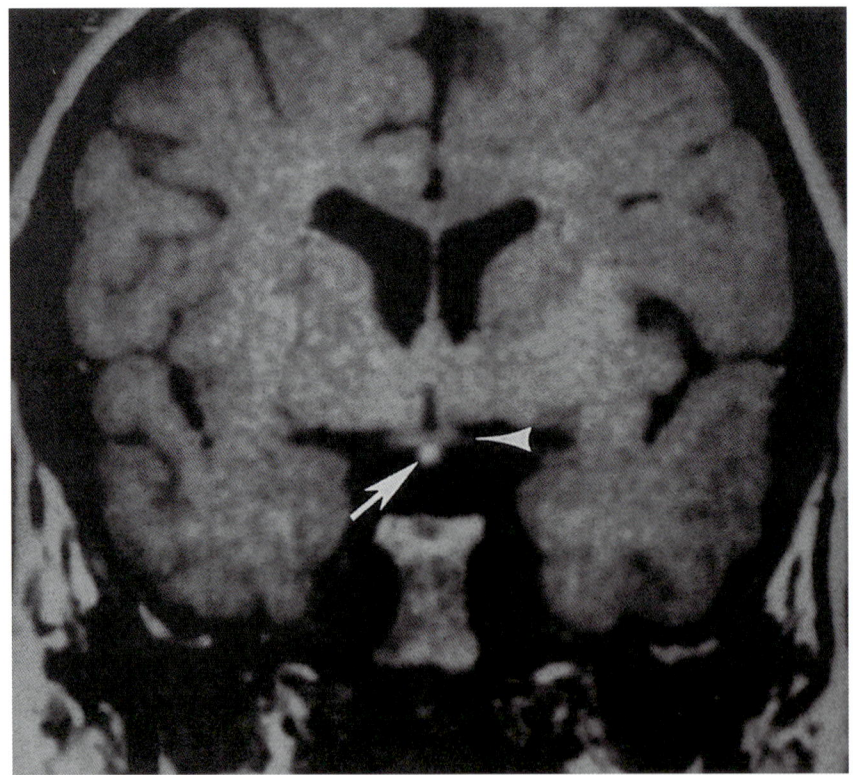

Figure 7–11. Posterior pituitary ectopia in a patient with bilateral optic nerve hypoplasia and endocrinologic dysfunction. T1-weighted coronal MRI reveals ectopic posterior pituitary gland (white arrow) located below the hypoplastic optic chiasm (white arrowhead). Note absence of the pituitary infundibulum. (Reprinted from Phillips PH, Spear C, Brodsky MC. Magnetic resonance diagnosis of congenital hypopituitarism in children with optic nerve hypoplasia. J AAPOS 5:275–280, figure 4, with permission from American Academy of Pediatric Ophthalmology & Strabismus.)

These hormonal abnormalities arise from hypothalamic dysfunction. De Morsier's syndrome comprises the triad of panhypopituitarism, bilateral optic disc hypoplasia, and midline brain abnormalities. It occurs in approximately 10% of children with bilateral optic nerve hypoplasia.[17]

7-1-3 *Superior Segmental Optic Hypoplasia.* At times, only a portion of the optic disc may be hypoplastic, and the patient may be unaware of congenital visual field defects. Such is the case in superior segmental optic hypoplasia, a funduscopic finding reported in the children of insulin-dependent diabetic mothers.[22] The presentation varies significantly, but the characteristic findings include (1) relative superior entrance of the central retinal artery, (2) pallor of the superior disc, (3) superior peripapillary halo, and (4) thinning of the superior nerve fiber layer. These disc changes are accompanied by inferior visual field defects, which can often be subtle (Fig. 7–12). The exact etiology remains unclear, but lower birth weight, shorter gestation time, and poorer control of maternal diabetes are all thought to contribute.[23]

7-1-4 *Hemioptic Hypoplasia.* Congenital hemispheric lesions and retrograde transsynaptic atrophy have led to the description of homonymous hemioptic hypopla-

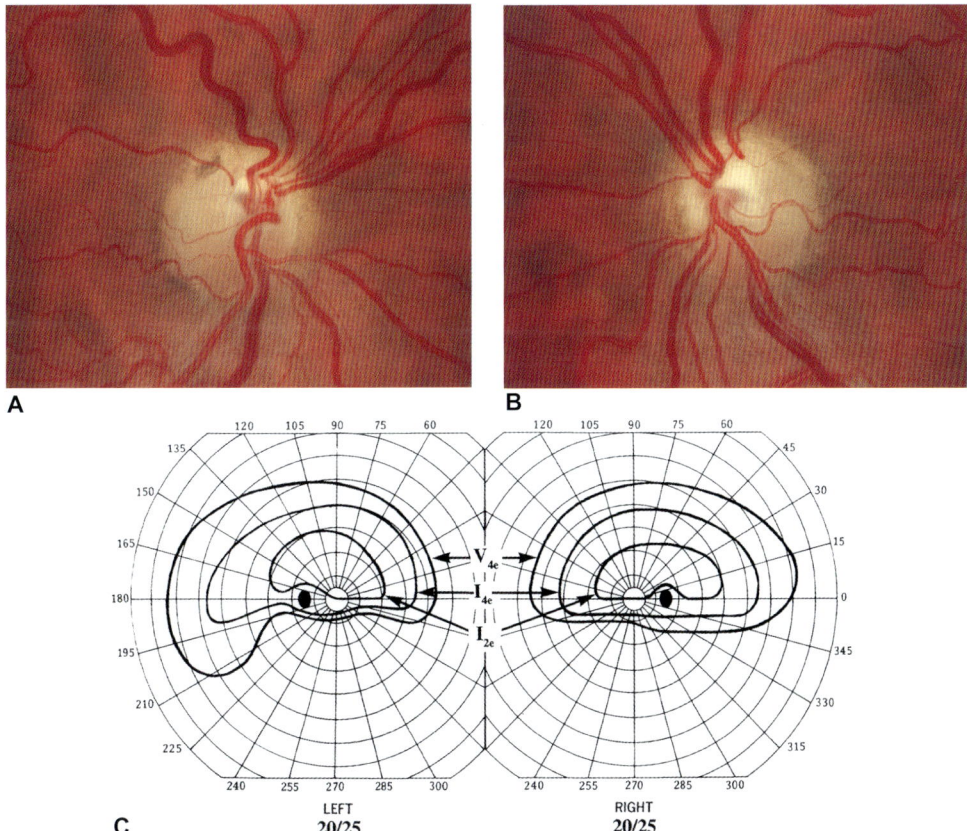

Figure 7–12. Superior segmental optic hypoplasia. (A) Right eye. (B) Left eye. (C) Bilateral inferior altitudinal visual field defects are present, but visual acuity is excellent.

sia.[24] This condition is characterized by "bowtie" or horizontal-band pallor of the disc contralateral to the damaged hemisphere and slight hypoplasia of the ipsilateral disc (Fig. 7–13). These patients also have congenital hemiplegia and hemianopia.

7-1-5 Coloboma. Colobomas are dysplastic excavations of the disc related to failure of the choroidal fissure to close during embryonic development. A coloboma may occupy the entire disc or involve only surrounding retinal pigment epithelium and choroid (Fig. 7–14). Optic disc coloboma can occur sporadically or be inherited in an autosomal dominant fashion.[19] It has been associated with choroidal or iris defects, CHARGE syndrome (coloboma, heart defects, atresia of the choanae, retardation of growth, genitourinary abnormalities, and ear abnormalities), PAX2 gene mutation in the renal-coloboma syndrome,[25,26] and malformations of the cerebral hemispheres.[27]

7-1-6 Optic Pit. Optic pits are small excavations occupying only a portion of the disc, usually inferior and temporal (Fig. 7–15). They result from defective closure of the embryonic fissure around gestational week 5.[28] Typically these lesions are nonprogressive, although they may be associated with an arcuate visual field defect that corresponds to the location of the pit.[29] Occasionally, an optic disc pit may lead to serous detachment of the macula with an accompanying decline in visual acuity.[30] The origin of the subretinal fluid has been proposed to be vitreous, or it may be cerebrospinal fluid. Treatment remains controversial.[31-33] On occasion, acquired pit-like changes may be seen in patients with chronic open-angle glaucoma associated with visual field defects close to fixation.[34]

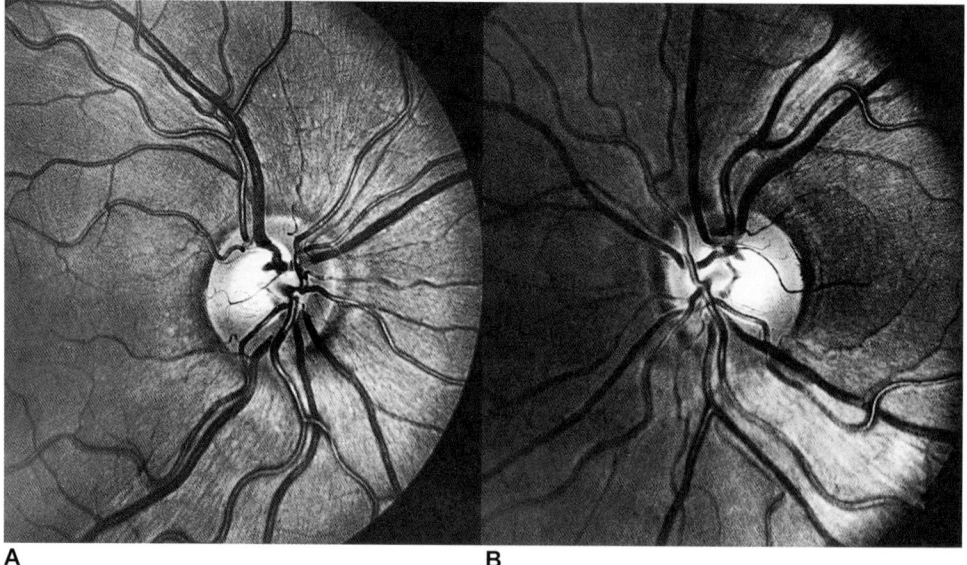

A   **B**

Figure 7–13. Hemioptic hypoplasia in patient with congenital left homonymous hemianopia. (A) Temporal pallor of right optic disc. (B) Band atrophy of left disc. There is loss of retinal nerve fiber layer in portions of each fundus corresponding to area of optic atrophy.(Courtesy of William F. Hoyt, MD.)

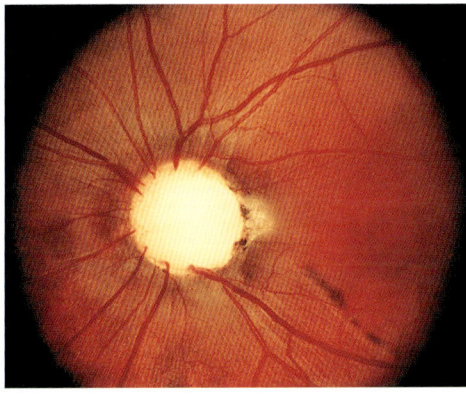

Figure 7–14. Coloboma of optic nerve.

7-1-7 Tilted Disc. The optic nerve head may have an oblique insertion into the globe, resulting in an oblique orientation of the disc when viewed ophthalmoscopically (Fig. 7–16). With the course of the nerve oblique inferiorly, there may be associated depigmentation of the retinal pigment epithelium and thinning of the underlying sclera (Fig. 7–17). Tilted discs may produce visual field defects that resemble temporal hemianopias. However, these differ from chiasmal temporal field defects in that they do not align along the vertical meridian (Fig. 7–18); and if any associated astigmatic refractive error is in place, the visual field defect disappears.

7-1-8 Morning-Glory Syndrome. In 1970, an unusual congenital anomaly of the optic disc was reported and termed *morning-glory syndrome* because of its similarity to the flower.[35] The anomaly consists of a unilaterally enlarged, funnel-shaped, excavated, and distorted optic disc surrounded by an elevated annulus of chorioretinal pigment disturbance (Fig. 7–19).

A few patients with morning-glory syndrome have good vision, but the vast majority suffer from marked visual loss, often with associated amblyopia. This optic disc anomaly may lead to retinal detachment, typically occurring around the deeply excavated disc and usually confined to the posterior pole of the retina. Of unknown causation, the morning-glory syndrome is typically an isolated ophthalmologic abnormality. However, it has been associated with basal encephalocele,[36,37] pituitary

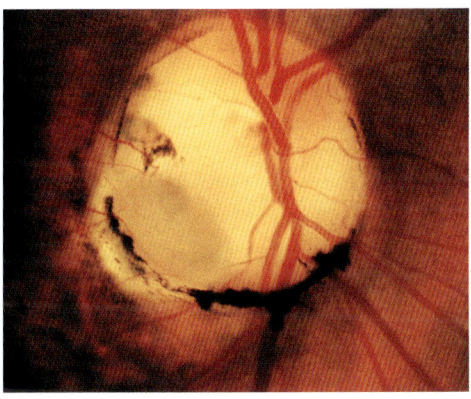

Figure 7–15. Optic pit in the inferotemporal portion of the right optic disc.

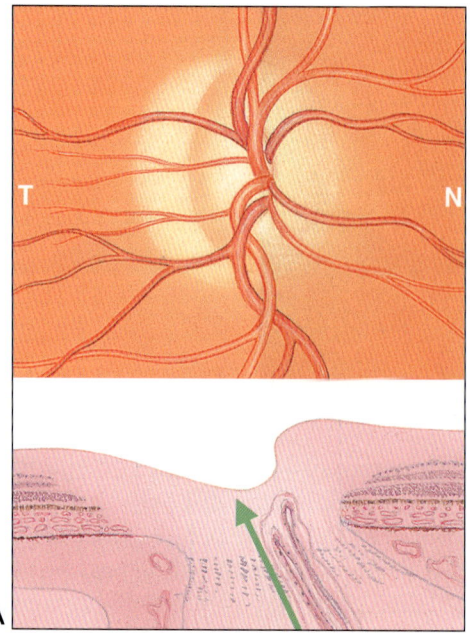

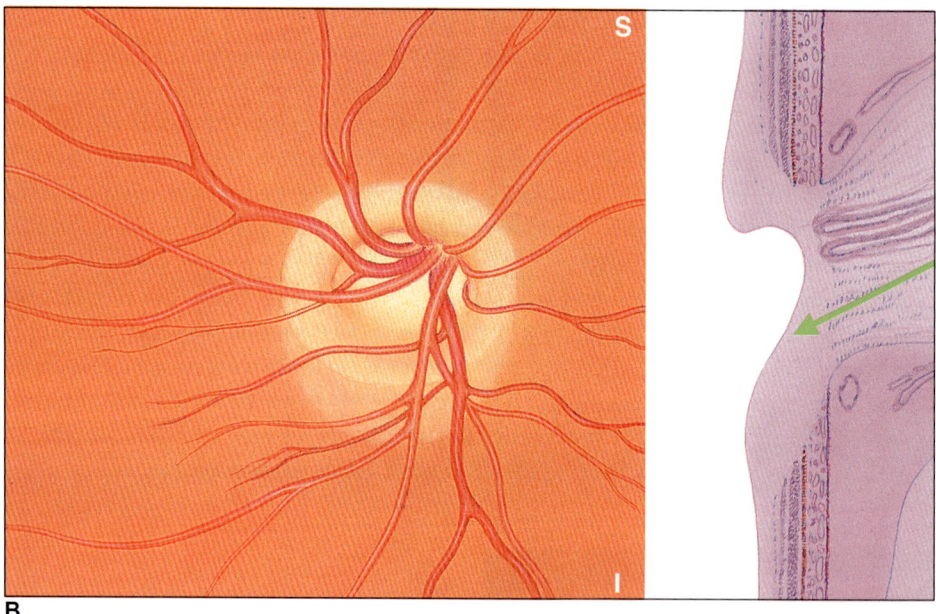

Figure 7–16. Axis of optic nerve (arrows) to globe may be oblique (A) to temporal side or (B) inferior, giving rise to altered appearance of optic nerve. T, temporal; N, nasal; S, superior; I, inferior. (Redrawn with permission from Hogan MJ, Alvarado JA, Weddell JE. Histology of the Human Eye: An Atlas and Textbook. Philadelphia: Saunders, 1971:531.)

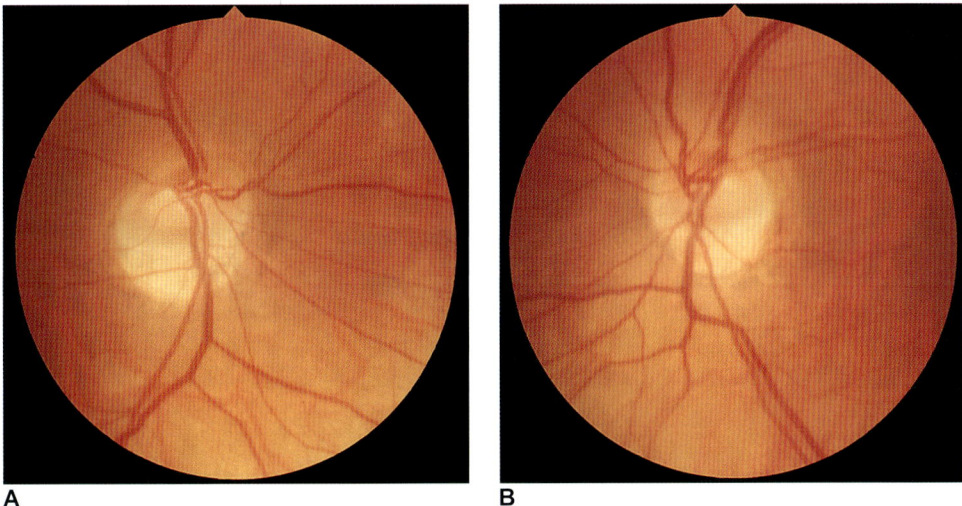

A   **B**

Figure 7–17. Tilted optic discs. Choroidal vessels in the inferior fundus are visible due to lack of pigmentation in the retinal pigment epithelium. (A) Right eye. (B) Left eye.

dwarfism,[38] and congenital anomalies of the internal carotid arteries (e.g., moyamoya disease).[37,39]

7-1-9 Astrocytic Hamartoma. Large, multilobulated deposits may form on the surface of the disc or retina in patients with tuberous sclerosis or, less frequently, in neurofibromatosis[40] and in normal individuals. Ophthalmoscopically, early lesions appear flat and translucent; with time, they gradually enlarge and become dome-shaped. Older lesions tend to undergo intralesional calcification, giving the a chalky-white, mulberry-like appearance (Fig. 7–20).

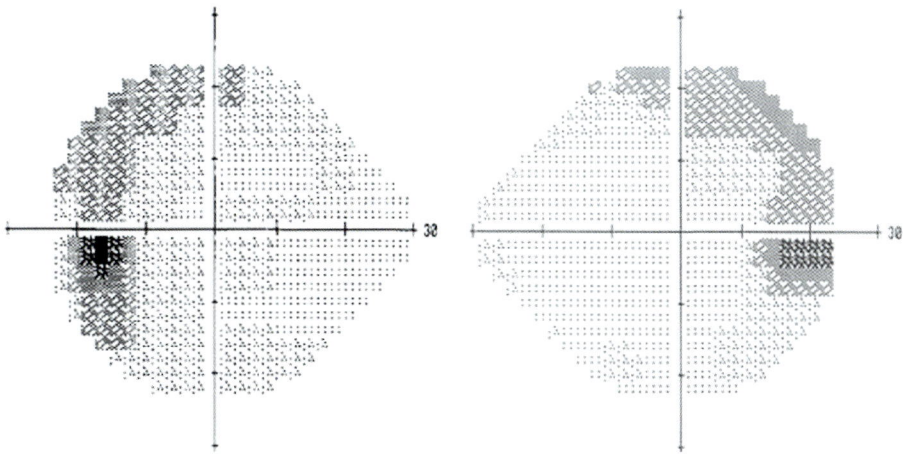

Figure 7–18. Visual fields of tilted optic discs. Note that the temporal field loss in each eye does not respect the vertical midline.

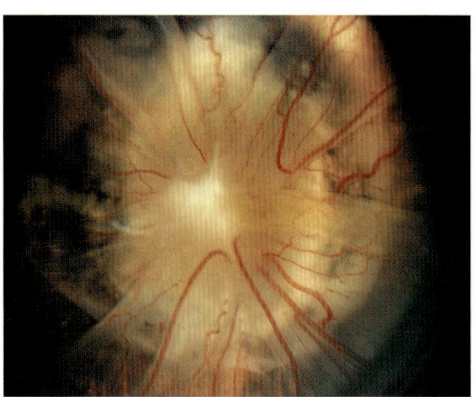

Figure 7–19. Morning-glory syndrome.

7-1-10 *Melanocytoma*. This pigmented tumor of the optic disc is benign, and about half the cases are reported in blacks.[41] Only rarely does melanocytoma cause significant visual loss, which is associated with an afferent pupillary defect and visual field abnormalities (e.g., enlarged blind spot, nerve-fiber-bundle defects).[42] The predominant cell type of this tumor—a plump, polyhedral nevus cell that is well differentiated—contains giant melanosomes located at the level of the lamina cribosa; it seems to be metabolically inactive. Melanocytoma has a deep black appearance and typically looks hypofluorescent on fluorescein angiography (Fig. 7–21). In contrast, juxtapapillary choroidal melanoma does not appear as black as melanocytoma, leads to progressive visual failure, and appears hyperfluorescent on fluorescein angiography (Fig. 7–22).[43] Patients with melanocytoma of the optic disc should still undergo periodic follow-up examinations, as less than 2% of these lesions have been reported to undergo malignant transformation.[44,45] Very rarely, a malignant melanoma may be totally confined to the optic nerve and simulate a melanocytoma.[46]

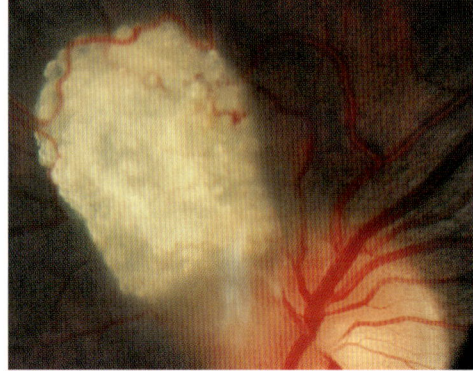

Figure 7–20. Astrocytic hamartoma overlying the optic disc in a patient with tuberous sclerosis.

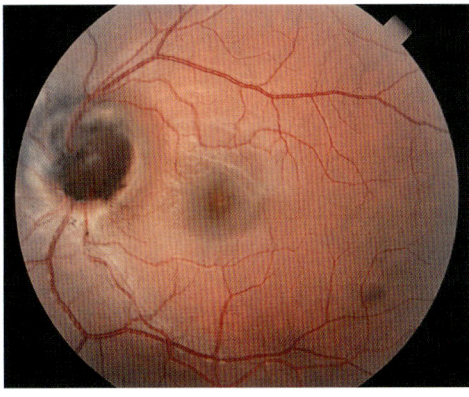

Figure 7–21. Melanocytoma of optic disc. (Courtesy of James A. Kimble, MD.)

7-2 HEREDITARY OPTIC NEUROPATHIES

The hereditary forms of optic nerve disease may occur as monosymptomatic deficits or may accompany other defects of the central nervous system. In addition, optic disc pallor may be a manifestation of hereditable neurolipid storage disorders, in which accumulation of abnormal material in retinal ganglion cells results in neuronal death. Because the literature dealing with optic nerve involvement in many of these disorders is large and somewhat confusing, the nosology of these optic neuropathies is unsettled. This section presents a clinical classification of heredofamilial optic neuropathies in an attempt to give the ophthalmologist a practical framework in which to approach these disorders.

7-2-1 *Dominant Optic Atrophy.* Dominant optic atrophy is the most common form of hereditary optic atrophy, with onset in the first decade of life. In general, it is associated with an imperceptible onset, a slowly progressive course, mild to moderate visual impairment, and absence of night blindness.[47]

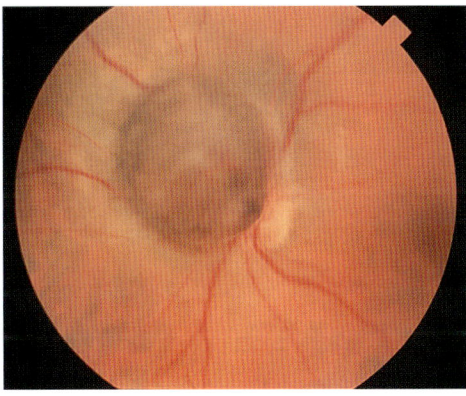

Figure 7–22. Juxtapapillary mushroom-shaped choroidal melanoma. (Courtesy Jerry A. Shields, MD.)

Diagnostic criteria that characterize dominant optic atrophy include the following[48]:

1. Autosomal dominant inheritance, established where possible by actual examination of even asymptomatic relatives.
2. Insidious onset, usually before 10 years of age.
3. Bilateral but possibly asymmetric visual loss.
4. Usually mild but occasionally moderate reduction in acuity (20/40 to 20/400).
5. Central or centrocecal scotomas.
6. Tritan (blue-yellow) dyschromatopsia has been described, although protan and deutan (red-green) axes may be superimposed, but severe generalized dyschromatopsia, regardless of acuity level, is the most common.[49]
7. Temporal disc pallor, often with a triangular area of temporal excavation. (Fig. 7–23).

The importance of examining relatives of a patient suspected of having dominant optic atrophy cannot be overemphasized. Because of a wide degree of intrafamilial and interfamilial variation, many apparently asymptomatic relatives may actually be mildly affected. Despite the variability in expression, the penetrance is approximately 98%.[50] Patients with dominant optic atrophy should undergo audiology testing because of the increased occurrence of associated sensorineural hearing loss.[51] In general, the visual prognosis is good, so that affected patients should be counseled to complete their education and obtain regular employment.

Histologic examination of the eyes and optic nerve of a patient with dominant optic atrophy has been reported.[52] Both eyes exhibited diffuse atrophy of the retinal ganglion cell layer, which is associated with atrophy and loss of myelin within the optic nerves. This finding suggests that dominant optic atrophy represents a primary degeneration of retinal ganglion cells. The most common genetic defects of dominant optic atrophy, OPA1 and OPA4, have been mapped to the 3q and 18q regions respectively. These genes are responsible for a protein involved in the formation and maintenance of mitochondria.[50,53–56]

7-2-2 *Recessive Optic Atrophy.* A rare form of hereditary optic nerve disease, recessive optic atrophy is usually discovered in the first 3 to 4 years of life.[57] It is character-

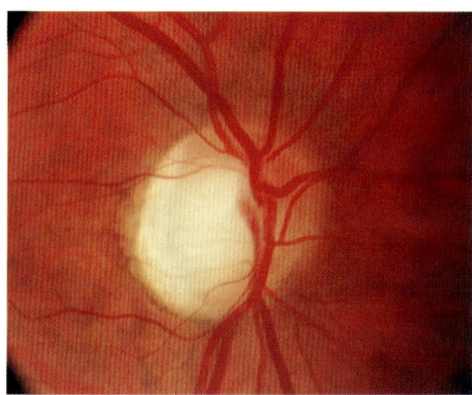

Figure 7–23. Dominant optic atrophy showing pallor and excavation of the temporal portion of the optic disc.

ized by severe visual impairment, frequently associated with searching nystagmus. Acuity is generally 20/400 or worse. Diffuse disc pallor and, at times, attenuation of retinal vessels, suggesting a tapetoretinal degeneration, are hallmarks of the condition. Electroretinography can help distinguish recessive optic atrophy from tapetoretinal degeneration. In most cases of recessive optic atrophy, consanguineous parentage has been found. The two most common syndromes associated with recessive optic atrophy are Wolfram's syndrome (diabetes insipidus, diabetes mellitus, optic atrophy, and deafness) linked to the WFS1 gene located on chromosome 4p[58] and Behr's syndrome (progressive encephalopathy, mental retardation, ataxia, nystagmus and pes cavus) linked to the OPA3 gene located on chromosome 19q (see section 7-2-4).[50,59]

7-2-3 *Leber's Hereditary Optic Neuropathy.* The clinical profile of Leber's hereditary optic neuropathy (LHON) has been well established since it was first described in 1871.[60] Rapid loss of central vision occurs primarily in males (80%–90%) during early adult years. Age of onset of visual dysfunction is usually between 15 and 35 years; however, it has been reported to occur between the ages of 2 and 80. Involvement of the second eye typically occurs within days to months. Color vision is affected early, and visual fields demonstrate central or centrocecal defects.

The classic ophthalmoscopic findings in acute LHON, shown in Fig. 7–24, are (1) circumpapillary telangiectatic microangiopathy, (2) swelling of the nerve fiber layer around the disc, and (3) absence of leakage from the disc or peripapillary region on fluorescein angiography.[61]

The diagnosis of Leber's disease is strongly supported by typical findings of circumpapillary telangiectatic microangiopathy in symptomatic or asymptomatic family members. However, some researchers have reported that the neurovascular abnormalities may not be present in acute LHON.[62] These authors concluded that the pathology of Leber's disease does not lie in the ophthalmoscopically visible microvasculature. This conclusion is also supported by the fact that the fundus changes may be visible long before vision is lost and are found in unaffected family members.[63] Therefore the microangiopathic findings are only an associated ophthalmoscopic marker for this disease.[64]

In some pedigrees of LHON, associated systemic features have been reported. These include cardiac abnormalities (preexcitation syndromes and hypertrophic

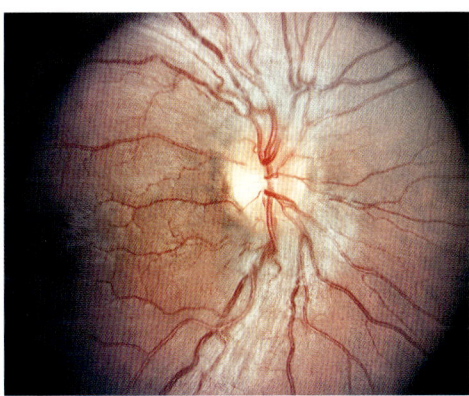

Figure 7–24. Leber's hereditary optic neuropathy.

cardiomyopathy),[65] reflex and sensory changes, Charcot-Marie-Tooth disease, and skeletal deformities.[66]

LHON is transmitted by non-Mendelian mitochondrial inheritance; thus there is no male-to-male transmission.[67–69] In 1988, a study identified a mitochondrial mutation causing LHON in 9 of 11 independent pedigrees.[70] A single nucleotide change at position 11778 in mitochondrial DNA converts codon 340 of NADH dehydrogenase subunit 4 from an arginine to a histidine. NADH dehydrogenase is the first enzyme in the electron-transfer pathway and leads to a reduced complex I function in oxidative phosphorylation (Fig. 7–25). This mitochondrial DNA mutation has been confirmed in other laboratories.[71–72]

Several other mutations of mitochondrial DNA have been proposed as causal in LHON. The primary mutations responsible for 95% of LHON cases are located at positions 11778, 3460, and 14484. Several others mutations have been identified and are also involved in encoding for complex I subunits.[73–79] None of these mutations occurs in the same gene affected by the 11778 mutation; rather they occur in other subunits of the same complex (I) in the respiratory chain.[56] Possibly the same clinical phenotype can arise from different mutations found in different subunits of the respiratory chain. Thus, a phenotype may not be the result of a specific enzyme defect but rather a reflection of a general reduction in mitochondrial energy production.

Mitochondrial DNA mutates at a much greater frequency than does nuclear DNA. A tissue that contains only one mitochondrial genotype is said to be homoplasmic (homoplasmic normal or homoplasmic mutant). A tissue that contains two or more mitochondrial genotypes (normal and mutant) is said to be heteroplasmic. Although investigators initially found LHON mutations to be homoplasmic, patients with 11778 mutations have subsequently been found to be heteroplasmic. One report of such a group of patients revealed varying proportions of normal and mutant mitochondrial DNA.[80] These investigators found that the relative proportion of mutant and normal mitochondrial DNA correlated with the risk of

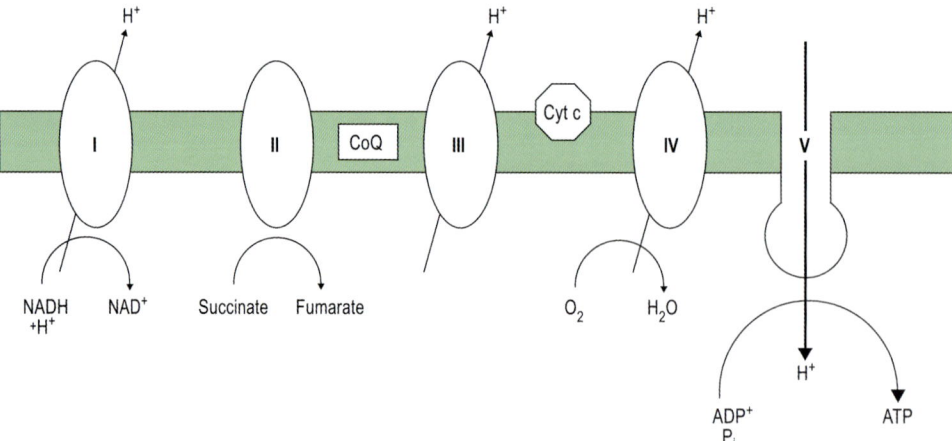

Figure 7–25. Major elements of the mitochondrial respiratory chain. Enzyme complexes are numbered I through V. CoQ, coenzyme Q; Cyt c, cytochrome c; ADP, adenosine diphosphate; ATP, adenosine triphosphate; NADH, reduced form of nicotinamide adenine dinucleotide; NAD+, oxidized form of nicotinamide adenine dinucleotide; Pi, orthophosphate.

developing clinical LHON. Another study demonstrated that, in one family, the proportion of mitochondrial DNA progressively increased from grandmother to mother to blind son. However, vision loss is not found in all patients with mutant homoplasmy.[73] The role of heteroplasmy in the pathophysiology or penetrance of this disease remains unclear.[50]

Much remains unexplained about the primary mitochondrial mutations and the cause of LHON.[81] Theories on the pathogenesis of LHON must be able to link the similar clinical presentation of sudden and bilateral optic nerve disease with the multiple discovered mitochondrial mutations. Traditional theories have hypothesized that environmental factors, nutritional deficiencies, systemic illnesses, or toxins may negatively influence mitochondrial metabolism, thus initiating the disease. However, one large case-controlled study showed that tobacco or alcohol consumption did not promote the expression of LHON in those who harbored known mutations.[82] Current leading theories on the pathogenesis of LHON include free radical formation triggering apoptosis of retinal ganglion cells and increased vulnerability of the unmyelinated, prelaminar portion of the optic nerve, which contains a high degree of mitochondrial respiratory activity.[56,83]

For most patients, the visual loss remains profound and permanent. However, there are well-documented instances of recovery of visual acuity years after visual deterioration.[63,84] The prognosis of spontaneous recovery does seem linked to mutation type. Less than 5% of patients with 11778 and 3460 experience recovery,[49,85] compared with 60% with 14484.[86] Recovery may be in one or both eyes and may occur as late as 10 years after onset of visual loss. Despite potential spontaneous recovery, there is no evidence for the efficacy of treatment to reverse vision loss in LHON.

7-2-4 Neurologic Syndromes. Hereditary forms of optic atrophy have been reported in association with a wide range of systemic and neurologic disorders (Fig. 7–26).[66] Although a complete discussion is beyond the scope of this chapter, the most commonly recognized syndromes are listed in Table 7–3.

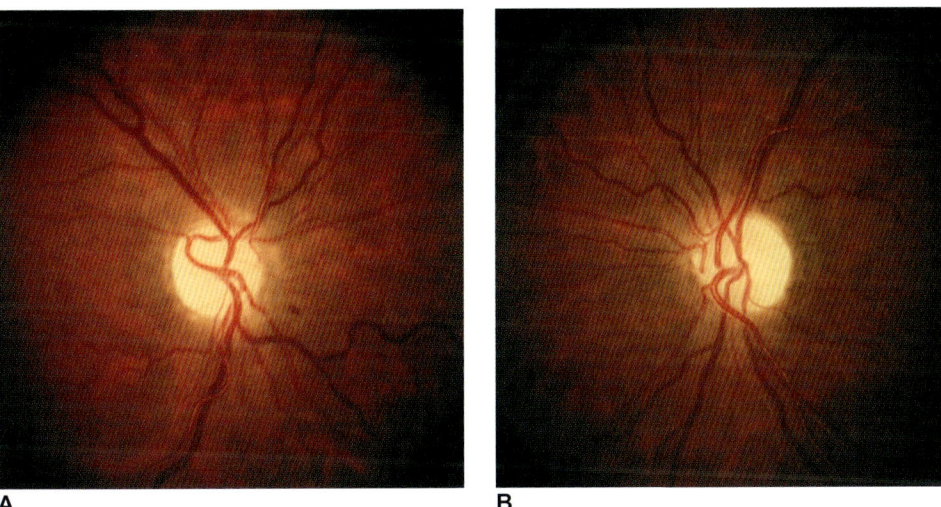

A   B

Figure 7–26. DIDMOAD syndrome in 19-year-old man (see Table 7–3). Visual acuity: 20/200 OU. (A) Right eye, (B) left eye.

Table 7–3 Hereditary Optic Atrophy Associated with Neurologic Disease

Neurologic Disorder	Inheritance
Congenital deafness	Dominant
Ataxia, deafness	Dominant
Diabetes mellitus, deafness	Recessive
DIDMOAD or Wolfram syndrome (diabetes insipidus, diabetes mellitus, optic atrophy, deafness)	Recessive
Behr's syndrome (pyramidal tract signs, mental retardation, ataxia, pes cavus)	Recessive
Hereditary ataxia	
Friedreich's	Dominant, recessive
Marie's	Dominant, recessive,
X-linked	
Charcot-Marie-Tooth disease (progressive muscular weakness, pes cavus, hammertoes)	Dominant, recessive, X-linked

7-2-5 Metabolic Disease. A lysosomal storage disease is defined as a pathologic condition resulting from a deficiency of a lysosomal hydrolytic enzyme, causing a metabolic block in the catabolism of one or more macromolecules normally requiring the missing enzyme for degradation. More than 100 such inherited metabolic diseases with ocular manifestations have been described. Those most frequently seen and associated with optic atrophy include the mucopolysaccharidoses and the lipidoses (Fig. 7–27).[66] These are summarized in Table 7–4.

In addition to the lysosomal storage diseases, clinicians must be aware of the neuronal ceroid lipofuscinoses (NCLs) as a cause of bilateral optic atrophy. NCLs are transmitted in an autosomal recessive pattern and may present with vision loss as the initial sign prior to seizures, motor disturbance, and dementia. The cause remains unknown and no treatment is available.[87–90]

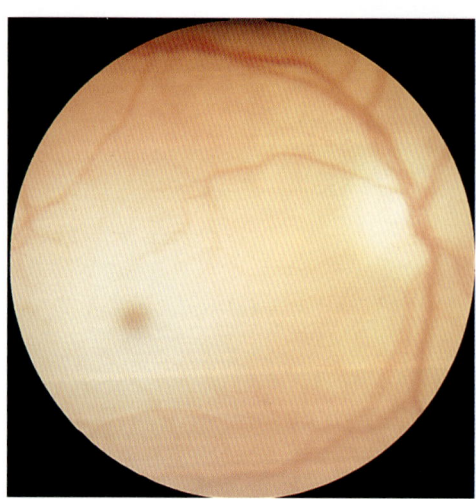

Figure 7–27. Cherry-red macula and optic atrophy in patient with Sandhoff's disease (GM$_2$–II gangliosidosis).

Table 7-4 Inborn Metabolic Disorders with Optic Atrophy

Disease	Enzyme Deficiency
Mucopolysaccharidoses	
Hurler (I-H)	α-L-iduronidase
Scheie (I-S)	α-L-iduronidas (partial)
Hunter A (IIA) (severe phenotype)	Iduronate sulfatase
Hunter B (IIB) (mild phenotype)	Iduronate sulfatase
Sanfilippo A (IIIA)	Heparan sulfate sulfatase
Sanfilippo B (IIIB)	N-acetyl-glucosaminidase
Morquio (IV)	N-acetyl-galactosamine sulfatase
Maroteaux-Lamy A (VIA) (severe phenotype)	Acrylsulfatase B
Lipidoses	
Generalized gangliosidosis (GM_1-I)	β-galactosidase A,B,C
Juvenile gangliosidosis (GM_1-II)	β-galactosidase B,C
Tay-Sachs (GM_2-I)	Hexosaminodase A
Sandhoff (GM_2-II)	Hexosaminodase A
Juvenile gangliosidosis (GM_2-III) (partial)	Hexosaminidase A
Niemann-Pick A (infantile)	Sphingomyelinase
Krabbe (globoid cell leukodystrophy)	Galactocerebroside β-galactosidase
Metachromatic leukodystrophy (infantile)	Acrylsulfatase A
Metachromatic leukodystrophy (juvenile and adult)	Acrylsulfatase A
Sulfatidosis, Austin variant (mucosulfatidosis)	Acrylsulfatase A,B,C

References

1. Apple DJ, Rabb MF, Walsh PM. Congenital anomalies of the optic disc. Surv Ophthalmol 1982;27:3–41.
2. Spencer TS, Katz BJ, Weber SW, et al. Progression from anomalous optic discs to visible optic disc drusen. J Neuroophthalmol 2004;24:297–298.
3. Rosen B, Barry C, Constable IJ. Progression of myelinated retinal nerve fibers. Am J Ophthalmol 1999;127:471–473.
4. Tso MO. Pathology and pathogenesis of drusen of the optic nerve head. Ophthalmology 1981;88:1066–1080.
5. Auw-Haedrich C, Staubach F, Witschel H. Optic Disc Drusen. Surv Ophthalmol 2002; 47:515–532.
6. Lorentzen SE. Drusen of the optic disc: a clinical and genetic study. Acta Ophthalmol 1966;90(suppl):7–180.
7. Rosenberg MA, Savino PJ, Glaser JS. A clinical analysis of pseudopapilledema. I: population, laterality, acuity, refractive error, ophthalmoscopic characteristics, and coincident disease. Arch Ophthalmol 1979;97:65–70.
8. Savino PJ, Glaser JS, Rosenberg MA. A clinical analysis of pseudopapilledema. II: visual field defects. Arch Ophthalmol 1979;97:71–75.
9. Wilkins JM, Pomeranz HD. Visual manifestations of visible and buried optic disc drusen. J Neuroophthalmol 2004;24:125–129.
10. Lee AG, Zimmerman MB. The rate of visual field loss in optic nerve head drusen. Am J Ophthalmol 2005;139:1062–1066.
11. Beck RW, Corbett JJ, Thompson HS, Sergott RC. Decreased visual acuity from optic disc drusen. Arch Ophthalmol 1985;103:1155–1159.

12. Grover S, Fishman GA, Brown J. Frequency of optic disc or peripapillary nerve fiber layer drusen in retinitis pigmentosa. Ophthalmology 1997; 104:295–298.

13. Brodsky MC. Septo-optic dysplasia: a reappraisal. Semin Ophthalmol 1991;6:227–232.

14. Frisén L, Holmegaard L. Spectrum of optic nerve hypoplasia. Br J Ophthalmol 1978; 62:7–15.

15. Parker KL, Hunold JJ, Blethen SL. Septo-Optic Dysplasia/Optic Nerve Head Hypoplasia: Data from the national cooperative growth study. J Pediatr Endocr Metab 2002: 15(suppl):697–700.

16. Hoyt WF, Kaplan SL, Grumbach MM, Glaser JS. Septo-optic dysplasia and pituitary dwarfism. Lancet 1970;1:893–894.

17. Siatkowski RM, Sanchez JC, Andrade R, Alvarez A. The clinical, neuroradiographic, and endocrinologic profile of patients with bilateral optic nerve hypoplasia. Ophthalmology 1997;104:493–496.

18. Sorkin JA, Davis PC, Meacham LR. Optic nerve hypoplasia: absence of posterior pituitary bright signal on magnetic resonance imagng correlates with diabetes insipidus. Am J Ophthalmol 1996;122:717–723.

19. Dutton GN. Congenital disorders of the optic nerve: excavations and hypoplasia. Eye 2004;18:1038–1048.

20. Phillips PH, Spear C, Brodsky MC. Magnetic resonance diagnosis of congenital hypopituitarism in children with optic nerve hypoplasia. J AAPOS 2001;5:275–280.

21. Lambert SR, Hoyt CS, Narahara MH. Optic nerve hypoplasia. Surv Ophthalmol 1987; 32:1–9.

22. Kim RY, Hoyt WF, Lessell S, Narahara MH. Superior segmental optic hypoplasia: a sign of maternal diabetes. Arch Ophthalmol 1989;107:1312–1315.

23. Landau K, Bajka JD, Kirchschlager BM. Topless optic discs in children of mothers with type 1 diabetes mellitus. Am J Ophthalmol 1998; 125:605–611.

24. Hoyt WF, Rios-Montenegro EN, Behrens MM, Eckelhoff RJ. Homonymous hemioptic hypoplasia: Br J Ophthalmol 1972;56:537–545.

25. Chung GW, Edwards AO, Schimmenti LA, et al. Renal-coloboma syndrome: report of a novel PAX2 gene mutation. Am J Ophthalmol 2001;132:910–914.

26. Eccles MR, Schimmenti LA. Renal-coloboma syndrome: a multi-system developmental disorder caused by PAX2 mutations. Clin Genet 1999;56:1–9.

27. Pagen RA. Ocular colobomas. Surv Ophthalmol 1981;25:223–236.

28. Meyer CH, Rodrigues EB, Schmidt JC. Congential optic nerve head pit associated with reduced retinal nerve fibre thickness at the papillomacular bundle. Br J Ophthalmol 2003;87:1300–1301.

29. Brown GC, Shields JA, Goldberg RE. Congenital pits of the optic nerve head, II: clinical studies in humans. Ophthalmology 1980;87:51–65.

30. Kranenburg EW. Crater-like holes in the optic disc and central serous retinopathy. Arch Ophthalmol 1960;64:912–924.

31. Yuen CH, Kaye SB. Spontaneous resolution of serous maculopathy associated with optic disc pit in a child: a case report. Journal of AAPOS 2002;6:330–331.

32. Yuen CH, Kaye SB. Congenital optic pit with serous maculopathy in childhood. Journal of AAPOS 2003;7:150.

33. Rutledge BK, Puliafito CA, Duker JS, Hee MR, Cox MS. Optical coherence tomography of macular lesions associated with optic nerve head pits. Ophthalmology 1996; 103:1047–1053.

34. Cashwell LF, Ford JG. Central visual field changes associated with acquired pits of the optic nerve. Ophthalmology 1995;102:1270–1278.

35. Kindler P. Morning glory syndrome: unusual congenital optic disk anomaly. Am J Ophthalmol 1970;69:376–384.

36. Goldhammer Y, Smith JL. Optic nerve anomalies in basal encephalocele. Arch Ophthalmol 1975;93:115–118.

37. Krishnan C, Roy A, Traboulsi EI. Morning glory disk anomaly, choroidal coloboma, and congenital constrictive malformations of the internal carotid arteries (moyamoya disease). Ophthal Genet 2000;21:21–24.

38. Eustis HS, Sanders MR, Zimmerman T. Morning glory syndrome in children: association with endocrine and central nervous system anomalies. Arch Ophthalmol 1994; 112:204–207.

39. Murphy MA, Perlman EM, Rogg JM, et al. Reversible carotid artery narrowing in morning glory disc anomaly. J Neuroophthalmol 2005;25:198–201.

40. Martyn LJ, Knox DL. Glial hamartoma of the retina in generalized neurofibromatosis (von Recklinghausen's disease). Br J Ophthalmol 1972;56:487–491.

41. Shields JA. Melanocytoma of the optic nerve head: a review. Int Ophthalmol 1978;1:31–37.

42. Osher RH, Shields JA, Layman PR. Pupillary and visual field evaluation in patients with melanocytoma of the optic disc. Arch Ophthalmol 1974;97:1096–1099.

43. Nicholson DH. Tumors of the optic disc. Trans Am Acad Ophthalmol Otolaryngol 1977;83:751–754.

44. Shields JA, Demirci H, Mashayekhi A, Shields CL. Melanocytoma of optic disc in 115 cases. Ophthalmology 2004;111:1739–1746.

45. Meyer D, Ge J, Blinder KJ, et al. Malignant transformation of optic disk melanocytoma. Am J Ophthalmol 1999;127:710–714.

46. De Potter P, Shields CL, Eagle RC, et al. Malignant melanoma of the optic nerve. Arch Ophthalmol 1996;114:608–612.

47. Kjer P. Infantile optic atrophy with dominant mode of inheritance: a clinical and genetic study of 19 Danish families. Acta Ophthalmol 1959;37(suppl 54):1–146.

48. Kline LB, Glaser JS. Dominant optic atrophy: the clinical profile. Arch Ophthalmol 1979;97:1680–1686.

49. Votruba M, Aijaz S, Moore AT. A review of primary hereditary optic neuropathies. J Inherit Metab Dis 2003;26:209–227.

50. Kerrison JB. Hereditary optic neuropathies. Ophthalmol Clin North Am 2001;14:99–107.

51. Hoyt CS. Autosomal dominant optic atrophy: a spectrum of disability. Ophthalmology 1980;87:245–251.

52. Johnston PB, Gaster RN, Smith VC, Tripathi RC. A clinicopathologic study of autosomal dominant optic atrophy. Am J Ophthalmol 1979;88:868–875.

53. Eiberg H, Kjer B, Kjer P, Rosenberg T. Dominant optic atrophy (OPA1) mapped to chromosome 3q region, I: linkage analysis. Hum Mol Genet 1994;3:977–980.

54. Delettre C, Lenaers G, Pelloquin L, et al. OPA1 dominant optic atrophy: a novel mitochondrial disease. Mol Genet Metab 2002;75:97–107.

55. Pesch UE, Fries JE, Bette S, et al. OPA1, the disease gene for autosomal dominant optic atrophy, is specifically expressed in ganglion cells and intrinsic neurons of the retina. Invest Ophthalmol Vis Sci 2004;45:4217–4225.

56. Newman NJ. Hereditary optic neuropathies: from the mitochondria to the optic nerve. Am J Ophthalmol 2005;140:517–523.

57. Waardenburg PJ. Different types of hereditary optic atrophy. Acta Genet 1957;7:287–290.

58. Cryns K, Sivakumaran TA, Van den Ouweland JM, et al. Mutational spectrum of the WFS1 gene in Wolfram syndrome, nonsyndromic hearing impairment, diabetes mellitus, and psychiatric disease. Hum Mutat 2003;22:275–287.

59. Newman NJ, Biousse V. Hereditary optic neuropathies. Eye 2004;18:1144–1160.

60. Leber T. Veber hereditare und congenitulangelegte Sehnervenleiden. Graefes Arch Ophthalmol 1871;17:249.

61. Smith JL, Hoyt WF, Susac JO. Ocular fundus in acute Leber optic neuropathy. Arch Ophthalmol 1973;90:349–354.

62. Lopez PF, Smith JL. Leber's optic neuropathy: new observations. J Clin Neuroophthalmol 1986;6:144–152.

63. Lessell S, Gise RL, Krohel GB. Bilateral optic neuropathy with remission in young men: variation on a theme by Leber? Arch Neurol 1983;40:2–6.

64. Rogers JA. Leber's disease. Aust J Ophthalmol 1977;5:111–119.

65. Sorajja P, Sweeney MG, Chalmers R, et al. Cardiac abnormalities in patients with Leber's hereditary optic neuropathy. Heart 2003;89:791–792.

66. Miller NR. The hereditary optic neuropathies. In: Walsh and Hoyt's Clinical Neuro-Ophthalmology. 4th ed. Baltimore: Williams & Wilkins; 1982.

67. Carroll WM, Mastalgia FL. Leber's optic neuropathy: a clinical and visual evoked potential study of affected and asymptomatic members of a six generation family. Brain 1979;102:559–580.

68. Seedorff T. The inheritance of Leber's disease: a genealogical follow-up study. Acta Ophthalmol 1985;63:135–145.

69. Nikoskelainen E. New aspects of the genetic, etiologic, and clinical puzzle of Leber's disease. Neurology 1984;34:1482–1484.

70. Wallace DC, Singh G, Lott MT, et al. Mitochondrial DNA mutation associated with Leber's hereditary optic neuropathy. Science 1988;242:1427–1430.

71. Yoneda M, Tsuji S, Yamauchi T, et al. Mitochondrial DNA mutation in family with Leber's hereditary optic neuropathy. Lancet 1989;1:1076–1077.

72. Parker WD Jr, Oley CA, Parks JK. A defect in mitochondrial electron-transport activity (NADH-coenzyme Q oxidoreductase) in Leber's hereditary optic neuropathy. N Engl J Med 1989;320:1331–1333.

73. Lott MT, Voljavec AS, Wallace DC. Variable genotype of Leber's hereditary optic neuropathy patients. Am J Ophthalmol 1990;109:625–631.

74. Huponen K, Vikki J, Aula P, et al. A new mtDNA mutation associated with Leber's hereditary optic neuropathy Am J Hum Genet 1991;48:1147–1153.

75. Johns DR, Neufield MJ. An ND-6 mitochondrial DNA mutation associated with Leber's hereditary optic neuropathy. Biochem Biophys Res Commun 1992;187:1551–1557.

76. Howell N, Kubacka I, Xu M, McCullough DA. Leber hereditary optic neuropathy: involvement of the mitochondrial ND1 gene and evidence for an intragenic suppressor mutation. Am J Hum Genet 1991;48:935–942.

77. Johns DR, Berman J. Alternative, simultaneous complex I mitochondrial DNA mutations in Leber's hereditary optic neuropathy. Biochem Biophys Res Commun 1991; 174:1324–1330.

78. Brown MD, Voljavec AS, Lott MT, et al. Mitochondrial DNA complex I and III mutations associated with Leber's hereditary optic neuropathy. Genetics 1992;130:163–173.

79. Johns DR, Heher KL, Miller NR, et al. Leber's hereditary optic neuropathy: clinical manifestations of the 14484 mutation. Arch Ophthalmol 1993;111:495–498.

80. Holt IJ, Miller DH, Harding AE. Genetic heterogeneity and mitochondrial DNA heteroplasmy in Leber's hereditary optic neuropathy. J Med Genet 1989;26:739–743.

81. Newman NJ. Leber's hereditary optic neuropathy. Ophthalmol Clin North Am 1991; 4:431–447.
82. Kerrison JB, Miller NR, Hsu F, et al. A case-control study of tobacco and alcohol consumption in Leber hereditary optic neuropathy. Am J Ophthalmol 2000;130:803–812.
83. Votruba M. Molecular genetic basis of primary inherited optic neuropathies. Eye 2004; 18:1126–1132.
84. Acaroglu G, Kansu T, Dogulu CF. Visual recovery patterns in children with Leber's hereditary optic neuropathy. Int Ophthalmol 2001;24:349–355.
85. Newman NJ, Lott MT, Wallace DC. The clinical characteristics of pedigrees of Leber's hereditary optic neuropathy with the 11778 mutation. Am J Ophthalmol 1991;111:750–762.
86. Riordan-Eva P, Sander MD, Govan GC, et al. The clinical features of Leber's hereditary optic neuropathy defined by the presence of pathogenic mitochondrial DNA mutation. Brain 1995;118:319–337.
87. Haltia M. The neuronal ceroid-lipofuscinoses. J Neuropathol Exp Neurol 2003;62:1–13.
88. Santavuori P, Lauronen L, Kirveskari E, et al. Neuronal ceroid lipofuscinoses in childhood. Neurol Sci 2000;21(suppl):35–41.
89. Bohra LI, Weizer JS, Lee AG, Lewis RA. Vision loss as the penetrating sign in juvenile neuronal ceroid lipofuscinosis. J Neuroophthalmol 2000;20:111–115.
90. Goebel HH. The neuronal ceroid-lipofuscinoses. Semin Pediatr Neurol 1996;3:270–278.

8

Toxic and Nutritional Optic Neuropathy

JOHN. B. KERRISON

Although the clinical profiles of patients with toxic optic neuropathy differ from the profiles of those with nutritional optic neuropathy, the pattern of visual loss is similar. It is characterized by decreased visual acuity with relative preservation of peripheral vision. Findings on examination are that of a bilateral optic neuropathy. Visual acuity characteristically ranges from 20/30–20/200. Significant dyschromatopsia is present, often disproportionate to the level of visual acuity.

Visual field testing shows central or centrocecal scotomas. Automated threshold perimetry of the central 30 degrees of vision may reveal depression of the entire tested field such that the central nature of field loss is not appreciated. Kinetic perimetry or confrontation visual fields may complement automated perimetry, clearly demonstrating the central nature of visual field loss. In other patients, a small central defect of only a few degrees may be associated with significant foveal threshold depression and an otherwise normal mean deviation. In this instance, testing of the central 10 degrees of vision is indicated.

Acuity loss, dyschromatopsia, and visual field defects are bilateral and symmetric. As such, a relative afferent pupillary defect is not generally present. On ophthalmoscopy, the optic nerve may be normal, mildly swollen, or pale. With acute ingestions, the optic disc is hyperemic and swollen, progressing to diffuse optic pallor with cupping.[1] With insidious vision loss, the optic nerve may appear normal or slightly hyperemic, progressing to pallor of the temporal optic nerve head with atrophy of the papillomacular bundle.

8-1 OPTIC NEUROPATHIES CAUSED BY TOXINS AND ADVERSE DRUG REACTIONS

A *toxin* is a substance that results in a harmful effect when ingested or inhaled. An *adverse drug reaction* is an unintended response to a drug that occurs *at doses usually used* for prophylaxis, diagnosis, or therapy of disease. Although a toxin may have an unintended harmful outcome, it is an expected result. Toxins are typically ingested accidentally. While toxic ingestions or inhalations typically present in an acute setting, adverse drug reactions resulting in vision loss often have an insidious course.

The evidence for establishing an agent as a cause of an optic neuropathy generally consists of clinical experience with individual cases. The criteria to establish causality include the following:

1. Temporal relationship of the cause to the proposed effect.
2. Absence of an alternative causation
3. Withdrawal leads to improvement and rechallenge leads to effect
4. Biologic plausibility that two factors could be related through a reasonable unifying mechanism
5. Analogy from previous animal or human experimental evidence
6. A specific and reproducible dose-response relationship of the proposed drug to the effect

Such rigorous criteria are often difficult to meet in a clinical setting. Furthermore, susceptibility may vary from one individual to another, and experimental evidence specifically investigating optic nerve toxicity is lacking. Thus, case reports are generally the most common source of information regarding toxic optic neuropathies.

8-1-1 *Clinical Presentations.* Patients with an optic neuropathy occurring as a result of a toxic ingestion often present to an emergency room with nausea, abdominal pain, and coma. Not until they have been resuscitated is it discovered that they have experienced visual loss.

Patients with optic neuropathy occurring as a result of an adverse drug reaction typically present with more insidious bilateral loss of vision. Other neurologic complaints may include numbness or tingling in their extremities due to a peripheral neuropathy. These patients generally have a chronic disease requiring prolonged medical therapy, often antimicrobial or cancer chemotherapy, for treatment or prophylaxis. A temporal association may be drawn between initiation of treatment and the start of symptoms. Of course, initiation of the drug has to precede vision loss, but it may be difficult in some cases to establish the onset of the vision loss because of its insidious nature or because of other confounding factors impairing vision, such as cataracts.

8-1-2 *Optic Neuropathies Caused by Toxins*

8-1-2-1 *Methanol.* Methanol is the best-characterized toxin affecting the optic nerve (Fig. 8–1).[1,2] It is a colorless, odorless liquid present in antifreeze, copying fluid, windshield washer fluid, and paint remover. It is generally ingested acciden-

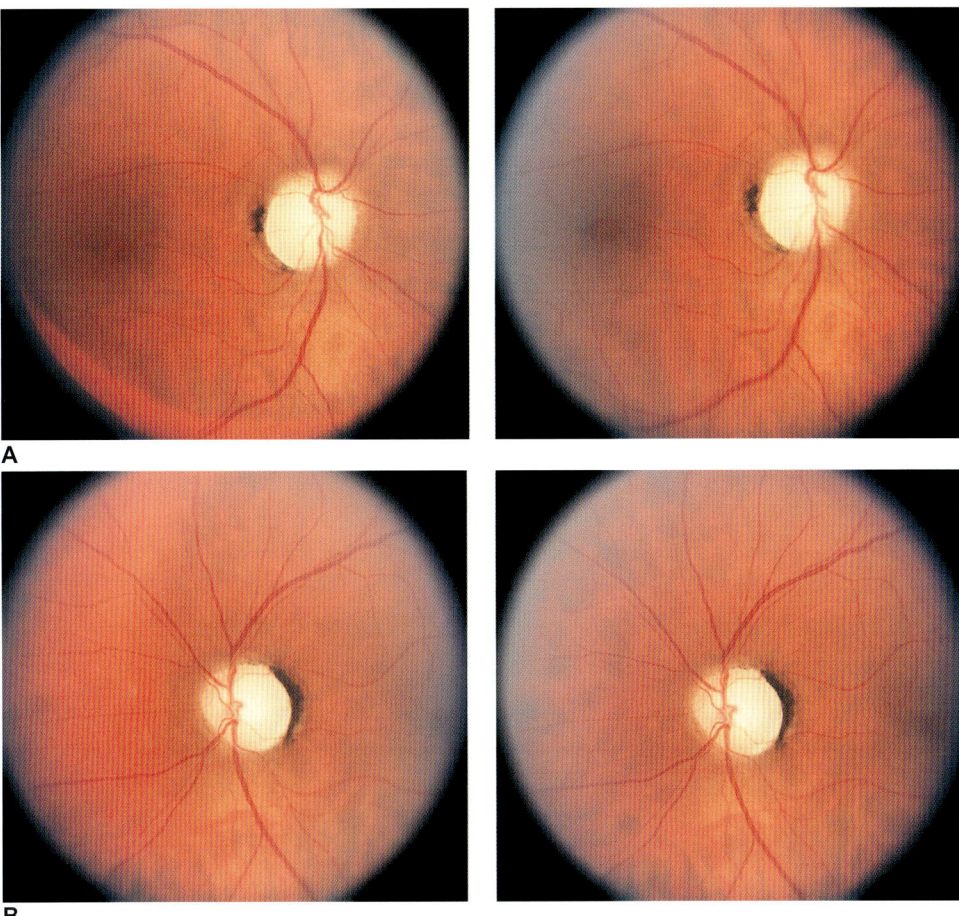

Figure 8–1. Toxic optic neuropathy. (A) Right and (B) left optic discs of patient with severe optic atrophy secondary to methanol toxicity. These are "free stereo" photographs and can be seen in stereo by crossing your eyes and fusing the central image.

tally when added to ethyl alcohol. It may also cause toxic vision loss from inhalation. Vision loss is typically profound, on the order of count fingers to no light perception. Patients present with nausea, abdominal pain, anion-gap metabolic acidosis, an osmolar gap, vision loss, and coma, often progressing to death. Magnetic resonance imaging (MRI) may show bilateral putaminal hyperintense lesions on T2-weighted images. Methanol is a substrate in the alcohol dehydrogenase pathway and is metabolized to formaldehyde and formic acid. Humans and nonhuman primates are uniquely sensitive to methanol-induced neurotoxicity because of the limited capacity of primate species to oxidize and thus detoxify formic acid. Formic acid is a mitochondrial toxin known to inhibit the essential mitochondrial enzyme cytochrome oxidase; thus it may act as a mitochondrial toxin to the retina and optic nerve. Electrophysiologic testing suggests that methanol affects the photoreceptors, Muller cells, and retrolaminar portion of the optic nerve. Postmortem studies have demonstrated bilateral central necrosis of the optic nerves from behind the lamina cribrosa to the orbital apex.

Medical treatment consists of ethanol, dialysis, and 4-methylpyrazole. High-dose intravenous steroids have been observed to be beneficial in the recovery of vision.[2] A beneficial effect of monochromatic red radiation projected onto the ocular fundus in a rodent model of methanol toxicity has been observed.[3,4] This potential treatment for vision loss is based on the observation that photobiomodulation by red to near-infrared radiation enhances mitochondrial activity and promotes cell survival in vitro by stimulating cytochrome oxidase activity.

8-1-2-2 *Ethylene Glycol.* Ethylene glycol poisoning, which is similar to methanol poisoning, results mainly from the ingestion of antifreeze. Severe cases present with metabolic acidosis and coma. Toxicity is related to the severity of metabolic acidosis resulting from the biotransformation of ethylene glycol into toxic metabolites. Oxalate crystals may be identified in the urine. Therapy consists of ethanol, hemodialysis, and intensive care support. Vision loss can occur as part of a general syndrome of neurotoxicity.

8-1-2-3 *Solvents (Toluene, Styrene, Others).* Exposure to solvents, particularly toluene and styrene, is associated with vision loss from an optic neuropathy.[5,6] Toluene is lipophilic and therefore absorbed and retained well by the lipid-rich central nervous system. Vision loss often occurs slowly with chronic abuse by inhalation or "glue sniffing." In fact, chronic occupational exposure to several solvents, metals, and other industrial chemicals can impair color vision in exposed workers. In one case, a 57-year-old owner of a dry-cleaning shop developed blindness following inhalation of perchloroethylene vapors.[7] This occurred after she ironed freshly dry-cleaned fabrics, causing the emission of vapors at a level five times above safe environmental concentrations.

8-1-2-4 *Carbon Monoxide.* Carbon monoxide poisoning may occur accidentally or from attempted suicide. Vision loss with electrophysiologic features consistent with an optic neuropathy has been observed.[8,9]

8-1-3 Medication-Induced Toxic Optic Neuropathies

8-1-3-1 *Antibiotics.* Ethambutol, widely used in the treatment of tuberculosis, may be one of the most commonly encountered drugs associated with an optic neuropathy (Figs. 8–2 and 8–3).[10] Patients are often treated with a combination of ethambutol and isoniazid, which may have an additive adverse effect.[11] Animal models demonstrate that toxicity begins in the optic chiasm. Cell-culture experiments suggest that the damage is mediated by increased calcium flux into the mitochondria of retinal ganglion cells.[12] Vision loss is dose related and more likely to occur in patients receiving 25 mg/kg/day or more. Patients with renal tuberculosis are more susceptible because of impaired renal excretion. Because vision loss is insidious, patients treated with ethambutol should undergo periodic examinations, including color vision and visual fields, to detect early damage and discontinue the drug if vision loss is detected.

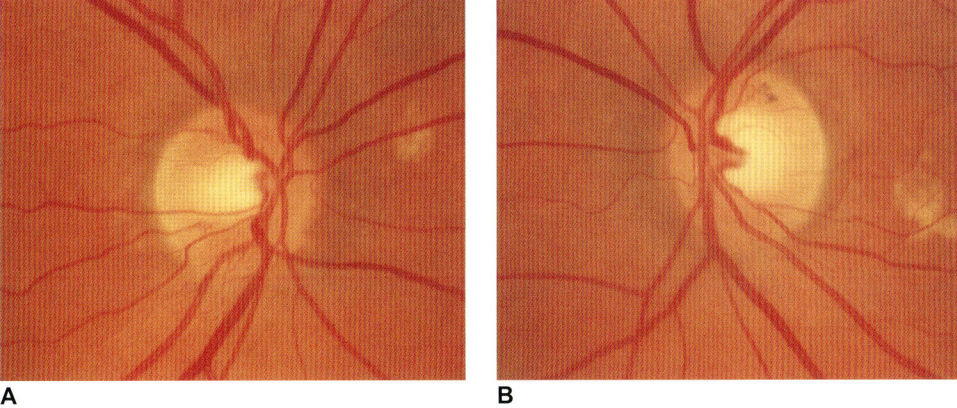

A   B

Figure 8–2. Ethambutol optic neuropathy. Normal appearance of (A) right and (B) left optic discs at onset of visual loss. Acuity 6/200 OU.

Halogenated hydroquinolones, such as clioquinol and iodochlorohydroxy-quinoline, have been used as amebicidal agents.[13] Toxic reactions to clioquinol may present with an acute encephalopathy; a combination of myelopathy, vision loss, and peripheral neuropathy; or an isolated optic neuropathy.[14] In one series, an isolated optic neuropathy occurred more commonly in children. The syndrome of subacute myelo-optic neuropathy (SMON) occurred in Japan in epidemic proportions between 1955 and 1970; it was attributed to the use of clioquinol as a gastrointestinal disinfectant.[13,15] Other antibiotics associated with an optic neuropathy include dapsone,[16] chloramphenicol,[17] and linezolid.[18–20]

8-1-3-2 *Immunosuppressants and Immunomodulators.* Both cyclosporine and tacrolimus (FK506) are widely used immunosuppressants. Cyclosporine neurotoxicity affects the optic nerves but may also cause other manifestations—including ophthalmoplegia, nystagmus, and ataxia—secondary to cerebellar neurotoxicity.[21]

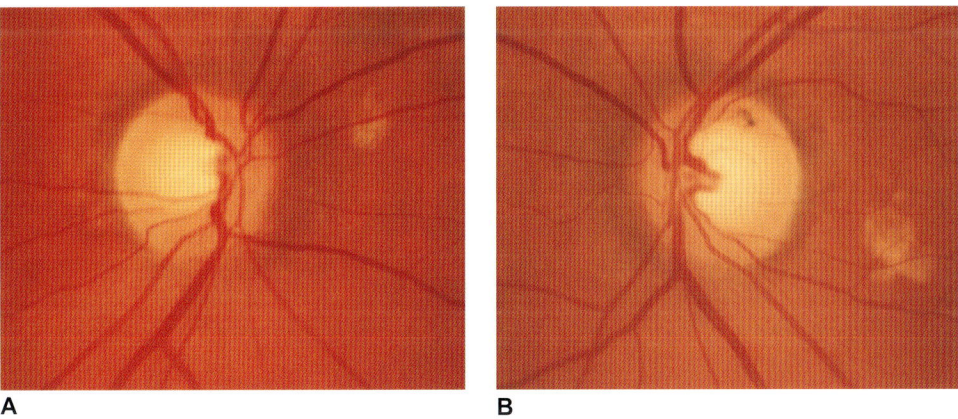

A   B

Figure 8–3. Ethambutol optic neuropathy. Same patient as in Figure 8–2. With recovery of vision to 20/25 OU, there is minimal optic atrophy bilaterally. (A) Right eye. (B) Left eye.

FK506 similarly may be associated with an optic neuropathy as well as other neurotoxicities.[22]

Alpha interferon–2b has also been associated with optic neuropathy.[23]

8-1-3-3 Chemotherapeutic Agents. Chemotherapeutic agents of note that have been associated with optic nerve toxicity include cisplatin and carboplatin, nitrosureas, and vincristine. These often cause neurotoxicity with symptoms of paresthesias, ataxia, nystagmus, and paresis. Nevertheless, vision loss secondary to an optic neuropathy may be the most prominent manifestation of toxicity. In addition, those patients who have been reported were often receiving multiple medications. Cisplatin and carboplatin are heavy metal alkylating agents used in treating a variety of cancers and are associated with a dose-limiting ototoxicity and peripheral neuropathy. These agents have also been reported to cause an optic neuropathy in addition to cortical blindness.[24] BCNU (carmustine), CCNU (lomustine), and methyl-CCNU (semustine), all nitrosoureas, are cell cycle–specific alkylating agents that bind DNA. Because they penetrate the blood-brain barrier, they are used in the treatment of several primary and recurrent central nervous system tumors. Vincristine is a vinca alkaloid that binds microtubules and arrests dividing cells in metaphase. It is widely used and causes a sensorimotor peripheral neuropathy. Although vision loss has been most often reported from an optic neuropathy, cortical blindness has been reported as well.[25] Another oncologic agent, 5-fluorouracil, has also been associated with optic neuropathy.[26]

8-1-3-4 Miscellaneous. Disulfiram is used in the treatment of alcoholism and may cause an acute optic neuropathy.[27] Because disulfiram interferes with the metabolism of acetaldehyde, a byproduct of ethanol metabolism, patients on disulfiram who ingest alcohol experience nausea and vomiting. Prognosis for visual recovery is generally good if the drug is discontinued.

Other drugs associated with an optic neuropathy include cimetidine,[28] benoxaprofen,[29] paclitaxel,[30] chlorpropamide,[31] and combined use of melatonin, sertraline, and a high-protein diet.[32]

Some drugs that are considered to cause a primary retinopathy have been observed to have an optic nerve findings as well. Deferoxamine, used to chelate iron, is associated with a macular toxicity but may also cause an optic neuropathy.[33] Vigabatrin, used to treat seizure is associated with gradual constriction of vision due retinal toxicity, has also produced findings consistent with optic nerve toxicity.[34,35]

8-1-3-5 Tobacco and Alcohol. What is the role of alcohol and tobacco in the development of an optic neuropathy? A direct role of alcohol has not been demonstrated in the development of a primary optic neuropathy. Although tobacco smoking is not considered to cause a primary optic neuropathy, it is a risk factor for vision loss in patients with nutritional deficiency (see below). The epidemic of optic neuropathy in Cuba demonstrated that, in addition to malnutrition, tobacco consumption, particularly in the form of cigars, was an independent risk factor for vision loss.[36] The toxicity from tobacco is attributed to elevated levels of cyanide-thiocynate in serum. A similar experience of optic neuropathy in Africa was associated with dietary cyanide from the consumption of food processed from the starchy roots of cassava.[37]

8-1-4 *Medication-Induced Optic Neuropathies Caused by a Nontoxic Mechanism.* The prior discussion features optic neuropathies, bilateral and painless, thought to be mediated by direct toxicity to the optic nerve. Other drugs have been associated with an acute optic neuropathy in which the vision loss is caused not by toxicity but by an alternative mechanism such as increased intracranial pressure, ischemia, or an autoimmune reaction.

Sildenafil (Viagra)-associated optic neuropathy presents with typical features of a nonarteritic anterior ischemic optic neuropathy (NAION), including a small cup-to-disc ratio, which is a primary risk factor for NAION.[38, 39] Sildenafil is postulated to influence the development of vision loss through a local effect on optic nerve perfusion or arterial hypotension. Tadalafil has also been associated with NAION.[40]

Infliximab is a chimeric IgG antibody, which is an antagonist of TNF-α.[41] A clinical syndrome of both retrobulbar[42] and anterior optic neuritis[41] has been associated with its use. In these instances, the toxicity is thought to be mediated by the effect of infliximab on the immune system, possibly by increasing the risk of demyelination.

A variety of medications have been associated with elevated intracranial pressure and papilledema with headaches and ocular motor nerve palsies. The best-recognized medications to be associated with this adverse reaction are vitamin A[43] and tetracycline derivatives.[44] Other medications include growth hormone,[45] cyclosporine,[46] OKT3 (a monoclonal murine IgG immunoglobulin used to treat acute cellular rejection of allografted organs),[47] oprelvekin (used in the treatment of radioimmunotherapy-induced thrombocytopenia),[48] lithium,[49] ketoconazole,[50]and nalidixic acid.[51]

8-1-5 *Amiodarone-Associated Optic Neuropathy.* Amiodarone is an anti-arrhythmic drug used to treat ventricular tachycardia and fibrillation and to reestablish sinus rhythm in atrial fibrillation. Amiodarone, known to cause a vortex epitheliopathy of the cornea and anterior subcapsular lens opacities, has been associated with a toxic optic neuropathy.[52–54] Patients taking amiodarone may develop a typical unilateral NAION. In this instance, the optic neuropathy is *not considered* to be an adverse drug event. In contrast, other patients develop an optic neuropathy that, in comparison with NAION, has a more insidious onset and slower progression. It is more often bilateral, and the disc swelling is more protracted, tending to stabilize within several months of discontinuing the medication. In this instance, the optic neuropathy is thought to be the result of a direct effect on the optic nerve, perhaps due to a chronic neurotoxic effect on the optic nerve via a drug-induced lipidosis.[55] In electronmicroscopic studies of postmortem optic nerve specimens from an asymptomatic patient on amiodarone, lamellar inclusions were found selectively in large axons and were taken as evidence of a drug-induced lipidosis.[55]

The existence of these two patterns of optic neuropathy and the potential for overlap can lead to diagnostic confusion and subsequent patient misunderstanding. Patients with a typical pattern of bilateral optic neuropathy considered to be a direct toxic effect of amiodarone on the optic nerve should be counseled in coordination with their cardiologist to discontinue the amiodarone or find an appropriate alternative. Patients on amiodarone who present with a clinical picture of NAION must be carefully informed about the possibility that amiodarone could cause optic nerve toxicity, especially because of the potential for second-eye involvement in NAION. If the optic nerve edema has a prolonged course, it may in fact be related to amiodarone. Such discussions should also include the cardiologist, so that an informed decision can be made.

8-2 DIFFERENTIAL DIAGNOSIS, WORKUP, TREATMENT

A clinically useful way to approach toxic and medication-induced optic neuropathies is based on the pattern of vision loss, whether primarily central or peripheral. Then, localization to the optic nerve or retina can be considered. In general, vision loss from an optic neuropathy is central. Vision loss from retinal toxicity may be primarily central or peripheral. There is considerable overlap among these categories.

The differential diagnosis for a bilateral, central pattern of vision loss from an optic neuropathy includes hereditary optic neuropathies, nutritional optic neuropathy, compressive lesions of the anterior visual pathways, inflammatory optic neuropathies, infiltrative optic neuropathies, or previous bilateral traumatic optic neuropathy. With regard to hereditary optic neuropathy, dominant optic atrophy is more likely to present with insidious loss of bilateral vision, in contrast with Leber hereditary optic neuropathy (LHON), which more commonly involves acute, bilateral, or sequential vision loss (see Chapter 7).

Bilateral loss of central vision may also occur from bilateral occipital lobe or bilateral macular disease. Bilateral occipital lobe lesions cause the same pattern of vision loss, with normal appearing optic nerves and normal pupillary reactions. Careful visual field testing may reveal a vertical step between hemifields. Bilateral macular disease from a variety of disorders (degenerative, toxic, hereditary, paraneoplastic) should not be overlooked. With some disease processes, the findings may be subtle. Furthermore, optic nerve pallor may be associated with retinal disease not only in retinitis pigmentosa but also with cone dystrophy.

Evaluation should be directed at careful questioning as to when a drug was ingested as well as family and dietary history. In addition to clinical history and examination, the workup should include neuroimaging with gadolinium-enhanced MRI of the brain and orbits and a laboratory evaluation including a complete blood count and serum levels of vitamin B_{12} and folate. In some cases, genetic testing for LHON or dominant optic neuropathy should be considered. In acute poisoning from methanol or ethylene glycol, the toxin or its metabolite may be measured.

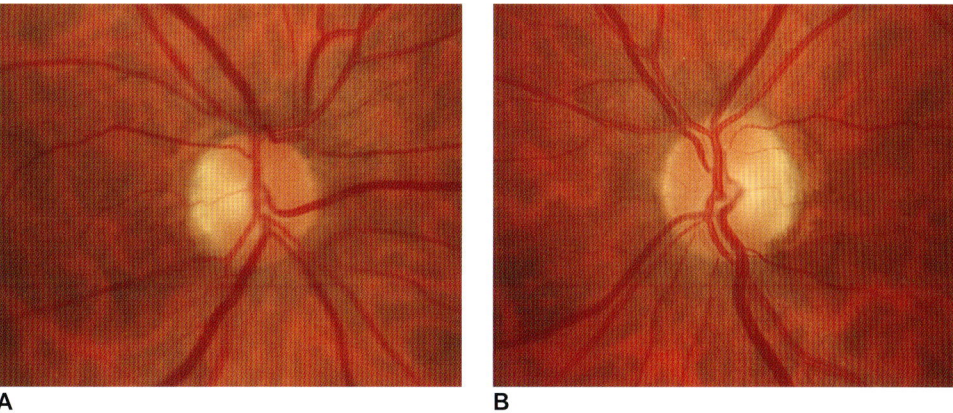

Figure 8–4. Nutritional optic neuropathy. This 74-year-old man was held prisoner during World War II. During captivity, he reported subacute loss of vision, which has persisted to the present. Vision is 20/400 OU, visual fields demonstrate bilateral centrocecal scotomas, and optic discs show temporal pallor. (A) Right eye. (B) Left eye.

8-3 OPTIC NEUROPATHIES CAUSED BY NUTRITIONAL DEFICIENCY

8-3-1 *Clinical Presentation.* Nutritional optic neuropathies are characterized by bilateral insidious vision loss occurring in association with dietary deficiency or malabsorption. A great deal of information came from studies of Allied prisoners of war of the Japanese during World War II.[56] As discussed, the epidemic of optic neuropathy in Cuba demonstrated that in addition to malnutrition, tobacco consumption was an independent risk factor for vision loss. Finally, nutritional optic neuropathies are often seen in patients who are chronic alcoholics and tobacco users (Fig. 8–4).

The clinical profile of all these groups is reasonably similar. At presentation, visual acuity is typically 20/40 to 20/200, bilateral, and symmetric. There may be a slow, insidious progression of vision loss. Color vision is reduced. Visual field defects include central, paracentral, and centrocecal scotomas. Initially, the optic nerves may appear normal, but hyperemia, swelling, and peripapillary hemorrhages

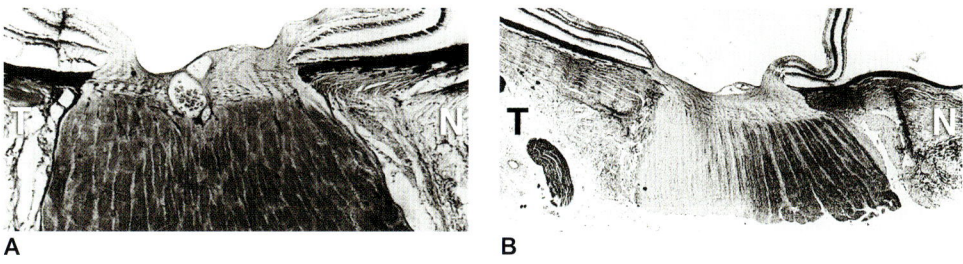

Figure 8–5. Sections through retina, nerve head, and optic nerve stained with hematoxylin and eosin (A) and for myelin (B). (A) Normal anatomic appearance. (B) With nutritional optic neuropathy, myelinated fibers are lost and fibrous tissue is increased in temporal parts of optic nerve. T, temporal aspect; N, nasal aspect. (Courtesy of Maurice Victor, MD.)

may be observed. Untreated, the disorder progresses and optic atrophy eventually develops.

In many individuals, other signs of malnourishment may be present, or patients may appear to have normal body mass. Be aware of the possibility of B_{12} deficiency in vegetarians and individuals who have undergone gastrointestinal surgery. Other neurologic manifestations may be present, as in the case of B_{12} deficiency, which affects the dorsal and lateral spinal columns, causing ataxia, paresthesias, and weakness.

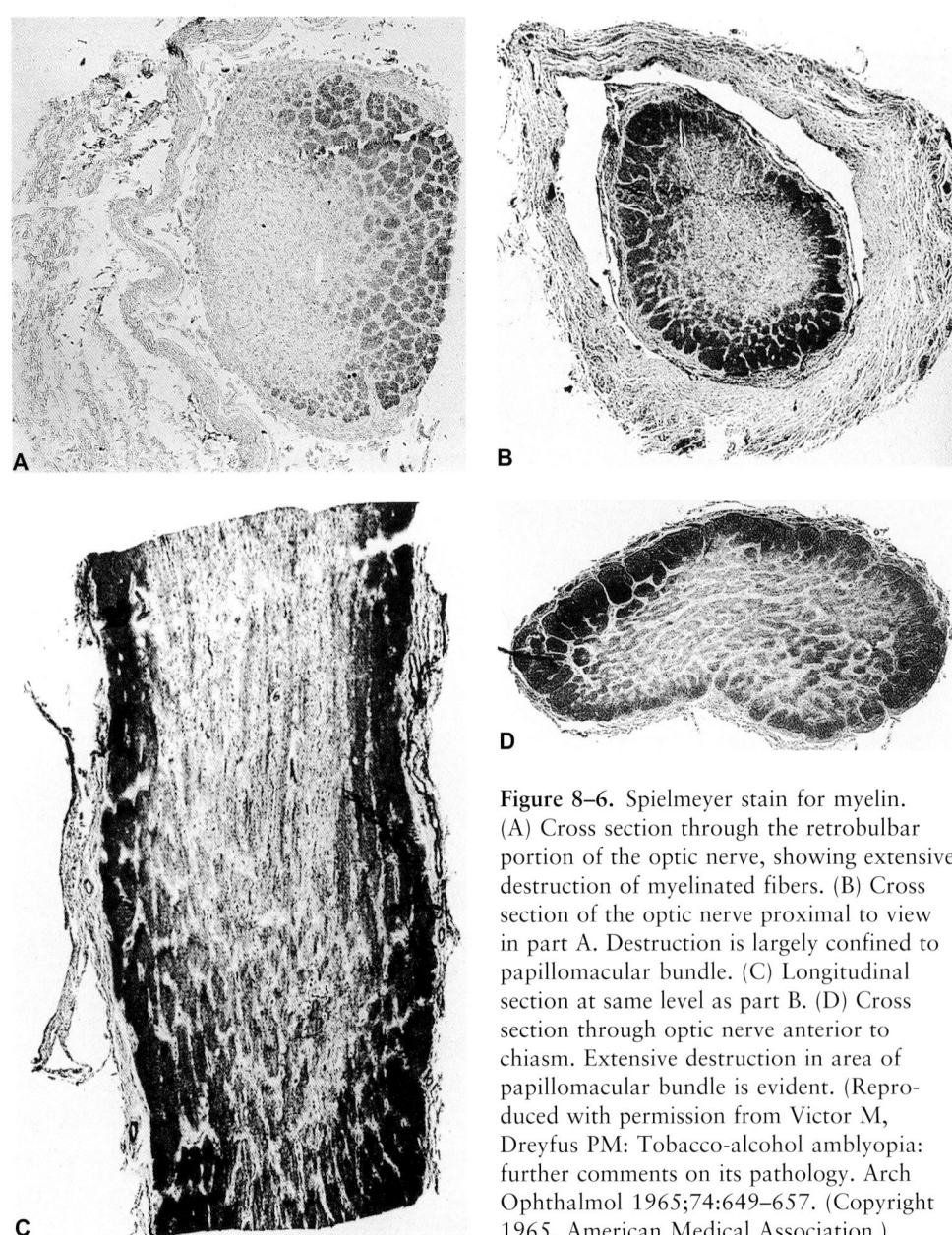

Figure 8–6. Spielmeyer stain for myelin. (A) Cross section through the retrobulbar portion of the optic nerve, showing extensive destruction of myelinated fibers. (B) Cross section of the optic nerve proximal to view in part A. Destruction is largely confined to papillomacular bundle. (C) Longitudinal section at same level as part B. (D) Cross section through optic nerve anterior to chiasm. Extensive destruction in area of papillomacular bundle is evident. (Reproduced with permission from Victor M, Dreyfus PM: Tobacco-alcohol amblyopia: further comments on its pathology. Arch Ophthalmol 1965;74:649–657. (Copyright 1965, American Medical Association.)

8-3-2 *Differential Diagnosis and Workup.* The differential diagnosis includes dominant optic atrophy, toxic optic neuropathy, macular degeneration, and dystrophies. Diagnosis is based on clinical history and examination. A complete blood count and serum levels of B_1, B_{12}, and folate should be evaluated. Workup should also include gadolinium-enhanced MRI of the brain and orbits to exclude a compressive disorder of the optic nerve. If B_{12} deficiency is identified, the patient should be evaluated for pernicious anemia.

8-3-3 *Pathology, Etiology, and Treatment.* The pathology of nutritional optic neuropathy includes degenerative changes in the optic nerve, chiasm, and tracts primarily confined to the papillomacular bundles. Such pathologic changes are associated with loss of retinal ganglion cells, particularly in the macula (Figs. 8–5 and 8–6).

The etiology of this disorder is a deficiency of B vitamins.[57] Specific vitamin deficiencies associated with vision loss include B_{12} and folate.[58] Some patients may present with the typical clinical picture of nutritional optic neuropathy yet have normal B_{12} and folate levels. The deficiency in these patients is often attributed to B-complex vitamins, particularly thiamine (B_1), and clinical improvement may occur with vitamin supplementation. However, emphasized in the literature, identification of a specific deficiency does not necessarily prove it to be the cause of the optic neuropathy. In addition, it is rare to find a deficiency in only one nutrient in the patient population at risk.

Treatment consists of thiamine, 100 mg orally twice a day; folate, 1 mg orally daily; and a daily multivitamin. If B_{12} deficiency is present, B_{12} in a dose of 1000 µg IM is administered monthly in coordination with an internist. Depending on the degree of optic atrophy, some improvement in vision can be anticipated.

References

1. Sharma M, Volpe NJ, Dreyer EB. Methanol-induced optic nerve cupping. Arch Ophthalmol 1999;117:286.
2. Sodhi PK, Goyal JL, Mehta DK. Methanol-induced optic neuropathy: treatment with intravenous high dose steroids. Int J Clin Pract 2001;55:599–602.
3. Eells JT, Henry MM, Lewandowski MF, Seme MT, Murray TG. Development and characterization of a rodent model of methanol-induced retinal and optic nerve toxicity. Neurotoxicology 2000;21:321–330.
4. Eells JT, Henry MM, Summerfelt P, et al. Therapeutic photobiomodulation for methanol-induced retinal toxicity. Proc Natl Acad Sci USA 2003;100:3439–3444.
5. Kiyokawa M, Mizota A, Takasoh M, Adachi-Usami E. Pattern visual evoked cortical potentials in patients with toxic optic neuropathy caused by toluene abuse. Jpn J Ophthalmol 1999;43:438–442.
6. Gobba F, Cavalleri A. Color vision impairment in workers exposed to neurotoxic chemicals. Neurotoxicology 2003;24:693–702.
7. Onofrj M, Thomas A, Paci C, Rotilio D. Optic neuritis with residual tunnel vision in perchloroethylene toxicity. J Toxicol Clin Toxicol 1998;36:603–607.
8. Fine RD, Parker GD. Disturbance of central vision after carbon monoxide poisoning. Aust N Z J Ophthalmol 1996;24:137–141.
9. Simmons IG, Good PA. Carbon monoxide poisoning causes optic neuropathy. Eye 1998;12:809–814.

10. Melamud A, Kosmorsky GS, Lee MS. Ocular ethambutol toxicity. Mayo Clin Proc 2003;78:1409–1411.

11. Boulanouar A, Abdallah E, el Bakkali M, Benchrifa F, Berraho-Hamani A. [Severe toxic optic neuropathies caused by isoniazid. Apropos of 3 cases]. J Fr Ophtalmol 1995;18: 183–187.

12. Heng JE, Vorwerk CK, Lessell E, et al. Ethambutol is toxic to retinal ganglion cells via an excitotoxic pathway. Invest Ophthalmol Vis Sci 1999;40:190–196.

13. Tateishi J. Subacute myelo-optico-neuropathy: clioquinol intoxication in humans and animals. Neuropathology 2000;20(Suppl):S20–S24.

14. Baumgartner G, Gawel MJ, Kaeser HE, et al. Neurotoxicity of halogenated hydroxy-quinolines: clinical analysis of cases reported outside Japan. J Neurol Neurosurg Psychiatry 1979;42:1073–1083.

15. Meade TW. Subacute myelo-optic neuropathy and clioquinol. An epidemiological case-history for diagnosis. Br J Prev Soc Med 1975;29:157–169.

16. Daneshmend TK, Homeida M. Dapsone-induced optic atrophy and motor neuropathy. Br Med J (Clin Res Ed) 1981;283:311.

17. Godel V, Nemet P, Lazar M. Chloramphenicol optic neuropathy. Arch Ophthalmol 1980;98:1417–1421.

18. Kulkarni K, Del Priore LV. Linezolid induced toxic optic neuropathy. Br J Ophthalmol 2005;89:1664–1665.

19. Lee E, Burger S, Shah J, et al. Linezolid-associated toxic optic neuropathy: a report of 2 cases. Clin Infect Dis 2003;37:1389–1391.

20. McKinley SH, Foroozan R. Optic neuropathy associated with linezolid treatment. J Neuroophthalmol 2005;25:18–21.

21. Walter SH, Bertz H, Gerling J. Bilateral optic neuropathy after bone marrow transplantation and Cyclosporin A therapy. Graefes Arch Clin Exp Ophthalmol 2000;238:472–476.

22. Brazis PW, Spivey JR, Bolling JP, Steers JL. A case of bilateral optic neuropathy in a patient on tacrolimus (FK506) therapy after liver transplantation. Am J Ophthalmol 2000;129:536–538.

23. Manesis EK, Petrou C, Brouzas D, Hadziyannis S. Optic tract neuropathy complicating low-dose interferon treatment. J Hepatol 1994;21:474–477.

24. Caraceni A, Martini C, Spatti G, Thomas A, Onofri M. Recovering optic neuritis during systemic cisplatin and carboplatin chemotherapy. Acta Neurol Scand 1997;96:260–261.

25. Norton SW, Stockman JA III. Unilateral optic neuropathy following vincristine chemotherapy. J Pediatr Ophthalmol Strabismus 1979;16:190–193.

26. Delval L, Klastersky J. Optic neuropathy in cancer patients. Report of a case possibly related to 5 fluorouracil toxicity and review of the literature. J Neurooncol 2002;60:165–169.

27. Dupuy O, Flocard F, Vial C, et al. [Disulfiram (Esperal) toxicity. Apropos of 3 original cases]. Rev Med Interne 1995;16:67–72.

28. Sa'adah MA, Al Salem M, Ali AS, Araj G, Zuriqat M. Cimetidine-associated optic neuropathy. Eur Neurol 1999;42:23–26.

29. Dodd MJ, Griffiths ID, Howe JW, Mitchell KW. Toxic optic neuropathy caused by benoxaprofen. Br Med J (Clin Res Ed) 1981;283:193–194.

30. Gianni L, Munzone E, Capri G, et al. Paclitaxel in metastatic breast cancer: a trial of two doses by a 3-hour infusion in patients with disease recurrence after prior therapy with anthracyclines. J Natl Cancer Inst 1995;87:1169–1175.

31. Wymore J, Carter JE. Chlorpropamide-induced optic neuropathy. Arch Intern Med 1982;142:381.

32. Lehman NL, Johnson LN. Toxic optic neuropathy after concomitant use of melatonin, zoloft, and a high-protein diet. J Neuroophthalmol 1999;19:232–234.

33. Lakhanpal V, Schocket SS, Jiji R. Deferoxamine (Desferal)-induced toxic retinal pigmentary degeneration and presumed optic neuropathy. Ophthalmology 1984;91:443–451.

34. Johnson MA, Krauss GL, Miller NR, Medura M, Paul SR. Visual function loss from vigabatrin: effect of stopping the drug. Neurology 2000;55:40–45.

35. Frisen L, Malmgren K. Characterization of vigabatrin-associated optic atrophy. Acta Ophthalmol Scand 2003;81:466–473.

36. Epidemic optic neuropathy in Cuba—clinical characterization and risk factors. The Cuba Neuropathy Field Investigation Team. N Engl J Med 1995;333:1176–1182.

37. Oluwole OS, Onabolu AO, Link H, Rosling H. Persistence of tropical ataxic neuropathy in a Nigerian community. J Neurol Neurosurg Psychiatry 2000;69:96–101.

38. Pomeranz HD, Smith KH, Hart WM, Jr., Egan RA. Sildenafil-associated nonarteritic anterior ischemic optic neuropathy. Ophthalmology 2002;109:584–587.

39. Egan RA, Fraunfelder FW. Viagra and anterior ischemic optic neuropathy. Arch Ophthalmol 2005;123:709–710.

40. Bollinger K, Lee MS. Recurrent visual field defect and ischemic optic neuropathy associated with tadalafil rechallenge. Arch Ophthalmol 2005;123:400–401.

41. ten Tusscher MP, Jacobs PJ, Busch MJ, de Graaf L, Diemont WL. Bilateral anterior toxic optic neuropathy and the use of infliximab. BMJ 2003;326:579.

42. Foroozan R, Buono LM, Sergott RC, Savino PJ. Retrobulbar optic neuritis associated with infliximab. Arch Ophthalmol 2002;120:985–987.

43. Colucciello M. Pseudotumor cerebri induced by all-trans retinoic acid treatment of acute promyelocytic leukemia. Arch Ophthalmol 2003;121:1064–1065.

44. Mochizuki K, Takahashi T, Kano M, Terajima K, Hori N. Pseudotumor cerebri induced by minocycline therapy for acne vulgaris. Jpn J Ophthalmol 2002;46:668–672.

45. Malozowski S, Tanner LA, Wysowski DK, Fleming GA, Stadel BV. Benign intracranial hypertension in children with growth hormone deficiency treated with growth hormone. J Pediatr 1995;126:996–999.

46. Cruz OA, Fogg SG, Roper-Hall G. Pseudotumor cerebri associated with cyclosporine use. Am J Ophthalmol 1996;122:436–437.

47. Strominger MB, Liu GT, Schatz NJ. Optic disk swelling and abducens palsies associated with OKT3. Am J Ophthalmol 1995;119:664–665.

48. Peterson DC, Inwards DJ, Younge BR. Oprelvekin-associated bilateral optic disk edema. Am J Ophthalmol 2005;139:367–368.

49. Alvarez-Cermeno JC, Fernandez JM, O'Neill A, Moral L, Saiz-Ruiz J. Lithium-induced headache. Headache 1989;29:246–247.

50. Or M, Akbatur H, Hasanerisoglu B, Bilgihan K, Cakir N. Ketoconazole induced papilledema. Acta Ophthalmol (Copenh) 1993;71:270–272.

51. Anderson EE, Anderson B Jr, Nashold BS. Childhood complications of nalidixic acid. JAMA 1971;216:1023–1024.

52. Macaluso DC, Shults WT, Fraunfelder FT. Features of amiodarone-induced optic neuropathy. Am J Ophthalmol 1999;127:610–612.

53. Nagra PK, Foroozan R, Savino PJ, Castillo I, Sergott RC. Amiodarone induced optic neuropathy. Br J Ophthalmol 2003;87:420–422.

54. Nazarian SM, Jay WM. Bilateral optic neuropathy associated with amiodarone therapy. J Clin Neuroophthalmol 1988;8:25–28.

55. Mansour AM, Puklin JE, O'Grady R. Optic nerve ultrastructure following amiodarone therapy. J Clin Neuroophthalmol 1988;8:231–237.
56. Bloom SM, Merz EH, Taylor WW. Nutritional amblyopia in American prisoners of war liberated from the Japanese. Am J Ophthalmol 1946;29:1248–1257.
57. Arnaud J, Fleites-Mestre P, Chassagne M, et al. Vitamin B intake and status in healthy Havanan men, 2 years after the Cuban neuropathy epidemic. Br J Nutr 2001;85:741–748.
58. Hsu CT, Miller NR, Wray ML. Optic neuropathy from folic acid deficiency without alcohol abuse. Ophthalmologica 2002;216:65–67.

9

Traumatic Optic Neuropathy

LANNING B. KLINE

Approximately 5% of all patients with head trauma manifest an injury to some portion of the visual system.[1] Traumatic optic neuropathy is most frequently seen in males, most often following motor vehicle and bicycle accidents.[2] The diagnostic challenge facing the clinician during the initial evaluation of such patients is considerable. The assessment of visual function is often difficult in an individual with an altered state of consciousness. If vision is found to be impaired, decisions must be made regarding further evaluation and management based on the site of injury.

In this chapter, traumatic optic neuropathy is classified into three categories: (1) evulsion, (2) direct injury, and (3) indirect injury.

9-1 OPTIC NERVE EVULSION

Optic nerve evulsion is the rarest form of traumatic optic neuropathy. This entity was first described in the early twentieth century as the "forceful backward dislocation of the optic nerve from the scleral canal without any break in the continuity of the adjacent coats of the globe."[3] The word evulsion comes from the Latin prefix "e" (out), plus the word "vellere" (to pluck). The word avulsion is derived from the Latin "a" (away), plus "vellere." These terms have been used interchangeably by most authors.

Total evulsion of the optic nerve occurs when the vitreous and retina separate from the optic disc; the retinal blood vessels are partly or totally interrupted, and the lamina cribrosa is ripped from its attachments to the choroid and sclera.[4] Partial evulsion involves a localized segment of the optic nerve, with partial disruption of the attachments of ocular tissues to the disc.[5]

Evulsions can be caused by penetrating and nonpenetrating injuries of the globe. Penetrating injuries are usually due to gunshot pellets, but other causes include wood and sharp metal objects such as a knife or an umbrella tip. More commonly, optic nerve evulsion is due to nonpenetrating injuries such as severe orbital trauma. Examples include an automobile accident, a blow from a fist, or a kick from a horse. In some reported cases, the external injury has been relatively minor. One such example is a finger jabbed into the orbit; such an injury causes minimal ocular damage but is a well-recognized cause of optic nerve evulsion. If self-induced, the term oedipism has been applied.[6]

Three mechanisms have been postulated as causes of optic nerve evulsion[7]:

1. When struck by an object, the globe may be compressed against the bony orbit and/or orbital contents. The ensuing elevation in intraocular pressure may be so high that the optic nerve is pushed out of the scleral canal.
2. With orbital trauma, a sudden rise in intraorbital pressure forces the globe forward, placing the optic nerve on stretch, with resultant tearing of the nerve axons.
3. With extreme rotation and displacement of the globe within the orbit, there is disruption of the lamina cribrosa and the laminar portion of the optic nerve.

The extent of the evulsion determines the visual prognosis. With partial evulsion, the patient may be able to see some of the Snellen optotypes; with complete evulsion, total blindness ensues.

Often, immediately after injury, the optic disc is obscured by an overlying vitreous hemorrhage. Associated ocular findings may include subconjunctival hemorrhage, limitation of extraocular movement, proptosis, and a dilated, fixed pupil. As the ophthalmoscopic view improves, either the optic disc contour is partly disrupted or the scleral canal can be seen totally devoid of the disc (Fig. 9–1). The defect is gradually filled in with gliotic tissue, which may extend into the vitreous. The differential diagnosis of this ophthalmoscopic appearance includes congenital optic pits, colobomas, staphylomas, and the morning-glory disc anomaly.

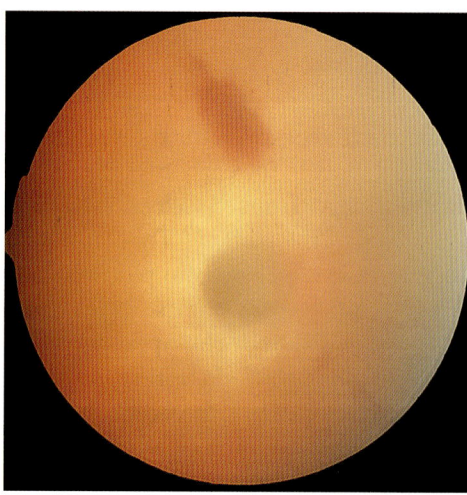

Figure 9–1. Evulsion of optic nerve following clearing of vitreous hemorrhage.

The clinical suspicion of optic nerve evulsion may be confirmed with orbital imaging techniques (Figs. 9–2 and 9–3).[8] These modalities may prove helpful when optic nerve evulsion is accompanied by vitreous hemorrhage and the diagnosis cannot be made initially by funduscopic examination.

In general, visual outcome in optic nerve evulsion is poor. Although medical therapy with megadose systemic corticosteroids might be employed, no studies to date have documented the efficacy of any form of therapy in optic nerve evulsion.

9-2 DIRECT OPTIC NERVE INJURY

Direct optic nerve injury is due to impact on the optic nerve or its sheath by a sharp or blunt object.[9] The injury may be caused by (1) a foreign object that has penetrated the globe, orbit, or cranium or (2) injury from a displaced fracture or spicule of bone in the region of the optic canal.

If the optic nerve is severed anterior to the entrance of the central retinal artery, the ophthalmoscopic picture is that of a central retinal artery occlusion, and loss of vision is instantaneous and complete. When the optic nerve is injured farther posteriorly, the fundus may appear normal or demonstrate mild retinal and optic disc edema due to axoplasmic flow stasis. Within 3–4 weeks, pallor of the optic disc occurs with diffuse loss of the retinal nerve fiber layer.

Immediate blindness after direct optic nerve injury is usually permanent.[10,11] Since the visual prognosis in these patients is so poor, case reports are rarely published. Yet there is a small series of cases in the literature with significant visual recovery. Optic nerve injury after shrapnel and gunshot wounds with initially no light perception has been reported.[12,13] Spontaneous recovery of vision occurred in both cases to counting fingers and 20/100, respectively.

Transethmoidal decompression of the canalicular portion of the optic nerve has led to dramatic visual improvement in instances of direct optic nerve injury. This surgical approach was employed following a stab wound to the orbital apex, with

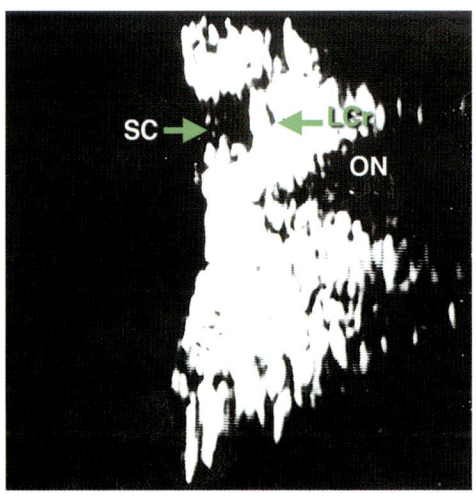

Figure 9–2. Optic nerve evulsion. Sagittal view of B-scan ultrasonogram shows the lamina cribrosa (LCr) posterior to the rest of sclera and the optic nerve (ON) shadow separated from scleral canal (SC).

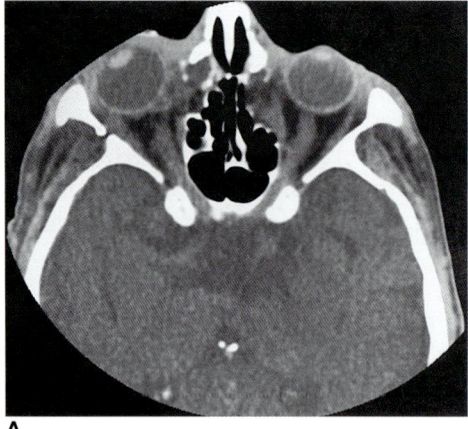

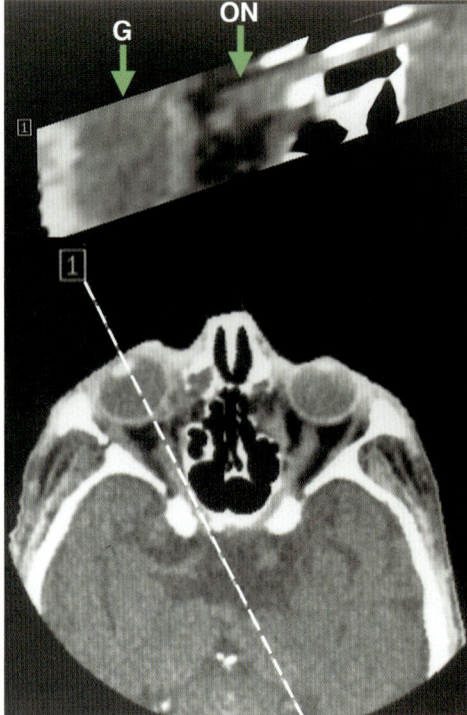

Figure 9–3. Orbital CT scan demonstrates displacement of the right intraorbital optic nerve as it attaches to globe. (A) Contrast-enhanced axial scan. (B) Reformatted image. G, globe; ON, optic nerve.

visual improvement to 20/50.[14] A similar surgical technique was used after an optic canal fracture, with final acuity of 20/20.[15]

The multiple pathophysiologic mechanisms leading to visual loss after direct optic nerve injury are listed in Table 9–1. Undoubtedly, many of these mechanisms occur simultaneously and are interdependent. For example, bony fracture of the optic canal may lead to vascular insufficiency and edema of the nerve; this edema may further compromise the vascular supply to the nerve, extending the area of the infarction. (A full description of potential mechanisms of injury can be found in section 9-3, which follows, dealing with indirect optic nerve injury.)

Evaluation of the depth, direction, and extent of orbital or eyelid wounds from sharp objects, no matter how minimal they appear superficially, is important in estimating the extent of orbital and possibly intracranial injury. Imaging studies should be routinely obtained (Fig. 9–4). Although the ocular damage may be assessed with ultrasonography, orbital and cranial injury is better delineated with computed tomography (CT) or magnetic resonance imaging (MRI) (Fig. 9–5). In general, MRI is superior to CT for the detection of nonmetallic foreign bodies. This is particularly true of radiolucent material such as dry wood, which may have the same CT density as orbital fat and air.[16] However, MRI is contraindicated when a ferromagnetic foreign body is suspected, as these foreign bodies may shift within the tissues subjected to a magnetic field and potentially cause visual loss.[17]

Because of the potential for intracranial brain injury, a neurologic examination is an essential part of the workup. The patient should be observed closely, even with no immediate evidence that the cranial cavity has been penetrated.

Table 9–1 Mechanisms of Direct Optic Nerve
Injury

Lacerations	*Vascular Insufficiency*
Incomplete	Ischemia
Complete	Infarction
Bone Deformation and/or Fracture	*Hemorrhage*
Optic canal	Nerve sheath
Orbital wall	Intraneural
Anterior clinoid process	

Treatment of patients with direct optic nerve injury is generally supportive. Patients must be evaluated individually to establish the extent of optic nerve injury. Not all such injuries result in permanent blindness, even in the setting of a nonrecordable visual evoked response immediately after trauma.[13]

9-3 INDIRECT OPTIC NERVE INJURY

Indirect optic nerve injury is the most common form of traumatic optic neuropathy.[18] Yet the literature has been confusing and controversial in both the understanding and the management of this condition. The following sections summarize current concepts of anatomic relationships, clinical findings, pathophysiologic mechanisms, and therapeutic modalities for patients with indirect optic nerve injury.

9-3-1 *Anatomic Considerations*. The intracanalicular portion of the optic nerve is the segment most apt to be damaged by indirect trauma (see Fig. 1–7). This portion of the optic nerve is 6–10 mm in length and 4 mm in cross section. The optic canal lies between the two bases of the lesser sphenoid wing. From the orbit, the canal extends posteriorly and medially and averages 9.22 mm in length (range 5.5–11.5 mm).[16] Contents of the optic canal include the optic nerve, meninges, the

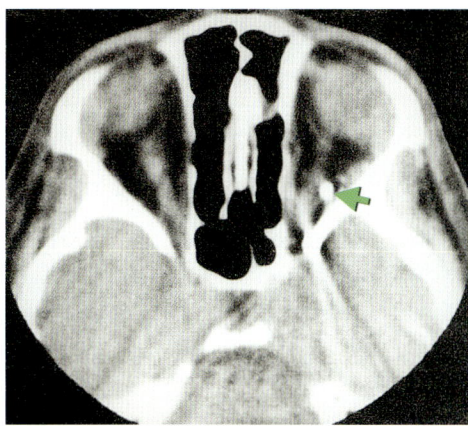

Figure 9–4. Axial orbital CT scan demonstrates shotgun pellet (arrow) lateral to the left optic nerve at the orbital apex.

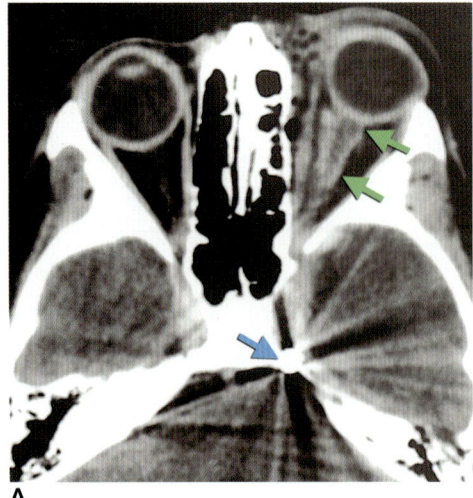 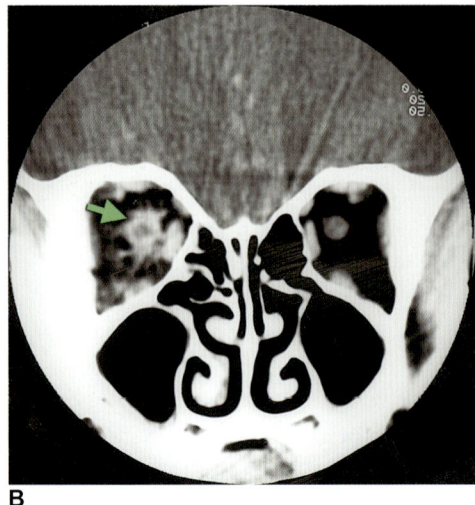

A   B

Figure 9–5. Accidental shooting of 14-year-old boy in left medial orbit. (A) Axial CT scan shows BB pellet (blue arrow) in the left parasellar region and effusion within the left optic nerve sheath (green arrows). (B) Coronal CT scan confirms trauma to the orbital portion of the left optic nerve (arrow).

ophthalmic artery, and the postganglionic sympathetic fibers. Within the canal, the optic nerve is immobilized by its dura, which is fixed to the surrounding periosteum and bone (see Fig. 1–7). Blood supply to the optic nerve is from penetrating pial branches arising from the ophthalmic and carotid arteries. The medial wall of the optic canal is on average 0.21 mm thick, and the distal portion of the canal (closest to the orbit) is the narrowest in cross section and has the thickest bony walls. About 4% of normal patients have no bone medially, and the nerve is separated from the sphenoid sinus only by sinus mucosa and dura.[19]

9-3-2 *Types of Indirect Injuries.* The intracanalicular portion of the optic nerve is the segment most frequently damaged following closed head trauma. Occasionally, the intraocular segment is damaged and ophthalmoscopic findings are then evident. In general, the intraorbital portion is spared because of its relative laxity within the orbit and the protection offered by surrounding orbital fat and extraocular muscles. Similarly, the intracranial portion of the nerve is rarely involved because of its relative mobility within the head.

From a practical standpoint, indirect optic nerve injuries can be divided into two categories: (1) anterior, in which the funduscopic abnormalities are present, and (2) posterior, in which the fundus initially appears normal.

9-3-2-1 *Anterior Indirect Injury.* Anterior injury denotes involvement of the intraocular optic nerve (optic disc) and that portion of the intraorbital segment containing the central retinal artery. In all instances, ophthalmoscopic abnormalities are visible. There may be a central retinal artery occlusion with an edematous retina, a pale optic disc, threadlike arterioles, visible sludging of blood flow in the retinal vasculature, and a cherry-red spot in the macula. In other instances, retinal vascular spasm without thrombosis has been observed.[20] Traumatic ischemic optic neuropathy with a diffusely swollen disc but the remainder of the fundus normal in appearance has also been reported.[21,22] Fluorescein angiography in these cases supports compromise of the posterior ciliary arterial circulation. Anterior marginal tears of the optic disc are characterized by optic nerve dysfunction, with a hemorrhage at the disc margin that rarely exceeds more than one-third of its circumference.[20] Within 2 weeks, the hemorrhage resolves, leaving a heavily pigmented scar at the disc margin; within 1 month, disc pallor (often mild) is evident. In general, there is good correlation between the visual field defect and the visible abnormality at the disc margin. Visual acuity is variable but usually poor.

9-3-2-2 *Posterior Indirect Injury.* The diagnosis of posterior optic nerve injury is based on evidence of optic nerve dysfunction in the absence of funduscopic abnormalities on initial examination and no evidence of chiasmal injury. From 4–8 weeks after head trauma, optic disc pallor and loss of the retinal nerve fiber layer become apparent. The lesion is presumed to lie somewhere between the entry of the central retinal artery into the optic nerve and the optic chiasm.

9-3-3 *Clinical Features.* Examination of the visual system after head trauma may be difficult or impossible. Nevertheless, every effort should be made to assess visual function. In alert and verbal patients, Snellen or Rosenbaum near card acuity should be recorded. Absence of light perception should be confirmed with the indirect ophthalmoscope as a light source in all quadrants. Pupillary responses are of critical importance and should be carefully tested. If possible, afferent pupillary defects should be graded with neutral density filters. After reviewing 22 cases of optic nerve injury following head trauma, one study concluded that pupillary response to light is the most reliable sign of the extent of optic nerve injury.[23] Visual field defects typically fall into two categories: central scotoma and nerve fiber bundle defects. Discovery of a hemianopic defect, either bitemporal or homonymous, establishes the site of injury posterior to the optic nerve. Direct and indirect ophthalmoscopy should be performed to rule out local eye trauma and direct optic nerve injury. Acutely, the optic nerve should appear normal in posterior indirect optic nerve trauma. Imaging of the retinal nerve fiber layer has documented decrements that correlate with the subsequent development of optic atrophy.[24]

Visual evoked responses (VERs) may be used adjunctively to document nerve-conduction delays, especially in unresponsive patients. Using a combination of electroretinogram and VER, a group of investigators examined 75 patients with acute head injury: 38 suffered optic nerve injury.[25] There was good correlation between the initial VER and the ultimate acuity. A more recent study also supported the value of flash VER as a predictor of visual outcome.[26] In comatose patients, VER can be used to assess optic nerve function accurately; unfortunately, the availability of VER testing is limited and it is not often practical to perform VER in a setting of acute head trauma.

The presence or absence of facial and optic canal fractures should be confirmed by high-resolution thin-section CT in both the coronal and the axial planes (Fig. 9–6). The incidence of canal fractures in patients with indirect optic nerve injury is highly variable, ranging from 1%–92%.[2,27–29]

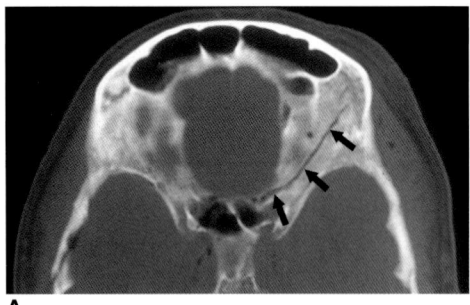
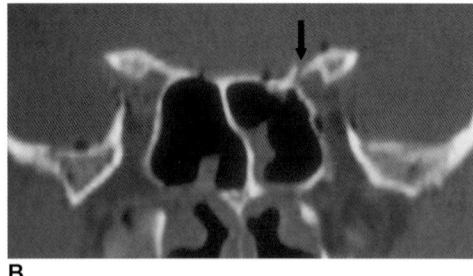

Figure 9–6. Thin-section CT scan demonstrates skull fracture (arrows) involving left optic canal on axial (A) and coronal (B) images. (Courtesy of Michael Vaphiades, DO.)

The presence or absence of fractures confirmed by CT helps direct therapy in instances of obvious bony-fragment compression of the nerve. CT may also demonstrate other abnormalities, including orbital lesions, foreign bodies, subperiosteal fluid collections, and optic nerve sheath hematomas, which may necessitate fenestration.

Although recognized as inferior to CT for evaluating bone, MRI is valuable in demonstrating the intracanalicular and intracranial segments of the optic nerve as well as soft tissue detail.

In the event of anterior optic nerve injury, the patient should also undergo orbital ultrasound. There have been reports of cases in which progressive visual loss after head trauma was associated with venous obstructive retinopathy and progressive enlargement of the optic nerve sheath on B-scan ultrasonography and CT.[30,31] In these cases, vision improved following sheath fenestration of the intraorbital optic nerve.

9-3-4 *Pathophysiology.* The sequence of events that leads to optic nerve damage following indirect injury is unsettled, but vascular insufficiency is common to many theories. A normal ophthalmoscopic examination in acute traumatic optic neuropathy rules out retinal ischemia and overt damage to the central retinal artery. Shearing forces may cause rupture, thrombosis, or spasm of small arterioles, hemorrhage, and infarction. Subsequently, edema of the nerve and compression within the optic canal develop. This compression further compromises vessels that supply nutrients. Alternatively, shearing forces on the nerve may cause edema, which in turn causes elevated intracanalicular pressure, compression, and ischemia without an intermediary vascular event. A postmortem examination of the optic nerve in one such case was done 4 days after injury; it revealed a totally infarcted nerve without evidence of vascular occlusion.[32] A histopathologic examination of 22 cases concluded that damage to small nutrient vessels is important in disease pathogenesis.[23]

Although the microscopic events outlined above probably occur in some form in almost all cases, certain optic nerve injuries may be less complex. Shearing forces may cause extensive hemorrhage into the optic nerve sheath, tearing or irreversible stress of nerve fibers, or contusion necrosis.

Hemorrhage also plays a role in certain cases of posterior indirect optic nerve injury. Hemorrhage may be within the nerve or within the sheath; when it occurs within the sheath, it may be intradural, subdural, or subarachnoid. The result is a hematoma causing optic nerve compression. One study reported decompression of intradural hemorrhage in two patients, resulting in minimal improvement of visual function in both.[33] Another report of four patients in whom a transfrontal approach was used found a hematoma of the optic nerve sheath in each.[34] All of the patients reportedly achieved complete recovery of vision after evacuation of the hematoma.

Holographic interferometry—an extremely sensitive technique in revealing surface perturbations on an object in response to surface loading—has been used to evaluate orbital and optic canal stress without fracture.[35] In using this technique, the investigators demonstrated that the forces applied to the frontal and malar eminences are transmitted to the area of the optic foramen. These forces alone, without fracture, were believed to be sufficient to cause compression, contusion, or stretching of the intracanalicular nerve. These data suggest that forces from frontal trauma may be transmitted to the optic nerve and its supporting structures and that deformation of surrounding bone without fracture is a potential mechanism for optic nerve injury.

No doubt vision is compromised by direct optic nerve compression from a fractured bony fragment in a small number of patients. In certain patients, resulting tears of the nerve or immediate contusion necrosis is unlikely to be amenable to treatment. Although compression by a bony fragment might be expected to be the most treatable form of indirect optic nerve trauma, only a small number of such cases have been documented in the literature.[15,32,36–38] Fractures may involve the optic canal, the anterior clinoid process, and the orbital roof. In one patient, the intracranial portion of the optic nerve was contused by a fractured and the displaced anterior clinoid process and vision did not improve after decompression.[36] Other investigations have documented cases of visual improvement after surgical removal of a compressive bony fragment.[15,39]

Although there are some reports of bony compression or hemorrhage leading to optic nerve injury, a significant number of patients fall into the category in which microscopic events subsequent to the injury induce optic neuropathy.

During the past decade, significant progress has been made in understanding the mechanisms of neuronal injury at a cellular and biochemical level. Of particular importance is the process of apoptosis, cellular death characterized by an orderly sequence of events.[40] These include DNA fragmentation, chromatin clumping, cell shrinkage, and membrane blebbing, with eventual formation of membrane–enclosed vesicles that are engulfed by neighboring cells without inciting inflammation. There is compelling evidence that apoptosis affects retinal ganglion cells after experimental optic nerve injury.[41,42] A number of pathways become active in apoptosis. (Fig. 9–7). Resultant injury is multifactoral and includes altered levels of glutamate and its excitotoxic effects, abnormal calcium fluxes, and lipid perioxidation due to free radical formation.[43] With a better understanding of these and other pathways yet to be elucidated, opportunities for therapy can be developed not only to inhibit pathways that initiate apoptosis but also to stimulate pathways that inhibit it. As may occur in stroke, there is a "penumbra" of still viable (optic nerve) axons following trauma, and being able to "rescue" this population of neurons may greatly improve the visual prognosis following traumatic optic neuropathy.

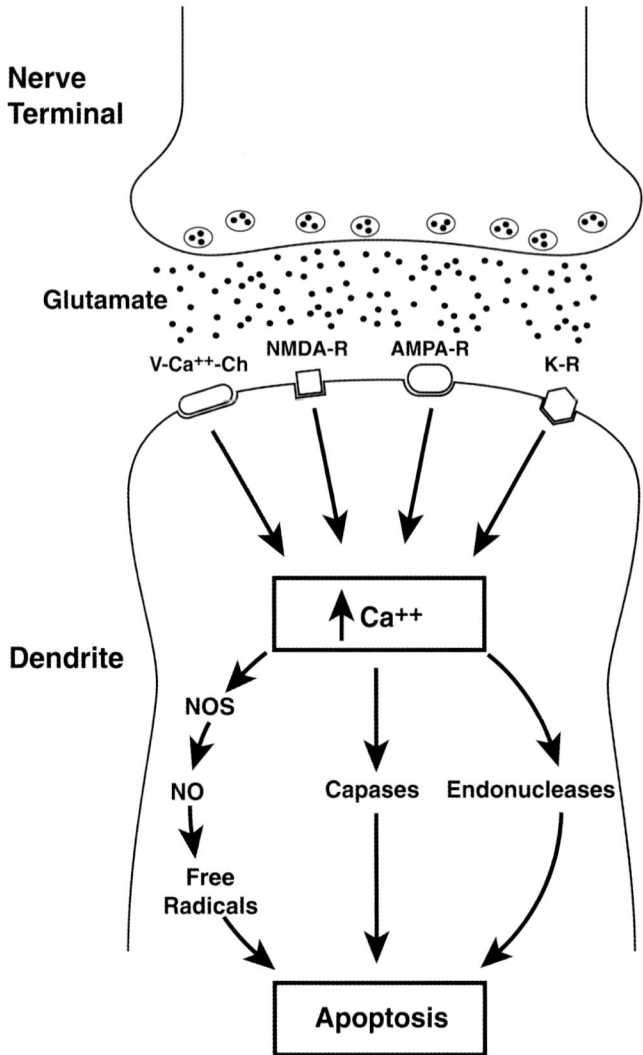

Figure 9–7. Diagram summarizing major postsynaptic intracellular pathways leading to neuronal injury and death. V-Ca++-Ch, voltage-gated calcium channel; NMDA-R, N-methyl diacetyl aspartate receptor; AMPA-R, alpha-amino-3-hydroxy-5-methyl-4-isoxazole propionate receptor; K-R, kainate receptor; CA++, calcium; NOS, nitric oxide synthetase; NO, nitric oxide.(Modified from Martin LJ. Neuronal cell death in nervous system development, disease and injury. Int J Mol Med 2001; 7: 455–478.)

9-3-5 *Management Options.* Multiple factors are operative in the development of indirect optic nerve injury. Because visual recovery occurs without intervention, it is difficult to evaluate the treatment modalities available, both medical and surgical. Tables 9–2 and 9–3 summarize reported nonsurgical and surgical results in the management of patients with indirect optic nerve trauma. It should be emphasized that none of these studies were done in a controlled fashion.

In the nonsurgical group, a significant number of patients improved spontaneously. Among the patients who underwent surgery, there was no clear trend to-

Table 9-2 Nonsurgical Therapy of Indirect Optic Nerve Injury

Study in Chronologic Order	Number of Patients	Number Improved	Number Not Improved	Comment
Davidson[44]	37	11	26	—
Turner[45]	46	23	23	—
Hooper[36]	17	5	12	—
Anderson et al.[35]	2	2	0	Megadose corticosteroids
Tang et al.[46]	13	5	8	No treatment
	5	1	4	Therapeutic dose of corticosteroids
	11	4	7	Megadose corticosteroids
Millesi et al.[47]	7	4	3	No specific treatment
	2	1	1	Intravenous corticosteroids
Lessell[2]	25	5	20	No specific treatment
	4	1	3	Corticosteroids (dosage not stated)
Wolin and Lavin[48]	4	4	0	Megadose corticosteroids in 3 patients
Seiff[49]	15	5	10	No specific treatment
	21	13	8	Megadose corticosteroids
Spoor et al.[50]	22	19	3	Megadose corticosteroids
Mauriello et al.[51]	16	9	7	Megadose corticosteroids
Chou[70]	10	0	10	—
	23	13	10	Corticosteroids
Yang[71]	18	8	10	Megadose corticosteroids
Rajmiganth[72]	44	10	34	Megadose corticosteroids
Levin[74]	9	5	4	—
	85	46	39	Corticosteroids
Tandon[76]	72	50	22	Corticosteroids

ward improved vision with one notable exception.[27] Although the exact indications and results of this study are difficult to interpret, virtually all of the 400 patients treated by transethmoidal surgical decompression of the optic nerve were stated to have improved vision. Only a few of these patients had no light perception before surgery, and most had only mildly impaired vision. The uniform improvement of the patients in this large series is unexplained.

In 1966, guidelines in considering surgical decompression of the optic nerve were proposed. The following general principles, which might add to our knowledge of unroofing the optic nerve, are now stated: (1) It should never be undertaken as an elective procedure on an unconscious patient. (2) If the loss of vision is associated with a nonreactive pupil and the loss occurred at the moment of impact, the procedure is probably contraindicated. (3) If the loss of vision or loss of pupillary response to light developed after the moment of impact, the possibility that an operation might improve the situation should be considered. (4) If it cannot be determined that the loss of vision or pupillary response to light was delayed sound judgment dictates that the best course would be to wait and watch for 4–6 days, because spontaneous improvement occurs in some such cases. If improvement does not occur, it might be reasonable to undertake the procedure.[61]

Table 9–3 Surgical Therapy of Indirect Optic Nerve Injury

Study in Chronologic Order	Number of Patients	Time Between Injury and Operation	Number Improved	Number Not Improved
Pringle[52]	3	2 to 4 weeks	0	3
Daum[53]	12	1 to 72 days	0	12
Hooper[36]	4	18 h to 18 months	1	3
Niho et al.[54]	7	5 to 263 days	5	2
Hughes[20]	5	20 hours to 2 months	0	5
Edmund and Godtfredsen[23]	6	—	1	5
Imachi et al.[37]	61	—	45	16
Niho et al.[54]	25	—	20	5
Schmaltz and Schurmann[39]	13	—	1	12
Hammer and Ambos[34]	4	Within 1 week	4	0
Fukado[27]*	400	<7 to >90 days	400	0
Goldware et al.[55]	2	36 hours to 10 weeks	2	0
Karnik et al.[56]	10	<1 week to >1 month	2	8
Brihaye[57]	56	—	7	49
Anderson et al.[35]*	4	12 to 48 hours	1	3
Tang et al.[46]	8	—	2	6
Fujitani et al.[58]	28	—	7	21
Waga et al.[59]	22	Within 21 days	11	11
Millesi et al.[47]	3	12 to 24 hours	0	3
Lessell[2]*	4	36 to 72 hours	3	1
Joseph et al.[60]*	14	1 to 5 days	11	3
Mauriello et al.[51]*	7	24 to 72 hours	3	4
Chou[70]	25*	2 to 54 days	15	10
Yang[71]	24*	—·	10	14
Rajmiganth[72]	30*	—·	11	19
Levin[74]	33*	Within 7 days	11	22
Tandon[76]	39*	3 weeks	22	17
Lubben[77]	52*	4 h to 14 days	30	22
Girard[78]	11	1 to 92 days	8	3

*Corticosteroids were used as well.

Surgical decompression can be accomplished in many ways, including transcranial, transorbital, transethmoidal, transantral-transethmoidal, and endonasal-transethmoidal approaches. The rationale for surgical treatment is simple: Visual loss from compressive optic neuropathy is reversible; therefore, to the extent that edema and swelling elevate pressure within the optic canal and on the nerve, there is a compressive component, and it is this compression that surgery attempts to relieve. In other situations, where a compressive hematoma or bony fragment is identified, evacuation or removal is required to relieve compression.

All of these approaches require microsurgical technique, and the techniques that do not require craniotomy are associated with less morbidity and mortality. The need for incision of the nerve sheath in addition to canal decompression is debated without consensus among surgeons performing these procedures.

In the 1980s, a randomized prospective double-blind study evaluated the use of megadose methylprednisolone (30 mg/kg bolus plus infusion at 5.4 mg/kg/h for 23 hours) within 8 hours of acute spinal cord injury.[62] Megadose corticosteroids were found to reduce the incidence of paralysis and other disabilities significantly. Further analysis of the data suggested that methylprednisolone treatment initiated more than 8 hours after spinal cord injury may be detrimental.[63]

However, experimental data has raised concerns about the effects of megadose steriods in the treatment of traumatic optic neuropathy. Ohlsson and colleagues[64] found neither a beneficial nor harmful effect due to methylprednisolone treatment following optic nerve crush injury in the rat. Steinsapir and coworkers[65] employed the optic nerve crush model in the cat and found that methylprednisolone exacerbated axonal loss. Taken together, this clinical and experimental evidence adds an element of uncertainty for the clinician in treating patients with traumatic optic neuropathy.

9-3-6 *Visual Prognosis.* Given the conflicting data on optimal treatment of traumatic optic neuropathy, recent reports have examined a variety of factors that may help assess visual recovery. In general, two seem to be of prime importance: (1) the level of visual acuity recorded immediately following trauma[69–72] and (2) the presence of skull fracture(s).[69–72] The absence of light perception and presence of orbital/optic canal fractures are associated with a poor visual outcome. Other factors that have less consistently been associated with a poor visual prognosis include institution of corticosteriod therapy beyond 7 days of trauma,[72] lack of improvement following 48 hours of intravenous steroids, age greater than 40 years, and loss of consciousness.[73] Further study may ultimately prove beneficial in identifying particular subgroups of patients with traumatic optic neuropathy who may benefit from specific forms of therapy.

An obvious need exists for a prospective study dealing with the management and treatment of indirect optic nerve injury. The International Optic Nerve Trauma Study (IONTS) was organized to answer the following question: Does treatment of traumatic optic neuropathy with intravenous corticosteroids followed by optic canal decompression improve the visual outcome, compared to treatment with intravenous corticosteroids alone? However, patient recruitment was insufficient and the study was converted to a comparative, nonrandomized interventional study.[74] Analysis consisted of 133 patients receiving steroid treatment alone, surgery with or without steroids, or no treatment. The study failed to find benefit for either corticosteroid therapy or optic canal decompression. The study concluded that there is currently no standard of care for traumatic optic neuropathy and recommended that individualized treatment decisions be made on a case-by-case basis. What does appear clear is that measures to avoid injury and research to establish better neuroprotective strategies offer the best hope for progress in dealing with traumatic optic neuropathy.[75]

References

1. Gjerris F. Traumatic lesions of the visual pathways. In: Vinken PJ, Bruyn GW, eds. Handbook of Clinical Neurology. Amsterdam: North-Holland, 1976;24:27–57.
2. Lessell S. Indirect optic nerve trauma. Arch Ophthalmol 1989;107:382–386.

3. Salzmann M. Die Ausreissung des Sehnerven (evulsio nervei optici). Z Augenheilkd 1903;26:489–505.

4. Williams DF, Williams GA, Abrams GW, et al. Evulsion of the retina associated with optic nerve evulsion. Am J Ophthalmol 1987;104:5–9.

5. Morris WR, Osborn FD, Fleming JC; Traumatic evulsion of the globe. Ophthalmol Plast Reconstr Surg 2002;18:261–267.

6. Patton N. Self-inflicted eye injuries: a review. Eye 2004;18:867–872.

7. Sanborn GE, Gonder JR, Goldberg RE, et al. Evulsion of the optic nerve: a clinicopathological study. Can J Ophthalmol 1984;19:10–16.

8. Kline LB, McCluskey MM, Skalka HW. Imaging techniques in optic nerve evulsion. J Clin Neuroophthalmol 1988;8:281–282.

9. Walsh FB, Hoyt WF. Ocular signs of craniocerebral trauma. Clinical Neuro-Ophthalmology. 3rd ed. Baltimore: Williams & Wilkins; 1969;3:2375–2380.

10. Runyan TE. Concussive and Penetrating Injuries of the Globe and Optic Nerve. St Louis: Mosby, 1975:143–164.

11. Walsh FB, Hoyt WF. Topical diagnosis of lesions of the optic nerves. Clinical Neuro-Ophthalmology. 3rd ed. Baltimore: Williams & Wilkins; 1969;1:66–68.

12. Marouf L, Azar DT. Reversible visual loss following optic nerve injury. Ann Ophthalmol 1985;17:582–584.

13. Feist RM, Kline LB, Morris RE, et al. Recovery of vision after presumed direct optic nerve injury. Ophthalmology 1987;94:1567–1569.

14. Spoor TC, Mathog RH. Restoration of vision after optic canal decompression. Arch Ophthalmol 1986;104:804–806.

15. Kennerdell JS, Amsbaugh GA, Myers EN. Transantral-ethmoidal decompression of optic canal fracture. Arch Ophthalmol 1976;94:1040–1043.

16. Specht CS, Varga JH, Jalali MM, Delstein JP. Orbitocranial wooden foreign body diagnosed by magnetic resonance imaging: dry wood can be isodense with air and orbital fat by computed tomography. Surv Ophthalmol 1992;36:341–344.

17. Kelly WM, Paglen PG, Pearson JA, et al. Ferromagnetism of intraocular foreign body causes unilateral blindness after MR study. Am J Neuroradiol 1986;7:243–245.

18. Steinsapir KD, Goldberg RA. Traumatic optic neuropathy. Surv Ophthalmol 1994;38:487–518.

19. Maniscalco JE, Habal MB. Microanatomy of the optic canal. J Neurosurg 1978;48:402–406.

20. Hughes B. Indirect injury of the optic nerves and chiasm. Bull Johns Hopkins Hosp 1963;11:98–126.

21. Hedges TR III, Gragoudas ES. Traumatic anterior ischemic optic neuropathy. Ann Ophthalmol 1981;13:625–628.

22. Wyllie AM, McLeod D, Cullen JF. Traumatic ischaemic optic neuropathy. Br J Ophthalmol 1972;56:851–853.

23. Edmund J, Godtfredsen E. Unilateral optic atrophy following head injury. Acta Ophthalmol 1963;41:693–697.

24. Medeiros FA, Moura FC, Vessani RM, et al. Axonal loss after traumatic optic neuropathy documented by optical coherence tomography. Am J Ophthalmol 2003;135:406–108.

25. Feinsod M, Auerbach E. Electrophysiological examinations of the visual system in the acute phase after head injury. Eur Neurol 1973;9:56–64.

26. Holmes MD, Sires BS. Flash visual evoked potentials predict visual outcome in traumatic optic neuropathy. Ophthalmol Plast Reconstr Surg 2004;20:342–346.

27. Fukado Y. Results in 400 cases of surgical decompression of the optic nerve. Mod Probl Ophthalmol 1975;14:474–481.

28. Kline LB, Morawetz RB, Swaid SN. Indirect injury of the optic nerve. Neurosurgery 1984;14:756–764.

29. Noble MJ, McFadzean R. Indirect injury to the optic nerves and chiasm. Neuroophthalmology 1987;7:341–348.

30. Hupp SL, Buckley EG, Byrne SF, et al. Posttraumatic venous obstructive retinopathy associated with enlarged optic nerve sheath. Arch Ophthalmol 1984;102:254–256.

31. Guy J, Sherwood M, Day AL. Surgical treatment of progressive visual loss in traumatic optic neuropathy: report of two cases. J Neurosurg 1989;70:799–801.

32. Ramsey JH. Optic nerve injury in fracture of the canal. Br J Ophthalmol 1979;63:607–610.

33. Niho S, Yasuda K, Sato T, et al. Decompression of the optic canal by the transethmoidal route. Am J Ophthalmol 1961;51:659–665.

34. Hammer VG, Ambos E. Das traumatische Optikusscheidenhämatom und seine operative Behandlungsmöglichkeit. Klin Monatsbl Augenheilkd 1971;159:818–819.

35. Anderson RL, Panje Gross CE. Optic nerve blindness following blunt forehead trauma. Ophthalmology 1982;89:445–455.

36. Hooper RS. Orbital complications of head injury. Br J Surg 1951;39:126–138.

37. Imachi J, Inoue K, Takahashi T. Clinical and pathohistological investigations of optic nerve lesions in cases of head injuries. Jpn J Ophthalmol 1968;12:70–85.

38. Obenchain TG, Killeffer FA, Stern WE. Indirect injury of the optic nerves and chiasm with closed head injury: report of three cases. Bull Los Angeles Neurol Soc 1973;38:13–20.

39. Schmaltz B, Schürmann K. Traumatische Optikusschäden: Probleme der Ätiologie und der operativen Behandlung. Klin Monatsbl Augenheilkd 1971;159:33–40.

40. Martin LJ. Neuronal cell death in nervous system development, disease and injury. Int J Mol Med 2001;7:455–478.

41. Quigley HA, Nickells RW, Kerrigen LA, ef al. Retinal ganglion cell death in experimental glaucoma after axotomy occurs by apoptosis. Invest Ophthalmol Vis Sci 1995;36:774–786.

42. Vorwede CK, Zurakowski D, McDermott LM, ed al. Effects of axonal injury on ganglion cell survival and glutamate homeostasis. Br Res Bul 2004;62:485–490.

43. Miller NR. Optic nerve protection, regeneration, and repair in the 21st century: LVII Edward Jackson Memorial Lecture. Am J Ophthalmol 2001:132:811–818.

44. Davidson M. The indirect traumatic optic atrophies. Am J Ophthalmol 1938;21:7–21.

45. Turner JWA. Indirect injuries of the optic nerves. Brain 1943;66:140–151.

46. Tang RA, Li HK, Regner LV, et al. Traumatic optic neuropathy: analysis of 37 cases. ARVO Abstracts (Suppl to Invest Ophthalmol Vis Sci.) Philadelphia: Lippincott, 1986:102.

47. Millesi W, Hollmann K, Funder J. Traumatic lesion of the optic nerve. Acta Neurochir 1988;93:50–54.

48. Wolin MJ, Lavin PJ. Spontaneous visual recovery from traumatic optic neuropathy after blunt head injury. Am J Ophthalmol 1990;109:430–435.

49. Seiff SR. High dose corticosteroids for treatment of vision loss due to indirect injury to the optic nerve. Ophthalm Surg 1990;21:389–395.

50. Spoor TC, Hartel WC, Lensink DB, Wilkinson MJ. Treatment of traumatic optic neuropathy with corticosteroids. Am J Ophthalmol 1990;110:665–669.

51. Mauriello JA, Deluca J, Kreiger A, et al. Management of traumatic optic neuropathy: a study of 23 patients. Br J Ophthalmol 1992;76:349–352.

52. Pringle JH. Atrophy of the optic nerve following diffused violence to the skull. Br Med J 1922;2:1156–1157.

53. Daum S. Quoted by Walsh FB, Hoyt WF. Clinical Neuro-Ophthalmology. 3rd ed. Baltimore: Williams & Wilkins; 1969:2381.

54. Niho S, Niho M, Niho K. Decompression of the optic canal by the transethmoidal route and decompression of the superior orbital fissure. Can J Ophthalmol 1970;5:22–40.

55. Goldware S, Sylvester R, Baker L. Delayed post-traumatic optic neuropathy with recovery after unroofing the optic canal. Neuroophthalmology 1980;1:77–78.

56. Karnik PP, Maskati BT, Kirtane MV, Tonsekar KS. Optic nerve decompression in head injuries. J Laryngol Otol 1981;95:1135–1140.

57. Brihaye J. Transcranial decompression of the optic nerve after trauma. In: Samii M, Janetta PJ, eds. The Cranial Nerves: Anatomy, Pathology, Pathophysiology. New York: Springer-Verlag; 1981:116–124.

58. Fujitani T, Inoue K, Takahashi T, et al. Indirect traumatic optic neuropathy: visual outcome of operative and nonoperative cases. Jpn J Ophthalmol 1986;30:125–134.

59. Waga S, Kubo Y, Sakakura M. Transfrontal intradural microsurgical decompression for traumatic optic nerve injury. Acta Neurochir 1988;91:42–46.

60. Joseph MP, Lessell S, Rizzo J, Momose KJ. Extracranial optic nerve decompression for traumatic optic neuropathy. Arch Ophthalmol 1990;108:1091–1093.

61. Walsh FB. Pathological-clinical correlations. I: Indirect trauma to the optic nerves and chiasm. II: certain cerebral involvements associated with defective blood supply. Invest Ophthalmol 1966;5:433–449.

62. Bracken MB, Shepard MJ, Collins WF, et al. A randomized, controlled trial of methylprednisolone or naloxone in the treatment of acute spinal-cord injury: results of the Second National Acute Spinal Cord Injury Study. N Engl J Med 1990;322:1405–1411.

63. Coleman WP, Benzel D, Cahill DW, et al. A critical appraisal of the reporting of the National Acute Spinal Cord Injury Studies of methylprednisolone in acute spinal cord injury. J Spinal Disord 2000;13:185–199.

64. Ohlsson M, Westerkind D, Langmoen IA, Svenson M. Methylprednisolone treatment does not influence axonal regeneration or degeneration following optic nerve injury in the adult cat. J Neurol Ophthalmol 2004;24:11–18.

65. Steinsapir KD, Goldberg RA, Sinha S, Hoyda DA. Methylprednisolone exacerbates axonal less following optic nerve trauma in rats. Rest Neurol Neurosci 2000;17:157–163.

66. Bracken MB, Collins WF, Freeman DF, et al. Efficacy of methylprednisolone in acute spinal cord injury. JAMA 1984;251:45–52.

67. Braughler JM, Hall ED. Current applications of "high dose" steroid therapy for CNS injury. J Neurosurg 1985;62:806–810.

68. Volpe NJ, Lessell S, Kline LB. Traumatic optic neuropathy: diagnosis and management. Int Ophthalmol Clin 1991;31:142–156.

69. Wang BH, Robertson BC, Girotto JA, et al. Traumatic optic neuropathy: a review of 61 patients. Plast Reconstr Surg 2001;107:1655–1664.

70. Chou PI, Sadun AA, Chen YC, et al. Clinical experience in the management of traumatic optic neuropathy. Neuroophthalmology 1996;16:325–336.

71. Yang WG, Chen CT, Tsay PK, et al. Outcomes for traumatic optic neuropathy; surgical versus nonsurgical treatment. Ann Plast Surg 2004;52:36–42.

72. Rajiniganth MG, Gupta AK, Gupta A, Bapuraj JR. Traumatic optic neuropathy: visual outcome following combined therapy protocol. Arch Otolaryngol Head Neck Surg 2003;129:1203–1206.

73. Carta A, Ferrigno L, Salvo M, et al. Visual progress after indirect traumatic optic neuropathy. J Neurol Neurosurg Psychiatry 2003;74:246–248.
74. Levin LA, Beck RW, Joseph MP, et al. The treatment of traumatic optic neuropathy. The international optic nerve trauma study. Ophthalmology 1999;106:1268–1277.
75. Sarkies N. Traumatic optic neuropathy. Eye 2004;18:1122–1125.
76. Tandon DA, Thakar A, Mahapatra AK, Gosh P. Trans-ethmoidal optic nerve decompression. Clin Otolayngol 1994;19:98–104.
77. Lubben B, Stoll W, Grenzebach U. Optic nerve decompression in the comatose and conscious patients after trauma. Laryngoscope 2001;111:320–328.
78. Girard BC, Bouzas EA, Lamas G, Soudant J. Visual improvement after transethmoid-sphenoid decompression in optic nerve injuries. J Clin Neuroophthalmol 1992;12:142–148.

10

Miscellaneous Optic Neuropathies

LANNING B. KLINE

S ome forms of optic nerve disease do not conform to any of the usual clinical categories. These disorders may be associated with a systemic disease (e.g., diabetes mellitus) or a therapeutic modality (e.g., radiation therapy) or may be of unknown cause (e.g., papillophlebitis). An understanding of these entities is important for the general ophthalmologist.

10-1 RADIATION OPTIC NEUROPATHY

Delayed necrosis of the optic nerves and chiasm is a well-recognized complication of radiotherapy. This was initially described following fractionated external beam radiotherapy and more recently after single-dose stereotactic radiosurgery.[1] Although most frequently seen after radiation for pituitary adenoma, radiation optic neuropathy (RON) has been reported after radiotherapy for a variety of other neoplasms, including meningioma, craniopharyngioma, metastatic carcinoma, hypothalamic glioma, and malignant tumors of the paranasal sinuses.

Review of the literature supports a consistent clinical profile of radiation optic neuropathy.[2–7] It occurs months or years following completion of radiation therapy, usually within 3 years, with a peak incidence of 1–1.5 years. Visual loss generally occurs in one eye and is acute in onset. Frequently, vision is lost in the other eye weeks or months later. The degree of visual loss is usually profound and may lead to total blindness. Although the pattern of visual field loss may implicate a chiasmal syndrome (bitemporal hemianopia), most patients develop field abnormalities typical of optic nerve involvement: central scotomas and defects of the nerve fiber bundle. Initial funduscopic examination rarely demonstrates optic disc edema.

Rather, the optic disc is either normal or appears pale due to preexisting compression of the anterior visual pathway. If it is initially normal in appearance, the affected optic nerve becomes pale within 8 weeks of visual loss.

The precise pathophysiologic mechanism of radiation optic neuropathy remains unclear. The primary pathologic finding is tissue ischemia secondary to progressive obliterative endarteritis of the microvasculature. Typically, blood vessels are thickened and have the waxy, hyaline appearance of fibrinoid necrosis. Endothelial proliferation is common, and occasionally these cells may actually occlude the vessel lumen. In addition to these vascular changes and areas of necrosis, demyelination and reactive gliosis are typically found.

Neuroimaging is essential in the diagnosis of radiation optic neuropathy, both to exclude potential tumor recurrence and to detect typical radiographic changes. Although computed tomography (CT) does not consistently image the entire anterior visual pathways, surrounding brain tissue may exhibit radiation damage. with minimal contrast enhancement, these damaged tissues are found to include areas of decreased density with or without mass effect. Reports of magnetic resonance imaging (MRI) in radiation optic neuropathy have revealed consistent findings of enlargement of the optic nerves and chiasm as well as focal enhancement following intravenous gadolinium (Fig. 10–1).[8,9]

A number of treatment parameters employed with external beam radiotherapy have been assessed for their potential role in the development of delayed cerebral radionecrosis. Risk factors include total dose, daily fractional dosage, time-dose fractionation factor, nominal standard dose, and adjunctive chemotherapy. Nevertheless, no single factor is predictive of this complication.

In a similar fashion, potential risk factors for RON have been examined with single-dose stereotactic radiosurgery. Even with improved visualization of intracranial structures using MRI (rather than CT) coupled with advanced computer software to delineate the boundaries of radiation effect, there remains a 1%–2% risk of RON.[10] Current literature suggests that the delivery doses higher than 10

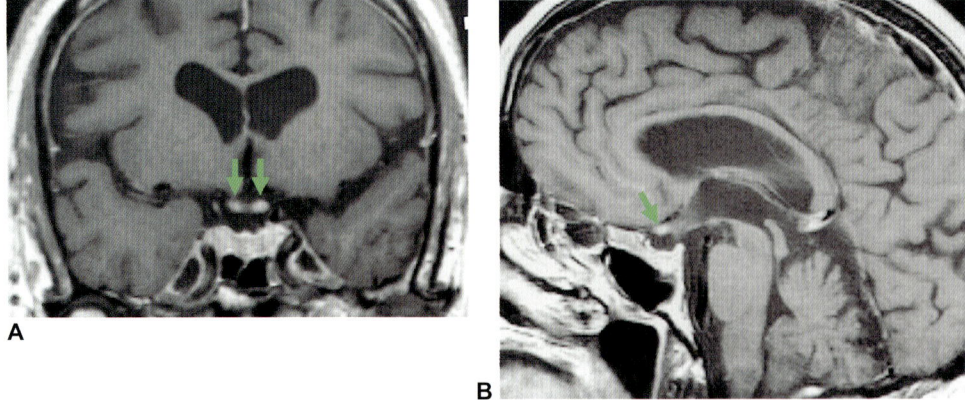

Figure 10–1. Radiation optic neuropathy. MRI scans following intravenous gadolinium. (A) Coronal scan demonstrates enhancement of intracranial optic nerves (arrows). (B) Sagittal scan shows enhancement of optic chiasm (arrow).

Gy in one fraction to the optic nerve or chiasm poses a significant risk of radiation damage.[11,12]

Treatment of delayed radionecrosis of the central nervous system has been generally unsuccessful. Although high-dose systemic corticosteroids and anticoagulants have been used, neither has led to visual improvement.[6] Hyperbaric oxygen has been reported to improve vision,[13,14] but other authors question the validity of these results.[7]

10-2 NEURORETINITIS

In 1916, Leber described patients with a triad of visual loss, optic disc edema, and macular star formation.[15] The majority of these patients recovered vision, and no identifiable cause could be found.

In the late 1970s, Gass, having demonstrated that neuroretinitis is an inflammatory optic neuropathy with secondary retinal changes, applied the term *neuroretinitis*.[16] He reported that the condition most frequently occurred in children and young adults, many of whom had had a viral illness, generally of the respiratory tract, a few weeks before the onset of visual symptoms. Subsequent reports[17–19] have shown that a large portion of cases of neuroretinitis are associated with a particular infectious agent (Table 10–1), whereas others remained unexplained. In the latter setting, the condition is called *Leber's idiopathic stellate neuroretinitis*.[20–23]

Acuity loss may be mild or severe, to the light perception level. Often the affected eye has an afferent pupillary defect, with central visual field loss. Up to one-third of cases may be bilateral. In general, the visual prognosis is excellent, with more than 90% of patients recovering acuity of 20/20 by 6 months. However, a small subgroup is left with more severe visual loss and associated optic atrophy. Neuroretinitis may rarely recur.[24]

In the acute phase, clinical examination reveals optic disc edema, ranging from mild disc swelling to severe engorgement with peripapillary retinal edema. Disc swelling is usually diffuse, although in some patients it is segmental. On initial examination, not all patients have a macular star, but it becomes apparent within the first 2 weeks of visual symptoms (Fig. 10–2). Disc edema generally resolves within 3 months, but the macular star may require 6–12 months for complete resolution. These fundus findings usually resolve with no sequelae, although two residual abnormalities have been reported: small subfoveal retinal pigment epithelial defects and optic disc pallor.

Stellate maculopathy is a nonspecific clinical finding that consists of a pattern of exudates radiating from the macula and ranging from discrete dots to dense divergent streaks. This star formation results from leakage of protein and lipid-rich exudate from deep capillaries of the optic disc into the subretinal space and outer plexiform layer of the retina.[16] Fluorescein angiography reveals dye leakage from optic nerve capillaries, but the retinal vasculature is normal.

Multiple focal chorioretinal lesions have been reported infrequently in idiopathic cases (Leber's stellate neuroretinitis).[22,23] The lesions appear as small, slightly elevated, and yellow-white at the level of the deep retina or Bruch's membrane and

Table 10–1 Causes of Neuroretinitis

Infectious

Bacterial
  Cat-scratch disease
  Syphilis
  Lyme disease
  Tuberculosis
Viral
  Influenza
  Rubella
  Measles
  Mumps
  Varicella
  Hepatitis B
  Herpes simplex
Nematode
  Toxocariasis
  Diffuse unilateral subacute neuroretinitis
Protozoan
  Leptospirosis
  Giardiasis
Fungal
  Coccidiomycosis
Chlamydial
  Psittacosis

Idiopathic—Leber's stellate neuroretinitis

Miscellaneous

Sarcoidosis
Behçet's disease

choriocapillaris. They leak dye during fluorescein angiography and slowly fade, resulting in small atrophic chorioretinal scars.

The evaluation of patients with neuroretinitis begins with a careful history. Questioning should include exposure to cats and dogs and a history of sexually transmitted disease, skin rash, and viral exanthem. Travel outside the country may provide a clue to etiology, and any known systemic inflammatory disorders should be discussed.

A variety of serologic tests should be performed, including tests for *Bartonella henselae* (cat-scratch disease), syphilis, Lyme disease, and toxoplasmosis. Currently, studies to detect specific viral nucleic acids or antibodies are not recommended; they are time-consuming, expensive, and have no implications for a particular form of therapy. On occasion, cerebrospinal fluid analysis may also be required. Testing for demyelinating disease appears to be unnecessary. Most studies have shown that the presence of a macular star in a patient with optic disc edema militates strongly against the subsequent development of multiple sclerosis.[25] However, on occasion, neuroretinitis may occur in patients with established multiple sclerosis.[26]

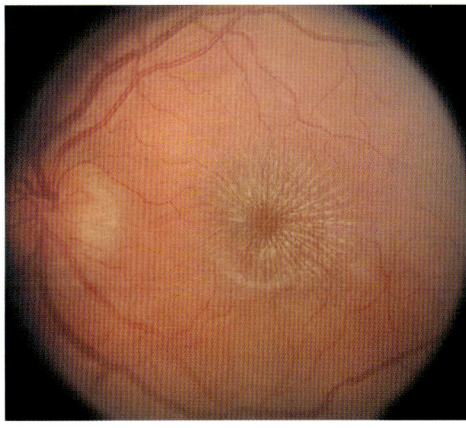

Figure 10–2. Leber's idiopathic stellate neuroretinitis. Mild optic disc edema and macular star formation in a 19-year-old man with acuity of 20/40.

Treatment of neuroretinitis depends on whether an underlying infection or inflammatory cause is identified. Appropriate antibiotic therapy is warranted when a causative organism is identified, and systemic corticosteroids or other immunosuppressive agents may be used in cases of sarcoidosis and Behçet's disease. In idiopathic cases, no treatment has proven to be of value. Periocular and systemic corticosteroids have been used, but their value remains unproven.

Neuroretinitis must be distinguished from a variety of conditions causing optic disc swelling with macular exudates. These include inflammatory papillitis, papilledema, and vascular disorders such as nonarteric ischemic optic neuropathy, diabetic eye disease, and hypertensive retinopathy.

10-3 CARCINOMATOUS OPTIC NEUROPATHY

Meningeal carcinomatosis is an unusual condition in which the meninges of the central nervous system are infiltrated by metastatic disease.[27] Such neoplastic involvement may occur as a complication of neoplasms arising within the central nervous system or as a metastatic process originating from a distant primary tumor. The clinical presentation of intracranial involvement usually includes severe headache and changes in mental status. Focal deficits may occur with cranial nerve palsies, while involvement of the spinal subarachnoid space results in spinal-root signs and symptoms, including back and extremity pain, urinary and bowel incontinence, and motor weakness.

Although the term *carcinomatous* is applied here, noncarcinomatous neoplasms may lead to an optic neuropathy, and are included under this rubric. Examples include lymphoma (Fig. 10–3), leukemia (Fig. 10–4), and melanoma. The two most common primary carcinoma sites are lung and breast.[28]

Blindness occurs in approximately one-third of reported cases of meningeal carcinomatosis[29] and may be the presenting feature.[30] When visual symptoms occur in the absence of systemic or neurologic signs, the diagnosis is usually not considered. Visual loss is typically due to tumor infiltration of the anterior visual pathways, particularly the optic nerves. Although the visual symptoms typically begin

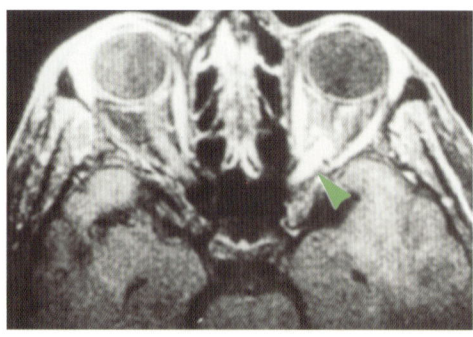

Figure 10–3. Fat-suppressed MR image with gadolinium showing enlargement and enhancement of left intraorbital and intra-canalicular optic nerve (arrowhead) in a patient with lymphoma. (Reproduced from Strominger MB, Schatz NJ, Glaser JS, Lymphomatous optic neuropathy. Am J Ophthalmol 1993;116:774–776. Published with permission from The American Journal of Ophthalmology. Copyright by The Ophthalmic Publishing Company.)

in one eye, both eyes are usually involved within a very short time. The clinical course is generally one of steady deterioration over a period of several weeks. Occasionally, total blindness may occur within a few days.

Clinical signs suggest optic nerve dysfunction, including an afferent pupillary defect, diminished color vision, and visual field changes with either a central scotoma or a defect of the nerve fiber bundle. Almost always, the optic disc appears normal at the onset of visual loss, with optic atrophy becoming apparent 6–8 weeks later. Rarely, there may be direct tumorous invasion of the optic disc, with optic disc edema (Fig. 10–5).[31,32]

Prompt diagnosis of carcinomatous optic neuropathy requires a high index of suspicion. A careful search must be made for other neurologic abnormalities. Although contrast-enhanced cranial CT may detect radiologic abnormalities, the current imaging study of choice is MRI with intravenous gadolinium. MRI can actually distinguish between invasion of the dura and invasion of the leptomeninges (arachnoid and pia).[33] Dural metastases appear as curvilinear contrast-enhanced segments underneath the inner table of the skull. The pattern of enhancement on MRI scans does

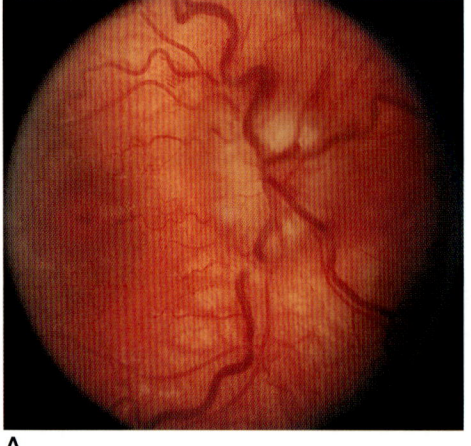

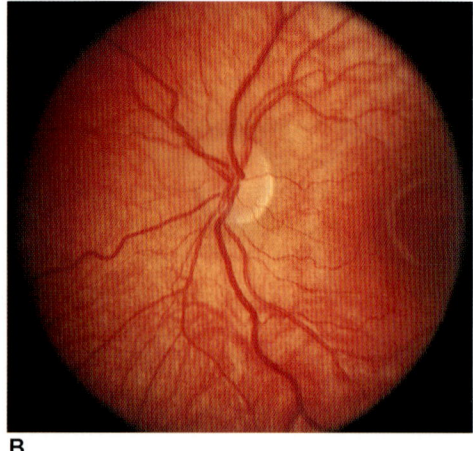

A   B

Figure 10–4. Leukemic optic neuropathy. A 9-year-old girl with acute lymphocytic leukemia reported decreased vision in her right eye. Visual acuity: 20/100 right eye, 20/20 left eye. Cerebrospinal fluid analysis detected leukemic cells and, following cranial radiotherapy and intrathecal chemotherapy, acuity returned to 20/20 in right eye. (A) Right eye, (B) left eye.

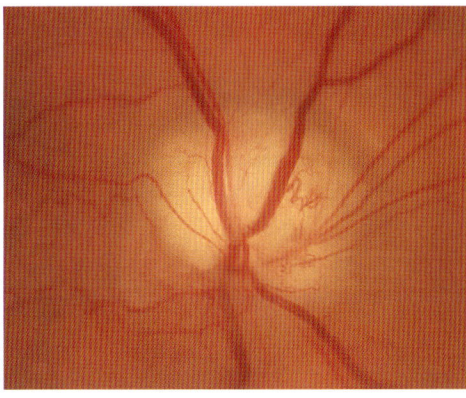

Figure 10–5. Carcinoma of lung metastatic to right optic disc. Patient presented with acuity of 20/25 and, on visual field examination, was shown to have a dense inferior altitudinal defect.

not follow the convolutions of the gyri. Conversely, leptomeningeal tumor can be diagnosed by the appearance of thin lines of contrast enhancement following the convolutions of the gyri or by small nodular deposits on the surface of the brain. In addition, MRI with gadolinium may detect thickening and abnormal enhancement of the orbital and canalicular segments of the optic nerve (see Fig. 10–3).[34]

The diagnosis of meningeal carcinomatosis can be confirmed with lumbar puncture. Cytologic examination of the cerebrospinal fluid may reveal malignant tumor cells. Characteristically, the glucose level in the spinal fluid is low and the protein level is often elevated. Yet this constellation of cerebrospinal fluid abnormalities is variable. In one series of 50 patients with leptomeningeal infiltration by systemic cancer, the yield of discovery of malignant cells in the cerebrospinal fluid increased from 45% on the first tap to 80% after several taps.[35] In this report, the cerebrospinal fluid in 1 patient yielded neoplastic cells only after the sixth spinal tap, and 2 patients never showed abnormal cells.

Precisely how the neoplasm reaches the meninges and spreads throughout them is not known. Speculation includes direct invasion of the cerebrospinal fluid through the choroid plexus and the leptomeningeal vessels or secondary invasion of spinal fluid from tumor in parenchyma or nerve roots. Other clinicopathologic studies suggest extension through the cranial and spinal foramina by way of perivascular and perineural lymphatics.[36]

Neither is it clear how leptomeningeal invasion with tumor produces neurologic signs and symptoms, including visual loss.[29,35] In some patients, there is unequivocal invasion of the underlying parenchyma of the brain, cranial nerves, spinal cord, and nerve roots; thus, direct destruction leads to neurologic findings. Yet in many of these patients, the destructive process is fairly minimal, while the clinical findings are profound. In some reported cases, there is marked meningeal tumor cuffing of blood vessels, suggesting that vascular compromise plays a role in the pathophysiology of this disorder. Hydrocephalus may develop during the clinical course of meningeal carcinomatosis, with elevation of intracranial pressure also contributing to neurologic deterioration.

Treatment of meningeal carcinomatosis is unsatisfactory.[28,35] Survival beyond 1 year of diagnosis is rare, but substantial palliation is possible with radiation therapy and chemotherapy. Caution is advised regarding empiric treatment of an optic neuropathy with a course of systemic corticosteroids; transient visual improvement may occur, only to give way ultimately to profound visual loss.[30]

Gadolinium-enhanced cranial MRI is the initial diagnostic procedure. If tumorous compression of the anterior visual pathways is excluded, the radiologist should search thoroughly for signs suggesting meningeal cancer. Since giant cell arteritis has been demonstrated to affect the retrobulbar portion of the optic nerve, patients of the appropriate age should be questioned regarding signs and symptoms of this disorder and a Westergren sedimentation rate obtained. Although retrobulbar optic neuritis should be considered in the differential diagnosis, the absence of periocular pain, the age of the patient (retrobulbar neuritis is unusual after age 50 years), and the progressive, relentless course of visual failure make this diagnosis unlikely. Lumbar puncture is a critical aspect of the patient's workup. Careful cytologic analysis of cerebrospinal fluid should be performed. Even if malignant cells are not found, other characteristics of the spinal fluid—particularly cell count, protein level, and glucose level—should be measured. Subsequent cerebrospinal fluid examinations may be required, and an evaluation for a primary source of cancer is necessary, although it may be negative.

10-4 DIABETIC PAPILLOPATHY

In 1971, a study described three patients with juvenile insulin-dependent diabetes mellitus who had optic disc swelling that was interpreted by some clinicians as papilledema.[37] This report and subsequent articles further characterized this particular entity with a variety of terms: *pseudopapilledema of juvenile diabetes mellitus*,[37] *diabetic papillitis*,[38,39] *optic neuritis in a diabetic patient*,[40] *acute disc swelling in juvenile diabetes*,[41] and *diabetic papillopathy*.[42]

Typical findings of this form of acquired disc edema in diabetes include the following:

1. Onset may occur from the second to eighth decade.
2. Individuals may have type I or type II diabetes of some chronicity.
3. The disc edema is commonly bilateral but may be unilateral.
4. The disc edema shows prominent surface telangiectatic changes without neovascularization (Fig. 10–6).
5. The edema has no correlation with the degree of diabetic retinopathy (although macular edema is often present) and is not a harbinger of progressive retinopathy or neovascularization of the disc.
6. Frequently there is no visual loss or only a modest drop in acuity to the 20/50 level. It is unusual for visual acuity to be severely impaired.
7. Visual field changes include an enlarged blind spot and an arcuate defect.
8. Generally, the visual prognosis is good, with return of normal acuity in 3 months to 1 year.
9. Visual improvement precedes the disappearance of disc swelling, usually by months.
10. The optic disc usually regains a normal appearance, although there may be diffuse or segmental atrophy.

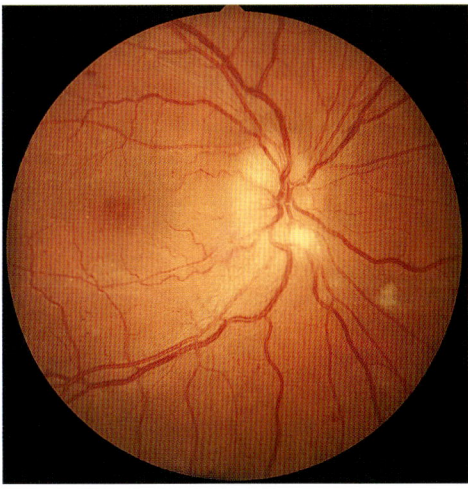

Figure 10–6. Diabetic papillopathy. Disc edema in a 32-year-old patient with juvenile-onset diabetes. Visual acuity: 20/25 with scattered nonproliferative diabetic retinopathy. (Courtesy of James A. Kimble, MD.)

The pathophysiologic mechanism of diabetic papillopathy is unknown. Currently, the favored hypothesis is microvascular disturbance of the superficial vessels of the disc, leading to impaired axoplasmic transport but not necessarily disrupted transmission of the visual impulse. Thus, the patient may retain good central acuity. Other possible contributors to this optic neuropathy include the size of the scleral canal, the "crowdedness" of the optic nerve head, and diabetes-specific factors such as prolonged hyperglycemia, failed glucose utilization, and chronic relative hypoxia.

To some degree, diabetic papillopathy is a diagnosis of exclusion. The two most common optic neuropathies to be considered in the differential diagnosis are optic disc neovascularization and papilledema associated with elevated intracranial pressure. In diabetic papillopathy, the dilated capillaries are within the disc and retina and have a radial orientation; neovascularization of the disc is preretinal, and new vessels follow a random course. Neovascularization of the disc usually appears in patients with more advanced diabetic retinopathy, whereas these signs are minimal in patients with diabetic papillopathy. Fluorescein angiography cannot be used to distinguish neovascularization of the disc from diabetic papillopathy because vessels in both conditions are permeable to fluorescein.

Differentiating diabetic papillopathy (particularly if bilateral) from papilledema may require a neurologic workup. In addition to careful neurologic examination, the patient requires neuroimaging studies to exclude an intracranial mass. If the intracranial contents appear normal, lumbar puncture with quantitation of opening pressure and cerebrospinal fluid analysis must be performed to exclude pseudotumor cerebri. Other optic nerve disorders to be considered include congenital pseudopapilledema, inflammatory optic neuritis, ischemic optic neuropathy, and autoimmune optic neuritis.

The visual prognosis of diabetic papillopathy is generally good.[42] Low-molecular-weight dextran, heparin, and systemic corticosteroids have all been tried,[37] but clear-cut efficacy for any of these agents has not been established. Recently, an uncontrolled observational study reported that the use of periocular corticosteroids may shorten the duration of diabetic papillopathy.[43]

The ophthalmologist should be able to recognize the condition of diabetic papillopathy and to counsel the patient appropriately. In addition, the ophthalmologist should alert colleagues in neurology and neurosurgery of its importance. Awareness of this entity may spare patients unnecessary neurologic evaluation.[41]

10-5 PAPILLOPHLEBITIS

In 1961, a study reported six patients with a benign, unilateral, and nearly asymptomatic venous occlusive disease in which edema of the optic disc was the outstanding feature.[44] The condition was termed *retinal vasculitis*.

Five years later, a second report described five additional patients and summarized the major clinical features[45]:

1. Unilateral disc edema
2. Young (usually under 50 years), healthy adults
3. Vague visual complaints (e.g., mistiness, grayness, black spots), with acuity usually no worse than 20/30
4. No relative afferent pupillary defect
5. Enlarged blind spot the only visual field abnormality
6. Striking dilation and tortuosity of retinal veins (Fig. 10–7)
7. Spontaneous, usually complete recovery within 6–18 months
8. Visible sequelae of perivenous sheathing of large veins in the posterior fundus and dilated venules over the surface of the optic disc (Fig. 10–8)

Both reports suggested that the major abnormality was impairment of venous drainage through the central retinal vein. Speculation arose that such an occlusion was probably initiated by a phlebitis of retinal veins in and about the optic nerve head. Thus, the designation *retinal vasculitis* was regarded as too general and the term *papillophlebitis* was proposed.[45]

Subsequently, a report on "retinal and papillary vasculitis" was published.[46] This study asserted a spectrum of severity in this group of conditions, with the poorer

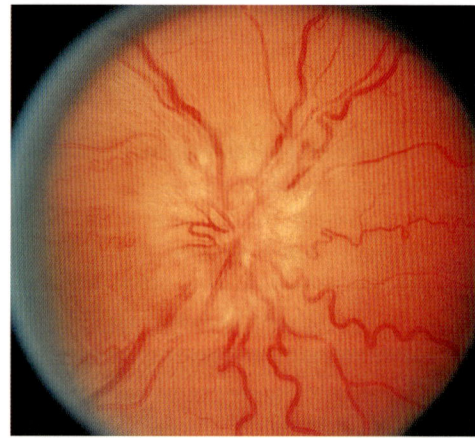

Figure 10–7. Papillophlebitis. Optic disc edema with engorgement and tortuosity of the retinal venous system in a 28-year-old woman. Visual acuity: 20/30.

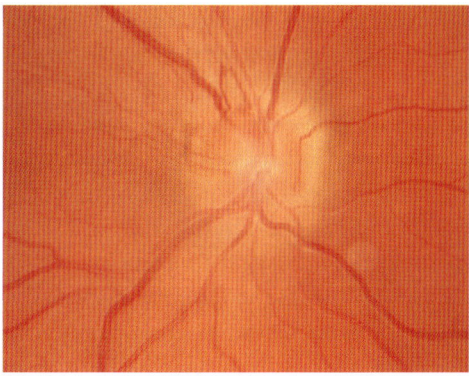

Figure 10–8. After resolution of optic disc edema in another patient with papillophlebitis, vascular changes of the optic nerve head and peripapillary retina persist. Visual acuity: 20/20.

visual prognosis occurring in patients who have associated systemic diseases such as hypertension. Other clinical and angiographic studies support this concept.[47]

Histopathologic studies in cases of papillophlebitis demonstrate an inflammatory component to this condition. Two investigations have shown round-cell infiltration of the venular walls.[46,48] These cells collect in the basement membrane of the vessel and show little tendency to exudate into adjacent tissue. In addition to an extensive phlebitis, there is occlusion of many small arterioles. The cause of this inflammatory process is unknown. In addition, papillophlebitis has been reported during pregnancy and in association with factor V Leiden and prothrombin G20210A mutations.[49]

The development of unusual vascular channels on the surface of the optic disc is probably related to the chronicity of impaired venous drainage. As one study demonstrated, some of the perioptic venous channels drain directly into the choroidal circulation (cilioretinal vein).[45] Although papillophlebitis is worrisome due to its clinical appearance and chronicity, the process is self-limited and usually with no functional residua. Therapy appears to be unnecessary; when corticosteroids and heparin have been used, they have not been convincingly effective.

10-6 OPTIC PERINEURITIS

Optic perineuritis (OPN), also known as perioptic neuritis, is a noninfectious inflammatory disorder involving the meninges of the optic nerve. It is felt to represent a form of idiopathic orbital inflammation, the specific target being the optic nerve sheath. Although most cases are isolated and of unknown cause, OPN may rarely be associated with a systemic inflammatory disease such as Wegener's granulomatosis and giant cell arteritis.[50]

Patients with OPN generally range from the third to seventh decades of life and complain of visual blurring associated with periocular pain.[51] At presentation, acuity is variably affected (20/20 to light perception), an afferent pupillary defect is present, visual field abnormalities are typically arcuate (nerve fiber bundle), but central or paracentral scotomas may be detected. The optic disc may appear swollen or normal. Visual decline generally occurs over several weeks. If the inflammatory process involves the extraocular muscles, ocular motility will be affected and the patient may complain of diplopia. Similarly, if inflammation involves the eyelids, ptosis may be found.

Neuroimaging of patients with OPN is essential in establishing the correct diagnosis.[51,52] MRI with orbital views, fat suppression, and gadolinium administration demonstrates a characteristic pattern of enhancement around the optic nerve (Fig. 10–9). On occasion, the nerve itself will enhance, presumably due to extension of the inflammatory process along intraneural pial septa. In addition, there may be subtle enhancement of the orbital fat and the extraocular muscles. CT scanning does not provide adequate spatial resolution to distinguish perineural from intraneural enhancement; indeed, before the advent of MRI, this limitation of CT created difficulty in distinguishing OPN from meningioma of the optic nerve sheath.[53]

Histopathologic study of specimens in patients with OPN reveals marked thickening of perioptic meninges.[51] Fibrosis is generally present, with a chronic, at times granulomatous cellular infiltrate. The inflammatory process may extend into the adjacent portion of the optic nerve and orbital fat. The cellular infiltrate is com-

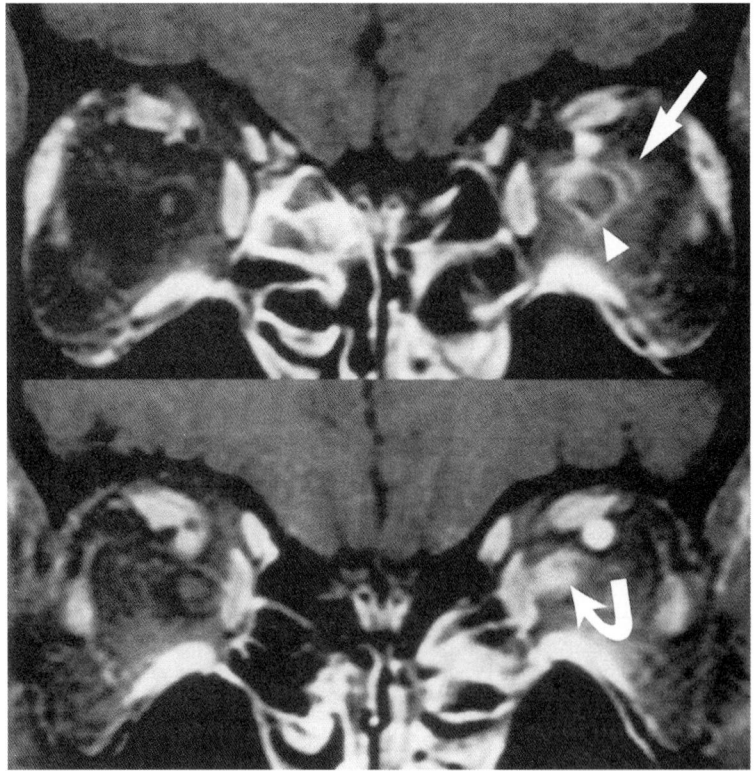

Figure 10–9. Optic perineuritis. Coronal projection of a contrast-enhanced T1-weighted MR image demonstrates abnormal enhancement of the left optic nerve sheath (arrowhead), perineural fat (straight arrow), and optic nerve (bent arrow, below). (Reproduced from Fay AM, Kane SA, Kazim M, et al. Magnetic resonance imaging of optic perineuritis. J Neuroophthalmol 1997;17:247–249.)

posed primarily of lymphocytes and may be associated with a vasculitis of small optic nerve vessels.

In almost all cases, patients with OPN respond promptly to systemic cortico-steroids. Initial therapy with high doses of corticosteroids are indicated. Periocular pain often resolves within hours to days. Visual function also dramatically improves; with rapid steroid tapering, however, relapses are common. Therefore therapy should be continued with gradual reduction over weeks to months to lessen the likelihood of recurrent attacks.

The visual prognosis in patients with OPN is generally excellent. The major factor affecting full visual recovery is the interval between the onset of visual loss and initiation of treatment. If attacks are recurrent, this too will worsen the visual out-come in patients with OPN.

The diagnosis of OPN is based on clinical and neuroimaging findings. An ini-tial salutary response of an optic neuropathy to corticosteroids may also be seen with infectious and neoplastic causes, including fungal infection, lymphoma, and meningeal carcinomatosis. In addition to appropriate patient evaluation, careful follow-up is mandatory to make certain one is indeed dealing with OPN.

The most likely misdiagnosis of patients with OPN is optic neuritis. Table 10–2 outlines important features to distinguish the two entities. These disorders have important prognostic and therapeutic differences. Patients with optic neuritis are at high risk of developing multiple sclerosis, while this is not the case with OPN. The use of corticosteroids has not been proven to be of any value in recovery of vision in patients with optic neuritis (see Chapter 4). Further, use of oral steroids alone increases the likelihood of subsequent attacks of optic neuritis. In contrast, steroid therapy is essential in OPN, and delay in beginning therapy may adversely affect ultimate visual recovery.

10-7 AUTOIMMUNE-RELATED RETINOPATHY AND OPTIC NEUROPATHY SYNDROME (ARRON)

The autoimmune-related retinopathy and optic neuropathy (ARRON) syndrome represents a group of patients with unexplained visual loss who demonstrate anti-bodies that are reactive with the optic nerve and/or retina.[54,55] The visual loss is typically bilateral and asymmetric, yet it may be unilateral in presentation.[55,56] In the literature, ARRON probably represents previous reported cases of steroid-responsive optic neuropathy or autoimmune-related retinopathy.[55,57]

ARRON patients present at an average age of 50 years with acute or more com-monly progressive visual loss. Acuity ranges from 20/20 to no light perception. The visual field ranges from mild to severe field constriction, and in some patients only one field is affected. The fundus is often normal in appearance. At times, optic at-rophy and retinal attenuation may be seen.

Patients with ARRON syndrome manifest electroretinographic changes similar to those of cancer-associated retinopathy, with a- and b-wave attenuation that is often detectable prior to the onset of visual failure.[54–56] The majority of ARRON patients have systemic immunologic diseases such as systemic lupus erythematosus,

Table 10-2 Features Distinguishing Optic Perineuritis from Optic Neuritis

Feature	Optic Perineuritis	Optic Neuritis
Age at onset	Broad range (36% are > 50 years old)	Usually young adults (only 15% are >50 y)
Visual field loss	Often paracentral or nerve fiber bundle defect	Usually central or nerve fiber layer defect
Time course	Progression over weeks	Progression over days
Natural history	Progressive visual loss	Spontaneous recovery
Response to corticosteroid	Prompt and dramatic; common relapse after brief treatment	Variable; uncommon relapse after stopping
Magnetic Resonance imaging scan findings	Perineural enhancement and "streaky" fat with or without extraocular muscle enhancement	Optic nerve enhancement with or without white matter brain lesions

Source: Modified from Purvin V, Kawasaki A, Jacobson DM: Optic perineuritis. Clinical and radiographic features. Arch Ophthalnol 2001; 119: 1299–1306.

rheumatoid arthritis, thyroid disease, celiac sprue, Sjögren's disease, psoriatic arthritis, and idiopathic thrombocytopenic purpura.[56]

Western blot analysis can be used to identify patients with ARRON syndrome, as many demonstrate autoantibodies reactive with a novel 22-kDa neuronal antigen present in the retina and/or optic nerve. It is yet unclear whether these antibodies are the cause of the visual loss or whether they are produced secondary to breakdown of retinal and optic nerve proteins.[54,55]

Because ARRON syndrome is newly described and often unrecognized, a consensus on treatment has yet to emerge. The basic tenet of therapy is suppression of the immune response, and multiple treatment regimens have been employed, including oral prednisone, intravenous methylprednisolone, immunosuppressive therapy, plasma exchange, and intravenous immunoglobulin. No single therapy has proven consistently effective. It is important to realize that acuity and field may not return to normal; often the most that can be expected is prevention of further visual deterioration.

10-8 NONGLAUCOMATOUS OPTIC DISC CUPPING

Glaucoma is the most common optic neuropathy encountered by the ophthalmologist. The diagnosis is not difficult when a patient presents with elevated intraocular pressure, arcuate and paracentral visual field defects, and an increased cup-to-disc ratio. In addition, the designation *normal-tension glaucoma* has been applied in patients who have no sign of increased intraocular pressure but do have cupped discs and progressive prechiasmal visual field loss with no other discernible cause for optic nerve disease.

Yet another clinical scenario involves acquired disc excavation due to other diseases of the optic nerve.[58] Several such examples have been collected under the rubric *pseudoglaucoma*, including cases of chiasmal tumors, syphilitic optic neuritis, congenital disc anomalies, and compression of the optic nerve by sclerotic carotid arteries.[59,60] This concept subsequently has been expanded to include other forms of ischemic[61] and compressive[62,63] optic neuropathy.

In addition to measuring intraocular pressure, the clinician can use several guidelines to distinguish glaucomatous from nonglaucomatous optic disc cupping. Some investigators have concluded that measuring Snellen acuity, pupillary reactions, and visual fields is essential in this clinical differentiation.[63] In general, visual acuity is spared until late in the course of advanced glaucoma. Thus, loss of acuity out of proportion to the extent of optic nerve cupping is suggestive of some other optic neuropathy. With asymmetric glaucomatous cupping, an afferent pupillary defect may be detected. But the presence of a Marcus Gunn pupil without asymmetric cupping suggests a nonglaucomatous rather than a glaucomatous causation. Visual field testing also contributes invaluable information regarding the potential cause of optic disc cupping. The same study found that most patients with nonglaucomatous damage had chiasmal field loss (bitemporal or junctional scotomas) rather than the arcuate or paracentral defects that are typical of glaucoma.[63] In compressive lesions of the anterior visual pathways, the loss of visual acuity is typically out of proportion to the extent of the field loss, and cupping of the optic disc is rarely advanced. This disparity should direct the clinician to a nonglaucomatous cause for the visual loss.

Two ophthalmoscopic features which may prove helpful in differentiating glaucomatous versus nonglaucomatous cupping are[62]:

1. Pallor of the neuroretinal rim, which indicates nonglaucomatous damage. This sign consists of pallor within the rim and outside the excavation—in other words, pallor of the nonexcavated rim (Fig. 10–10).
2. Focal or diffuse obliteration of the neuroretinal rim (i.e., cupping that extends to the margin of the optic disc), which is seen only in glaucoma.

In a further attempt[64] to determine which patients with optic nerve cupping yet normal intraocular pressure may require neuroimaging, the following factors may suggest a neurologic cause:

1. age younger than 50 years
2. visual acuity poorer than 20/40
3. hemianopic (vertically aligned) visual field defects
4. optic nerve pallor in excess of cupping

Histopathologic study of nonglaucomatous optic disc cupping is limited. In one study, disc cupping was caused by an aneurysm arising at the junction of the ophthalmic and internal carotid arteries.[65] Compression of the distal optic nerve led to atrophy of the axons and sufficient collapse of glial support to cause a vertically elongated cup resembling glaucomatous change. However, glial cell loss, which frequently accompanies glaucomatous damage, was not seen.

In summary, the clinician must be alert to the occurrence of nonglaucomatous disc cupping, which may occur with inflammatory, ischemic, or compressive optic

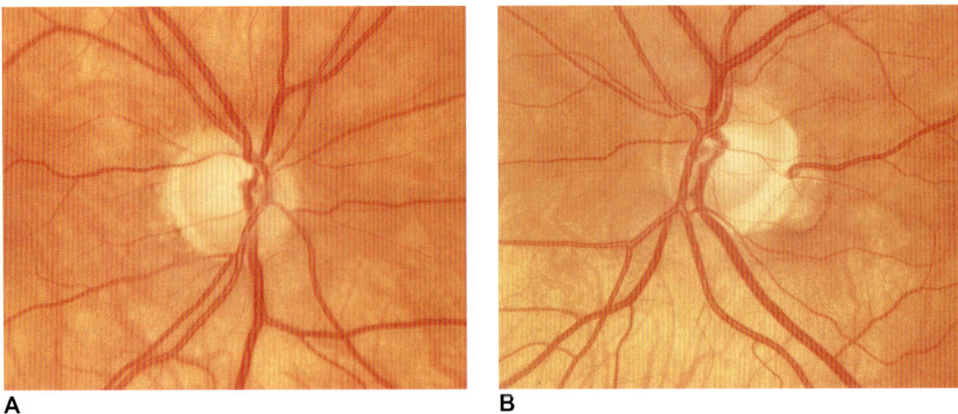

A   **B**

Figure 10–10. Nonglaucomatous optic disc cupping. (A) Optic disc cupping and temporal pallor in the right eye of a 47-year-old woman with a right internal carotid–ophthalmic artery aneurysm. (B) The left optic nerve appears to be normal. Visual acuity: 20/40 right eye, 20/20 left eye.

nerve disorders. Careful ophthalmoscopic evaluation is essential, looking at the contours of the neuroretinal rim and for the presence of pallor extending beyond the region of cupping. In addition, Snellen acuity, pupillary reactions, and visual field findings must be assessed. Only after all this information is considered can a diagnosis be formulated and appropriate patient evaluation instituted.

References

1. Girkin CA, Comey CH, Lunsford LD, et al. Radiation optic neuropathy after stereotactic radiosurgery. Ophthalmology 1997;104:1634–1643.
2. Schatz NJ, Lichtenstein S, Corbett JJ. Delayed radiation necrosis of the optic nerves and chiasm. In: Glaser JS, Smith JL, eds. Neuro-ophthalmology. (Symposium of University of Miami and Bascom Palmer Eye Institute.) St Louis: Mosby, 1975;8:131–139.
3. Harris JR, Levene MB. Visual complications following irradiation for pituitary adenomas and craniopharyngiomas. Radiology 1976;120:162–171.
4. Atkinson AB, Allen IV, Gordon DS, et al. Progressive visual failure and acromegaly following external pituitary irradiation. Clin Endocrinol 1979;10:469–479.
5. Hammer HM. Optic chiasmal radionecrosis. Trans Ophthalmol Soc UK 1983;103:208–211.
6. Kline LB, Kim JY, Ceballos R. Radiation optic neuropathy. Ophthalmology 1985;92:1118–1126.
7. Roden D, Bosley TM, Fowble B, et al. Delayed radiation injury to the retrobulbar optic nerves and chiasm: clinical syndrome and treatment with hyperbaric oxygen and corticosteroids. Ophthalmology 1990;97:346–351.
8. Guy J, Mancuso A, Quisling RG, et al. Gadolinium-DTPA-enhanced magnetic resonance imaging in optic neuropathies. Ophthalmology 1990;97:592–599.
9. Zimmerman CF, Schatz NJ, Glaser JS. Magnetic resonance imaging of radiation optic neuropathy. Am J Ophthalmol 1990;110:389–394.
10. Stafford SL, Pollock BE, Leavitt JA, et al. A study on the radiation tolerance of the optic nerves and chiasm after stereotactic radiosurgery. Int J Radiat Oncol Biol Phys 2003;55:1177–1181.

11. Leber KA, Bergloff J, Pendl G. Dose-response tolerance of the visual pathways and cranial nerves of the cavernous sinus to stereotactic radiosurgery. J Neurosurg 1998;88:43–50.

12. Ove R, Kelman S, Amin PP, Chin LS. Preservation of visual fields after peri-sellar gamma-knife radiosurgery. Int J Cancer 2000;90:343–350.

13. Guy J, Schatz NJ. Hyperbaric oxygen in the treatment of radiation-induced optic neuropathy. Ophthalmology 1986;93:1083–1088.

14. Borruat FX, Schatz NJ, Glaser JS, et al. Visual recovery from radiation-induced optic neuropathy: the role of hyperbaric oxygen therapy. J Clin Neuroophthalmol 1993;13:98–101.

15. Leber T. Die pseudonephritischen Netzhauterkrankungen, die Retinitis stella: die Purtschersche Netzhautaffektion nach schwerer Schadelverletzung. In: Graefe AC, Saemisch T, eds. Graefe-Saemisch Handbuch der Gesamten Augenheilkunde, 2nd ed. Leipzig: Engelmann,; 1916:chap 10.

16. Gass JD. Diseases of the optic nerve that may simulate macular disease. Trans Am Acad Ophthalmol Otolaryngol 1977;83:763–770.

17. Maitland CG, Miller NR. Neuroretinitis. Arch Ophthalmol 1984;102:1146–1150.

18. Golnik KC, Marotto ME, Fanous MM, et al. Ophthalmic manifestations of *Rochalimaea* species. Am J Ophthalmol 1994;118:145–151.

19. Newsom RW, Martin TJ, Wailasaukas B. Cat-scratch disease diagnosed serologically using an enzyme immunoassay in a patient with neuroretinitis. Arch Ophthalmol 1996;114:493–494.

20. François J, Verriest G, De Laey JJ. Leber's idiopathic stellate retinopathy. Am J Ophthalmol 1969;68:340–345.

21. Papastratigakis B, Stavrakas E, Phanouriakis C, Tsamparlakis J. Leber's idiopathic stellate maculopathy. Ophthalmologica 1981;183:68–71.

22. Carroll DM, Franklin RM. Leber's idiopathic stellate retinopathy. Am J Ophthalmol 1982;93:96–101.

23. Dreyer RF, Hopen G, Gass JD, Smith JL. Leber's idiopathic stellate neuroretinitis. Arch Ophthalmol 1984;102:1140–1145.

24. Purvin VA, Chioran G. Recurrent neuroretinitis. Arch Ophthalmol 1994;112:365–371.

25. Parmley VC, Schiffman JS, Maitland CG, et al. Does neuroretinitis rule out multiple sclerosis? Arch Neurol 1987;44:1045–1048.

26. Williams KE, Johnson LN. Neuroretinitis in patients with multiple sclerosis. Ophthalmology 2004;111:335–341.

27. Pavlidis N. The diagnostic and therapeutic management of leptomeningeal carcinomatosis. Ann Oncol 2004;15 (Suppl 4):iv285–iv291.

28. Little JR, Dale AJ, Okazaki H. Meningeal carcinomatosis: clinical manifestations. Arch Neurol 1974;30:138–143.

29. Altrocchi PA, Reinhardt PH, Eckman PB. Blindness and meningeal carcinomatosis. Arch Ophthalmol 1972;88:508–512.

30. Susac JO, Smith JL, Powell JO. Carcinomatous optic neuropathy. Am J Ophthalmol 1973;76:672–679.

31. Allen RA, Straatsma BR. Ocular involvement in leukemia and allied disorders. Arch Ophthalmol 1961;66:490–508.

32. Ellis W, Little HL. Leukemic infiltration of the optic nerve head. Am J Ophthalmol 1973;75:867–871.

33. Sze G. Diseases of the intracranial meninges: MR imaging features. Am J Roentgenol 1993;160:727–733.

34. Strominger MB, Schatz NJ, Glaser JS. Lymphomatous optic neuropathy. Am J Ophthalmol 1993;116:774–776.

35. Olson ME, Chernik NL, Posner JB. Infiltration of the leptomeninges by systemic cancer: a clinical and pathologic study. Arch Neurol 1974;30:122–137.

36. Gonzalez-Vitale JC, Garcia-Bunuel R. Meningeal carcinomatosis. Cancer 1976;37:2906–2911.

37. Lubow M, Makley TA Jr. Pseudopapilledema of juvenile diabetes mellitus. Arch Ophthalmol 1971;85:417–422.

38. Topilow A, Bisland T. Diabetes mellitus as a cause of papillitis. Am J Ophthalmol 1952;35:855–858.

39. Freund M, Carmon A, Cohen AM. Papilledema and papillitis in diabetes. Am J Ophthalmol 1965;60:18–20.

40. Skillern PG, Lokhart G. Optic neuritis and uncontrolled diabetes mellitus in 14 patients. Ann Intern Med 1959;51:468–475.

41. Barr CC, Glaser JS, Blankenship G. Acute disc swelling in juvenile diabetes: clinical profile and natural history of 12 cases. Arch Ophthalmol 1980;98:2185–2192.

42. Regillo CD, Brown GC, Savino PJ, et al. Diabetic papillopathy: patient characteristics and fundus findings. Arch Ophthalmol 1995;113:889–895.

43. Mansour AM, El-Dairi MA, Shehab MA, et al. Periocular corticosteroids in diabetic papillopathy. Eye 2005;19:45–51.

44. Lyle TK, Wybar K. Retinal vasculitis. Br J Ophthalmol 1961;45:778–788.

45. Lonn LI, Hoyt WF. Papillophlebitis: a cause of protracted yet benign optic disc edema. Eye Ear Nose Throat Mon 1966;45:62–68.

46. Cogan DC. Retinal and papillary vasculitis. In: Cant JS, ed. William MacKenzie Centenary Symposium on the Ocular Circulation in Health and Disease. St Louis: Mosby, 1969:249–269.

47. Hart CD, Sanders MD, Miller SJ. Benign retinal vasculitis: clinical and fluorescein angiographic study. Br J Ophthalmol 1971;55:721–733.

48. Appen RE, de Venecia G, Ferwerda J. Optic disk vasculitis. Am J Ophthalmol 1980;90:352–359.

49. Charakidas A, Brouzas D, Andrioti E, et al. Papillophlebitis associated with coexisting factor V Leiden and prothrombin 20210A mutations. Retina 2001; 22:239–240.

50. Nassani S, Cocito L, Arcuri T, Favale E. Orbital pseudotumor as a presenting sign of temporal arteritis. Clin Exp Rheumatol 1995;13:367–369.

51. Purvin V, Kawasaki A, Jacobson DM. Optic perineuritis. Clinical and radiographic features. Arch Ophthalmol 2001;119:1299–1306.

52. Fay AM, Kane SA, Kazim M, et al. Magnetic resonance imaging of optic perineuritis. J Neuroophthalmol 1997;17:247–249.

53. Dutton JJ, Anderson RL. Idiopathic inflammatory perioptic neuritis simulating optic nerve sheath meningioma. Am J Ophthalmol 1985; 100:424–430.

54. Keltner JL, Thirkill CE. The 22-kDa Antigen in optic nerve and retinal diseases. J Neuroophthalmol 1999;19:71–83.

55. Keltner JL. Paraneoplastic retinopathies vs. (non-cancer) autoimmune related retinopathy and optic neuropathy (ARRON syndrome). North American Neuro-Ophthalmology Society course syllabus. 2003:293–306.

56. Keltner JL, Thirkill CE, Huynh PM. Autoimmune-related retinopathy and optic neuropathy (ARRON) syndrome (abstract). J Neuroophthalmol. 2002;22:160–161.

57. Mizener JB, Kimura AE, Adamus G, et al. Autoimmune retinopathy in the absence of cancer. Am J Ophthalmol 1997;123(5):607–618.

58. Ambati BK, Rizzo JF. Nonglaucomatous cupping of the optic disc. Int Ophthalmol Clin 2001;41:139–149.

59. Dalsgaard-Nielsen E. Glaucoma-like cupping of the optic disc and its etiology. Acta Ophthalmol 1937;15:151–178.
60. Blazar HA, Scheie HG. Pseudoglaucoma. Arch Ophthalmol 1950;44:499–513.
61. Quigley H, Anderson DR. Cupping of the optic disc in ischemic optic neuropathy. Trans Am Acad Ophthalmol Otolaryngol 1977;83:755–762.
62. Trobe JD, Glaser JS, Cassady J, et al. Nonglaucomatous excavation of the optic disc. Arch Ophthalmol 1980;98:1046–1050.
63. Kupersmith MJ, Krohn D. Cupping of the optic disc with compressive lesions of the anterior visual pathway. Ann Ophthalmol 1984;16:948–953.
64. Greenfield DS, Siatkowski M, Glaser JS, et al. The cupped disc. Who needs neuro-imaging? Ophthalmology 1998;105:1866–1874.
65. Portney GL, Roth AM. Optic cupping caused by an intracranial aneurysm. Am J Ophthalmol 1977;84:98–103.

Index

Acquired immunodeficiency syndrome (AIDS), optic neuritis in, 77–78, 78f
ACTH-secreting tumors, 120–121, 122
Actin, 17
Acute disseminated encephalomyelitis (ADEM), 74
Adenomas
  chromophobe, 118
  pituitary. *See* Pituitary adenomas
Adenosine triphosphate (ATP), 18
Adrenoleukodystrophy, 77
Adverse drug reaction
  definition of, 178
  optic neuropathy from, 180–184, 181f
AIDS (acquired immunodeficiency syndrome), optic neuritis in, 77–78, 78f
AION. *See* Arteritic anterior ischemic optic neuropathy; Nonarteritic anterior ischemic optic neuropathy
Alcohol-induced toxic optic neuropathy, 182–183
Amiodarone-induced nonarteritic anterior ischemic optic neuropathy, 91–92, 183–184
Amsler grid screening, 27
Aneurysms. *See* Intracranial aneurysms
Animal model, of papilledema, 41, 42f
Annulus of Zinn, 9
Anterior clinoid process meningiomas, 125
Anterior communicating artery aneurysm, 133
Anterior ischemic optic neuropathy (AION)
  with giant cell arteritis. *See* Arteritic Anterior ischemic optic neuropathy
  without systemic arteritis. *See* Nonarteritic anterior ischemic optic neuropathy

Anterior visual pathway compression, 104t. *See also* Compressive optic neuropathy
Antibiotics, toxic optic neuropathy from, 180–181, 181f
Anticardiolipin antibodies, 79–80
Antifreeze ingestion, ethylene glycol poisoning from, 180
Apoptosis, postsynaptic intracellular pathways, 199, 200f
Arcuate optic nerve fiber bundles, 6, 12, 13f
ARRON (autoimmune-related retinopathy and optic neuropathy syndrome), 221–222
Arteriosclerosis, posterior ischemic optic neuropathy and, 96
Arteritic anterior ischemic optic neuropathy
  causes of, 93
  clinical features, 85, 94, 94f
  giant cell arteritis and, 94
  serologic markers, 94
  treatment, 94–95
  vs. NAION, 95t
  vs. nonarteritic anterior ischemic optic neuropathy, 94, 95t
Astrocytes, in lamina choroidalis, 6, 6f
Astrocytic hamartoma, 163, 164f
Ataxia and deafness, with hereditary optic atrophy, 170t
ATP (adenosine triphosphate), 18
Autoimmune disease, with optic neuritis, 79–80
Autoimmune-related retinopathy and optic neuropathy syndrome (ARRON), 221–222

Autoregulation, 14–15
Avonex (interferon beta-1a), for multiple
    sclerosis prevention, 73
Axonal transport
    anterograde or orthograde, 16–17, 17f, 18f,
        19
    fast, 17–18
    in glaucoma, 18–19
    retrograde, 16, 17, 19
    slow, 17

"Band or bowtie" optic atrophy
    in compressive optic neuropathy, 106, 108f
    in hemioptic hypoplasia, 160, 160f
BCNU (carmustine) neurotoxicity, 182
B$_{12}$ deficiency. See Vitamin B$_{12}$ deficiency
BDNF (brain-derived neurotrophic factor), 19
Behr's syndrome, 167, 170t
Bilateral optic nerve hypoplasia (BONH), 157,
        158f
Biopsy
    of chiasmal glioma, 114–115
    of optic nerve or chiasmal mass, 113
    temporal artery, for giant cell arteritis, 95
Bitemporal hemianopia, 119
"Blackouts," in papilledema, 47
Blindness
    in meningeal carcinomatosis, 213
    rapid, in papilledema, 48
Blind spot enlargement, in papilledema, 48
BONH (bilateral optic nerve hypoplasia), 157,
        158f
Borrellia burgdorferi antibody titer, 78
"Bowtie or band" optic atrophy
    in compressive optic neuropathy, 106, 108f
    in hemioptic hypoplasia, 160, 160f
Brain-derived neurotrophic factor (BDNF),
        19
Brightness comparison, evaluation of, 27–28
Bromocriptine, for prolactinoma, 121
B-scan echography, 31

Carbergoline, for prolactinoma, 121
Carbon monoxide poisoning, 180
Carboplatin neurotoxicity, 182
Carcinomatous optic neuropathy
    causes, 213, 214f, 215f
    clinical signs, 214, 215f
    diagnosis, 214–216, 215f
    treatment, 215–216
    visual loss, 213–214
Carmustine (BCNU) neurotoxicity, 182
Carotid-opthalmic artery aneurysm, 103
Carotid-paraophthalmic artery aneurysms, 131,
        132f
Cataract extraction, postoperative nonarteritic
    anterior ischemic optic neuropathy, 91
CCNU (lomustine) neurotoxicity, 182
Central cup obliteration, in chronic
    papilledema, 46, 48f

Cerebral angiography, of intracranial
    aneurysms, 133–135, 134f, 135f
Cerebral venous sinuses
    anatomy, normal, 55f
    obstruction or thrombosis, papilledema from,
        53, 54, 55f
Cerebrospinal fluid
    absorption rate reduction, papilledema from,
        53, 55f
    cytology, in carcinomatous optic neuropathy,
        215
    diversion, in chronic papilledema, abrupt
        vision loss from, 50
"Champagne cork" appearance, in chronic
        papilledema, 46, 48f
CHAMPS (Controlled High-Risk Subjects
        Avonex MS Prevention study) trial, 73
Charcot-Marie-Tooth disease, with hereditary
        optic atrophy, 170t
CHARGE syndrome, 160
Chemotherapeutic agents, neurotoxicity of, 182
Chemotherapy
    for chiasmal glioma, 116
    for craniopharyngioma, 118
    for meningiomas, 126–127
Chiasm. See Optic chiasm
Chiasmal neuritis, 75, 75f
Children, optic neuritis in, 73–74
Choroid plexus tumors, 54
Chromophobe adenomas, 118
Cialis (tadalafil), nonarteritic anterior ischemic
    optic neuropathy and, 92, 183
Cilioretinal arteries, 14, 14f
Circle of Willis, saccular aneurysms in, 131,
        131f–132f
Circle of Zinn-Haller, 14
Circumferential retinal folds (Paton's lines), in
        fully-developed papilledema, 43, 47f
Cisplatin neurotoxicity, 182
Clioquinol-induced optic neuropathy, 181
Collagen, in lamina cribrosa, 7
Colobomas, 160, 161f
Color desaturation, 27
Color Doppler imaging, 31, 32f
Color vision
    deficits
        in compressive optic neuropathy, 110t
        in nonarteritic anterior ischemic optic
            neuropathy, 87
        in optic neuritis, 66
        in pituitary adenomas, 119
    testing, 27
Compressive optic neuropathy
    causes, 101, 104t
        chiasmal glioma and, 111–112, 113–116,
            115f
        craniopharyngioma, 116–118, 118f
        intracranial aneurysm. See Intracranial
            aneurysms
        meningiomas. See Meningiomas

optic nerve glioma and, 111–113, 112f, 114f
pituitary adenoma, 118–122, 119f, 120f
thyroid-associated orbitopathy. *See*
  Thyroid-associated orbitopathy
patient evaluation, 111
physical examination, 111
signs of, 105–106, 198, 107f–109f, 110t
symptoms, 101–105, 104f, 105f
Computed tomography (CT)
of compressive optic neuropathy, 104f, 111
of meningiomas, 125, 125f
of optic disc drusen, 33, 33f
for optic nerve glioma, 112
of optic nerve sheath meningioma, 125f 128
of optic neuritis, 69–70, 70f
of radiation optic neuropathy, 210
vs. magnetic resonance imaging, 31, 112
Computed tomography angiography (CTA),
  intracranial aneurysms, 134–135, 134f
Congenital deafness, with hereditary optic
  atrophy, 170t
Connective tissue disorders, 96
Contrast sensitivity thresholds, 28–29
Corticosteroids
for giant cell arteritis, 94–95
for indirect optic nerve injury, 203
for optic neuritis, 72, 73
for thyroid-associated orbitopathy, 140
Cotton-wool spots, in papilledema, 43, 44f–45f, 47f
Cranial surgery for chronic papilledema, abrupt
  vision loss from, 50
Craniopharyngioma
clinical features, 116, 118f
compressive optic neuropathy and, 103
diagnosis, clinical example of, 36–37, 38f
histopathology, 116–117
incidence/prevalence, 116
management, 117–118
neuroradiologic criteria for, 116, 118f
pathophysiology, 116, 117f
C-reactive protein (CRP), in giant cell arteritis, 94
CT. *See* Computed tomography
CTA (computed tomography angiography),
  intracranial aneurysms, 134–135, 134f
Cup-to-disc ratio, nonarteritic anterior ischemic
  optic neuropathy risk and, 86
CVST (cerebral venous sinus thrombosis),
  papilledema from, 53, 54, 55f
Cyclosporine neurotoxicity, 181
Cytoskeleton, anterograde axonal transport and,
  16, 17f, 18f

Decompression
for indirect optic nerve injury, 201–203, 202t
of optic nerve sheath
  for nonarteritic anterior ischemic optic
    neuropathy, 89
  for papilledema, 60, 61f, 62f
transethmoidal of canalicular portion of optic
  nerve, 193–194

Deferoxamine-induced optic neuropathy, 182
DeMorsier's syndrome, 159
Demyelinating disorders
differentiation, from optic neuritis, 76
multiple sclerosis. *See* Multiple sclerosis
Developmental optic nerve disorders, 151–
  165
anomalous elevation of optic nerve. *See*
  Pseudopapilledema
astrocytic hamartoma, 163, 164f
colobomas, 160, 161f
hemioptic hypoplasia, 159–160, 160f
melanocytoma, 164, 165f
morning-glory syndrome, 161, 163, 164f
optic nerve hypoplasia, 156–157, 159, 157f–
  159f
optic pits, 160, 161f
superior segmental optic hypoplasia, 159,
  159f
tilted discs, 161, 162f, 163f
Devic's disease (neuromyelitis optica), 74
Diabetes mellitus. *See also* Diabetic papillopathy
with deafness and hereditary optic atrophy,
  170t
nonarteritic anterior ischemic optic
  neuropathy risk and, 86–87
Diabetic papillopathy
diagnosis, 217
nonarteritic anterior ischemic optic
  neuropathy and, 93
optic disc edema in, 216, 217f
pathophysiology, 217
treatment, 217–218
visual prognosis, 217
Diaphragma sellae meningiomas, 125
DIDMOAD (Wolfram's syndrome), 167, 170t
Diplopia
in compressive optic neuropathy, 105
in papilledema, 49
Disulfiram-induced optic neuropathy, 182
Dominant optic atrophy, 165–166, 166f
"Double-ring sign," 156, 158f
Drugs. *See also specific drugs*
adverse reactions
  definition of, 178
  optic neuropathy from, 180–184, 181f
Drusen
diagnosis, clinical tests for, 33–34, 33f
in pseudopapilledema, 153, 155–156, 155f,
  156f
symptoms of, 33–34
vs. early papilledema, 154t
Dynein, 18
Dyschromatopsia
acquired, 27
in compressive optic neuropathy, 106
in nonarteritic anterior ischemic optic
  neuropathy, 87
in optic neuritis, 66
in toxic optic neuropathy, 177

Elastin, in lamina cribrosa, 7, 8*f*
Electrophysiology, 30–31
Embolic occlusion, nonarteritic anterior
 ischemic optic neuropathy and, 89, 92,
 92*f*
Empty sella, 122, 123*f*
Endovascular embolization, of intracranial
 aneurysms, 136, 137*f*
Enophthalmos, in compressive optic neuropathy,
 106
En plaque meningioma, 123
Erythrocyte sedimentation rate (ESR), in giant
 cell arteritis, 94
Ethambutol-induced optic neuropathy, 180,
 181*f*
Ethylene glycol poisoning, 180
Evaluation, patient
 assessment of findings, 31–37, 33*f*, 35*f*–38*f*,
  31–38
 brightness comparison, 27–28
 color vision, 27
 in compressive optic neuropathy, 111
 contrast sensitivity testing, 28–29
 electrophysiology, 30–31
 history taking, 25–26
 imaging studies, 31, 32*f*
 nutritional optic neuropathy, 185–186
 ophthalmoscopy, 29–30
 in papilledema, 54, 56–57
 photostress recovery test, 28
 pupillary testing, 28
 toxic optic neuropathy, 184
 visual acuity, 26
 visual field testing, 26–27
Evulsion, optic nerve
 diagnosis, 192–193, 192*f*, 193*f*
 mechanisms of, 192
 total *vs.* partial, 191
Extraocular muscles
 enlargement, nonthyroid causes of, 139*t*
 movement abnormalities, in compressive optic
  neuropathy, 106
Exudates, in fully-developed papilledema, 43,
 45
Eyelid abnormalities
 in compressive optic neuropathy, 106
 in thyroid-associated orbitopathy, 136
Eye pain, in compressive optic neuropathy,
 105

Farnsworth-Munsell 100-hue test, 27
FK506 (tacrolimus) neurotoxicity, 181–182
Foster Kennedy syndrome
 clinical features, 50–51, 52*f*
 in compressive optic neuropathy, 108
Friedreich's ataxia, with hereditary optic
  atrophy, 170*t*
Functional visual loss, diagnosis of, 34, 37*f*
Funduscopy, in compressive optic neuropathy,
 110*t*

Fungal infections
 of optic nerve, 77–78, 78*f*
 posterior ischemic optic neuropathy and, 96

Ganglion cell axons, 11
Ganglion cells, 5, 16
Giant cell arteritis (GCA)
 with anterior ischemic optic neuropathy. *See*
  Arteritic anterior ischemic optic
  neuropathy
 arteritic anterior ischemic optic neuropathy
  in, 94, 94*f*
 clinical features, 94
 incidence/prevalence, 93
 pathogenesis, 93
 posterior ischemic optic neuropathy and, 96
 serologic markers, 94
 symptoms of, 26
 temporal artery biopsy, 95
 treatment, 94–95
Glaucoma
 axonal transport in, 18–19
 normal-tension, 222
 optic disc cupping in, 222–224, 224*f*
Glial cells, in nerve fiber layer, 4
Glioma
 chiasmal, 111–112, 113–116, 115*f*
  clinical features, 113–114, 115*f*
  management, 114–116, 115*f*
  natural history, 114
  neurofibromatosis type 1 and, 111–112
 optic nerve, 111–113, 112*f*, 114*f*
  of adulthood, 103
  clinical features, 112–113, 112*f*
  histopathology, 113
  juvenile, 103
  management, 113
  natural history, 113
  neurofibromatosis type 1 and, 111–112
  terminology, 111
"Glue sniffing," optic neuropathy from, 180
Goldmann perimetry, 27
"Grayouts," in papilledema, 47
Growth hormone-secreting tumors, 120. *See
 also* Pituitary adenomas
 treatment, 122

Hamartomas, astrocytic, 163, 164*f*
Hardy-Rand-Rittler test (HRR), 27
Headache
 in compressive optic neuropathy, 105
 in intracranial hypertension, Valsalva's
  maneuver and, 52, 58
 in papilledema, 52
Hemioptic hypoplasia, 159–160, 160*f*
Hemiparesis, in papilledema, 52
Hemisensory deficits, in papilledema, 52
Hemorrhage
 flame-shaped or cotton-wool spots, 43, 44*f*–
  45*f*, 47*f*

in fully-developed papilledema, 43, 45, 47*f*
intratumoral, in pituitary adenoma, 120,
    120*f*
posterior indirect optic nerve injury and, 198–
    199
Hereditary optic neuropathies, 165–171
    dominant optic atrophy, 165–166
    Leber's hereditary optic neuropathy, 167–169,
        167*f*, 168*f*
    metabolic disease and, 170, 171*t*
    neurologic syndromes, 169, 170*t*
    recessive optic atrophy, 166–167
Herpes zoster ophthalmicus, 96
History taking, 25–26
Holographic interferometry, 199
HRR (Hardy-Rand-Rittler test), 27
Humphrey automated bowl perimetry
    description of, 27
    in optic neuritis, 67, 68*f*
Hyaline bodies. *See* Drusen
Hyaloid remnants, in pseudopapilledema, 152, 153*f*
Hydrocephalus
    in carcinomatous optic neuropathy, 215
    in chiasmal glioma, 114
    communicating, 53
    noncommunicating, 53
    papilledema from, 53, 54*f*
Hydroquinolones, halogenated, 181
Hypercholesterolemia, nonarteritic anterior
        ischemic optic neuropathy risk and, 86–87
Hyperopia, in pseudopapilledema, 153
Hyperostosis, 123
Hypertension
    intracranial. *See* Intracranial hypertension
    nonarteritic anterior ischemic optic
        neuropathy risk and, 86–87
Hypoplasia, optic nerve
    bilateral, 157, 158*f*
    magnetic resonance imaging, 157, 159, 158*f*
    ophthalmoscopic features, 156–157, 157*f*, 158*f*
Hypotension, nonarteritic anterior ischemic
        optic neuropathy and, 92
Hypothalamus, chiasmal glioma in, 114, 115*f*

ICP. *See* Intracranial pressure
Idiopathic intracranial hypertension (IIH)
    associated disorders, 58, 58*t*–59*t*
    benign, 59
    diagnostic criteria, 57–58, 58*t*
    recurrences, 59
    treatment, 56*f*–57*f*, 59–60
Immunomodulator-induced optic neuropathy,
    181–182
Immunosuppressant-induced optic neuropathy,
    181–182
Infectious agents, causing optic neuritis, 76–78, 78*f*
Inferonasal fiber projections, 12
Infliximab, optic neuropathy and, 183
Interferon beta-1a (Avonex), for multiple
    sclerosis prevention, 73

International Optic Nerve Trauma Study
    (IONTS), 203
Intracanalicular nerve, 10
Intracranial aneurysms
    asymptomatic, 130–131
    categories, 129
    clinical features, 131, 133, 132*f*, 133*f*
    fusiform, 130
    incidence, 130
    management, 135–136, 136*f*, 137*f*
    mortality, 130
    mycotic, 130
    neuroimaging, 133–135, 134*f*, 135*f*
    saccular, 130, 131*f*–132*f*
    size, 130
    symptomatic, 131
Intracranial hypertension
    headache from, 52
    idiopathic, papilledema from, 54, 56*f*–57*f*,
        57
Intracranial pressure (ICP)
    elevation, with optic disc swelling. *See*
        Papilledema
    increased, mechanisms of, 53–54, 53*f*–55*f*
    lowering, for papilledema management, 60,
        61*f*, 62*f*
Intraocular inflammation, optic neuritis and,
    7878
Intraocular pressure (IOP)
    changes, 4
    elevated, laminar beam movement and, 8, 8*f*
    elevation, axonal transport and, 18
Intrapapillary refractile bodies, in optic nerve
        sheath meningioma, 128
Intrasellar meningiomas, 125
Intraventricular tumor, papilledema from, 53,
    53*f*
IONDT (Ischemic Optic Neuropathy
    Decompression Trial), 86, 87, 89–90
IONTS (International Optic Nerve Trauma
    Study), 203
IOP. *See* Intraocular pressure
Ischemic optic neuropathy
    arteritic anterior, 93–95, 94*f*, 95*t*
    associated conditions, 86*t*
    classification of, 85
    nonarteritic anterior. *See* Nonarteritic anterior
        ischemic optic neuropathy
    posterior, 95–96
Ischemic Optic Neuropathy Decompression
    Trial (IONDT), 86, 87, 89–90
Ishihara test, 277

Junctional syndrome, 119
Juxtapapillary choroidal melanoma, 164, 165*f*

Kinesin, anterograde axonal transport and, 18

Lamina choroidalis, 6, 6*f*, 14
Lamina cribrosa (lamina scleralis), 7–8, 8*f*

Leber's hereditary optic neuropathy (LHON)
  associated systemic features, 167–168
  clinical features, 167
  diagnosis, ophthalmoscopic, 167, 167f
  mimicking of optic neuritis, 81
  mitochondrial DNA mutations in, 168–169,
    168f
  pathogenesis, 168–169, 168f
  prognosis, 169
Leber's idiopathic stellate neuroretinitis, 211
Leptomeningeal metastases, compressive optic
    neuropathy from, 103, 105f, 111
Leukemic optic neuropathy, 213, 214f
LHON. See Leber's hereditary optic neuropathy
Lipidoses, hereditary optic neuropathies and,
    171t
Luminance (magnocellular) pathway, 16
Lyme disease, 78
Lymphoma, optic neuropathy of, 213, 214f
Lysosomal storage diseases, hereditary optic
    neuropathies and, 170, 171t

Macula
  nerve fibers, 11
  pigmentary disturbances, following
    papilledema resolution, 47, 51f
Macular disease, differentiation from optic
    neuropathy, photostress recovery test for,
    28
Macular star, 78, 80f
Magnetic resonance angiography (MRA),
    intracranial aneurysms, 134–135, 134f
Magnetic resonance imaging (MRI)
  of compressive optic neuropathy, 105f, 109f,
    111, 111f
  of intracranial aneurysms, 133–135, 134f
  of meningiomas, 125–126, 126f
  of optic nerve glioma, 112, 112f
  of optic nerve sheath meningioma, 109f,
    128
  of optic neuritis, 69–70, 70f
  of optic neuritis, multiple sclerosis prediction
    and, 72
  of optic perineuritis, 220, 220f
  with orbital with fat suppression, 109f, 111
  of papilledema, 54, 55f, 56f
  of pituitary adenomas, 119f, 120f, 121
  of posterior pituitary ectopia, with bilateral
    optic nerve hypoplasia, 157, 158f
  of radiation optic neuropathy, 210, 210f
  vs. computed tomography, 31, 112
Magnetic resonance venography (MRV), of
    papilledema, 54
Magnocellular (luminance) pathway, 16
MAP1C (microtubule-associated protein 1C),
    18
Marie's hereditary ataxia with hereditary optic
    atrophy, 170t
Medication-induced toxic optic neuropathy,
    180–184, 181f

Medications. See specific medications
Melanocytoma, 164, 165f
Meningeal carcinomatosis, 213
Meningioma
  intrasellar, 125
  optic nerve sheath. See Optic nerve sheath
    meningioma
  suprasellar
    clinical features, 123–125, 124f
    histologic patterns, 123
    incidence/prevalence, 122–123
    locations, 122–125, 124f
    management, 126–127, 127f
    neuroimaging, 125–126, 125f, 126f
Metabolic disease, hereditary optic neuropathies
    and, 170, 171t
Methanol toxicity, optic neuropathy from, 178–
    180, 179f
Methyl-CCNU (semustine) neurotoxicity, 182
Methylprednisolone
  for giant cell arteritis, 94–95
  for indirect optic nerve injury, 202–203
  for optic neuritis, 72, 73
Microtubule-associated protein 1C (MAP1C),
    18
Microtubules, 16, 17, 18f
Migraine, ischemic optic neuropathy and, 93
Monocular visual deficit, 25–26
Morning-glory syndrome, 161, 163, 164f
Motility defects, in pituitary adenomas, 119–
    120
MRA (magnetic resonance angiography),
    intracranial aneurysms, 134–135, 134f
MRI. See Magnetic resonance imaging
Mucocele, 102, 104f
Mucopolysaccharidoses, hereditary optic
    neuropathies and, 171t
Multiple sclerosis
  CHAMPS trial, 73
  optic neuritis in, 70–71, 71f
  prevention, CHAMPS trial and, 73
  risk prediction, cranial MRI and, 72
  vision loss in, 66

NAION. See Nonarteritic anterior ischemic
    optic neuropathy
Nausea, in papilledema, 52
Nerve fiber bundles, traversing optic nerves and
    chiasm, 12, 13f
Nerve fiber layer, of optic nerve head, 4–6, 4f
  papillomacular fibers, 5, 5f
  thickness of, 4–5
  topographical zones, 5
Neuritis
  optic. See Optic neuritis
  perioptic. See Optic perineuritis
Neurofibromatosis
  history, compressive optic neuropathy and,
    105
  type 1, gliomas and, 111–112

Neurofilaments, 16, 17, 18*f*

Neuroimaging. *See also* Computed tomography; Magnetic resonance imaging
  abnormalities, in optic neuritis, 69–70, 70*f*
  of compressive optic neuropathy, 111

Neurologic diseases, with hereditary optic atrophy, 169, 170*t*

Neuromyelitis optica (Devic's disease), 74

Neuroretinitis
  causes, 212*t*
  idiopathic or Leber's idiopathic stellate, 211–212
  macular star and, 78, 80*f*
  serologic tests, 212
  treatment, 213

Neutral density filters (NDF), to quantify RAPD, 28, 29*f*

NMO (neuromyelitis optica; Devic's disease), 74

Nonarteritic anterior ischemic optic neuropathy (NAION)
  age of incidence, 90
  amiodarone-induced, 91–92, 183–184
  atypical features, 90
  clinical characteristics, 87–89, 87*f*, 88*f*
  clinical example, 90
  differential diagnosis, 81, 90
  drug-induced, 183
  idiopathic, 86
  incidence of, 86
  pathophysiology, 85–86
  progressive, 89
  recurrent, 89
  risk factors, 86–87
  secondary, causes of, 91–93
  sequential, 89
  treatment, 89–90
  visual acuity, outcome, 89
  visual field defects, 90
  vs. arteritic anterior ischemic optic neuropathy, 95*t*

Nonglaucomatous optic disc cupping, 222–224, 224*f*

Normal-tension glaucoma, 222

Null-cell tumor, 118

Nutritional optic neuropathies
  clinical presentation, 185, 185*f*
  differential diagnosis, 185–186
  etiology, 186
  pathology, 186, 186*f*, 187*f*
  patient evaluation/workup, 185–186
  treatment, 186

Nystagmus, in chiasmal glioma, 114

Occipital lobe lesions, bilateral, 184

Ocular motility disturbances, in papilledema, 52

Olfactory groove meningioma, 105, 124–125

Oncocytoma, 118

ONSM. *See* Optic nerve sheath meningioma

ONTT (Optic Neuritis Treatment Trial), 67, 71–73, 76

Ophthalmic artery
  anatomy, 12, 14, 14*f*
  aneurysm, 131

Ophthalmoscopy
  description of, 29–30
  in glaucomatous *vs.* nonglaucomatous optic disc cupping, 223, 224*f*
  of papilledema, 42–43, 42*f*
    early, findings in, 43, 45*f*, 46*f*
    retinal nerve fiber layer in, 43, 44*f*–45*f*

OPN. *See* Optic perineuritis

Optic atrophy
  "band or bowtie"
    in compressive optic neuropathy, 106, 108*f*
    in hemioptic hypoplasia, 160, 160*f*
  in compressive optic neuropathy, 106, 107*f*
  diagnosis of, 34, 36*f*
  dominant, 165–166, 166*f*
  in Foster Kennedy syndrome, 50–51, 52*f*
  hereditary, 169, 170*t*
  postpapilledema, 46–47, 49*f*, 50*f*
  recessive, 166–167

Optic canal
  fractures, optic nerve injury from, 197–198, 198*f*, 199
  meningioma of, 125

Optic chiasm
  anatomic rules of, 12
  lesions, causing optic atrophy, 110*t*
  magnetic resonance imaging of, 102*f*–103*f*
  neuritis, 75, 75*f*

Optic disc
  abnormalities
    in compressive optic neuropathy, 106, 108, 107*f*–109*f*
    in optic neuritis, 67, 69, 69*f*
  congenitally full, 151–152, 152*f*
  cupping
    glaucomatous, 222–224, 224*f*
    neurologic cause, signs of, 223
    nonglaucomatous, 222–224, 224*f*
  drusen. *See* Drusen
  edema
    in compressive optic neuropathy, 106, 109*f*
    in diabetes, 216, 217*f*
    in papillophlebitis, 218, 218*f*
    vs. papilledema, 41
  pallor
    in hemioptic hypoplasia, 160, 160*f*
    in NAION, 88, 88*f*
    in optic nerve sheath meningioma, 128
  size, NAION risk and, 86
  swelling
    causes of, 19
    with elevated intracranial pressure. *See* Papilledema

Optic disc (*continued*)
    in nonarteritic anterior ischemic optic
      neuropathy, 87–89, 88*f*
    in optic nerve sheath meningioma, 128
    with optic neuritis. *See* Papillitis
  tilted, 161, 162*f*, 163*f*
Optic nerve. *See also specific optic nerve
    disorders*
  anatomy, 3–4
    of intracanalicular segment, 10, 10*f*
    of intracranial segment, 10–11, 11*f*
    of intraocular segment, 4–8, 4*f*–6*f*, 8*f*, 9*f*
    of intraorbital segment, 8–10
    magnetic resonance of, 102*f*–103*f*
  anomalous elevation. *See* Pseudopapilledema
  axonal physiology, 16–19, 17*f*
  blood supply, 12, 14–16, 15*f*
  energy demands, 16
  enlargement, in optic nerve sheath
    meningioma, 128, 129*f*
  evulsion. *See* Evulsion, optic nerve
  functional tests. *See* Testing, clinical
  glioma. *See* Glioma, optic nerve
  hypoplasia. *See* Hypoplasia, optic nerve
  inflammation. *See* Optic neuritis
  injury. *See* Optic nerve injury
  intracanalicular segment
    anatomy of, 10, 10*f*, 195–196
    blood supply of, 15–16
  intracranial segment, 10–11, 11*f*, 16
  intraocular segment
    anatomy of, 4–8, 4*f*–6*f*, 8*f*, 9*f*
    blood supply of, 12, 14–15, 14*f*
  intraorbital segment, 8–10, 15, 15*f*
  lesions, causing optic atrophy, 110*t*
  topographical organization of, 11–12, 13*f*
  trauma. *See* Optic nerve injury
Optic nerve head
  capillaries of, 14–15
  lamina choroidalis, 6, 6*f*
  lamina cribrosa or lamina scleralis, 7–8, 8*f*
  nerve fiber layer of, 4–6, 4*f*
Optic nerve injury
  direct, 193–195, 194*f*, 195*t*
  indirect, 195–203
    anatomic considerations, 195–196
    anterior, 196–197
    clinical features, 197–198, 198*f*
    nonsurgical management, 200–201, 201*t*
    pathophysiology, 198–199, 200*f*
    posterior, 197
    surgical management, 201–203, 202*t*
    visual prognosis, 203
Optic nerve sheath decompression. *See*
    Decompression, of optic nerve sheath
Optic nerve sheath meningioma (ONSM)
  clinical features, 127–128
  differential diagnosis, 81
  management, 128–129

neuroimaging, 109*f*, 125*f*, 128, 129*f*
optic disc edema from, 106, 109*f*
Optic neuritis, 65–81
  causes of, 76–78, 77*t*, 78*f*
  chiasmal, 75, 75*f*
  in children, 73–74
  clinical features, 65–67, 69–70, 66*f*–69*f*
    neuroimaging abnormalities, 69–70, 70*f*
    optic disc abnormalities, 67, 69, 69*f*
    Uhthoff's symptom, 67
    visual evoked response abnormalities, 67,
      69, 69*f*
  collaborative studies
    CHAMPS, 73
    Optic Neuritis Treatment Trial, 67, 71–
      73
  diagnosis, 65, 81
    clinical example of, 35–36, 38*f*
    criteria for, 76
  differential diagnosis, 76–80, 78*f*–80*f*
    from mimickers, 81
    NAION and, 90
    optic perineuritis and, 221, 222*t*
  infectious agents, 76–78, 78*f*
  in multiple sclerosis, 70–71, 71*f*
  neuromyelitis optica or Devic's disease, 74
  optic tract, 76, 75*f*
  positive visual phenomena in, 66
  retrobulbar, 65
  symptoms, 26, 65–66, 66*f*
  terminology, 65
Optic Neuritis Treatment Trial (ONTT), 67,
    71–73, 76
Optic neuropathy
  from adverse drug reactions. *See* Toxic optic
    neuropathy
  anterior ischemic
    with giant cell arteritis. *See* Arteritic
      Anterior ischemic optic neuropathy
    without systemic arteritis. *See* Nonarteritic
      anterior ischemic optic neuropathy
  autoimmune-related retinopathy and optic
    neuropathy syndrome, 221–222
  carcinomatous, 213–216, 214*f*, 215*f*
  compressive. *See* Compressive optic
    neuropathy
  diabetic papillopathy, 216–218, 217*f*
  differentiation from macular disease,
    photostress recovery test for, 28
  infiltrative, 103
  inflammatory, with secondary retinal changes.
    See Neuroretinitis
  neuroretinitis, 211–213, 212*t*, 213*f*
  nonglaucomatous optic disc cupping, 222–
    224, 224*f*
  optic perineuritis, 219–221, 220*f*
  papillophlebitis, 218–219
  radiation-induced, 209–211, 210*f*
  toxin-induced. *See* Toxic optic neuropathy

Optic perineuritis (OPN)
  causes, 78, 219
  clinical features, 78, 79f, 219–220
  differential diagnosis, 221, 222t
  neuroimaging, 220, 220f
  treatment, 221
Optic pits, 160, 161f
Optic tract
  anatomy, 102f–103f
  lesions, causing optic atrophy, 110t
  neuritis, 76, 75f
Optociliary shunt vessels
  in compressive optic neuropathy, 106, 109f
  diagnosis of, 34, 35f
Orbit
  anatomy of, 102f
  decompression surgery, for thyroid-associated
      orbitopathy, 138f–139f, 140
  signs, in compressive optic neuropathy, 106
Orbital apex, anatomy of, 102f

Papilledema, 41–62
  associated clinical features, 47–49, 51f, 52f
  associated disorders, 58, 58t–59t
  axoplasmic flow obstruction and, 19
  causes, 53–54, 53f–55f, 56t
  classification
    chronic, 46, 48f, 49f
    early, 43, 45f, 46f
    fully-developed, 43, 45, 46f, 47f
    postpapilledema optic atrophy, 46–47, 49f,
        50f
  in compressive optic neuropathy, 106
  definition of, 41
  early, vs. optic disc drusen, 154t
  in Foster Kennedy syndrome, 50–51, 52f
  in idiopathic intracranial hypertension, 57–
      60
  management, 60, 61f, 62f
  pathogenesis
    animal model of, 41, 42f
    ophthalmoscopic findings and, 42–43, 42f
  patient evaluation, 54, 56–57, 55f–57f
  symptoms
    neurologic, 52
    retinal nerve fiber layer elevation, 43, 44f
    visual, 47
  visual prognosis, 49–50
  vs. optic disc edema, 41
Papillitis, 65
Papillophlebitis, 218–219, 218f
Paraclinoid arteriovenous malformation, 135f
Paraophthalmic aneurysm, 137f
Parvocellular pathway, 16
Paton's lines (circumferential retinal folds), in
      fully-developed papilledema, 43, 47f
PAX2 gene mutations, 160
Perchloroethylene vapor inhalation, optic
      neuropathy from, 180

Pericytes, 15
Perioperative posterior ischemic optic
      neuropathy, 96
Periopic neuritis. See Optic perineuritis
Peripapillary capillaries, 14, 14f
Peripapillary nerve fiber layer opacification, in
      papilledema, 43, 45f
Phosphenes (positive visual phenomena), in
      optic neuritis, 66
Photophobia, in pituitary adenomas, 119
Photostress recovery test, 28
Pia mater, 9
Pial plexus, 16
PION (posterior ischemic optic neuropathy),
      95–96
Pituitary adenomas
  clinical features, 118–121, 120f
    endocrine signs, 120–121
    visual signs, 119–120
  management, 121–122
    adverse outcomes, 122, 123f
  neuroimaging, 119f, 120f, 121
Pituitary apoplexy, 102
Pituitary gland
  dysfunction, in compressive optic neuropathy,
      105
  embryology, 116, 117f
Planum sphenoidale, meningiomas of, 124–125
Platelet count, in giant cell arteritis, 94
Pneumosinus dilatans, 123
Polyarteritis nodosa, 96
Postcataract extraction, nonarteritic anterior
      ischemic optic neuropathy and, 91
Posterior ischemic optic neuropathy (PION),
      95–96
Postpapilledema optic atrophy, 46–47, 49f, 50f
Postvaccination optic neuritis, 77
Postviral syndrome, optic neuritis in, 77
Prednisone, oral, for optic neuritis, 72
Pregnancy, meningiomas in, 123
Prolactinoma, treatment, 121
Prolactin-secreting tumors, 120. See also
      Pituitary adenomas
Proptosis, in compressive optic neuropathy, 106
Protein synthesis, in axon, 18
Pseudodrusen, in chronic papilledema, 46, 48f
Pseudo-Foster Kennedy syndrome, 51, 108
Pseudoglaucoma, 222–223
Pseudoisochromatic color-plate tests, 27
Pseudopapilledema, ophthalmoscopic features,
      151–152, 152f, 152t
  congenitally full optic discs, 151, 152f
  hyaline bodies or drusen, 153, 155–156, 155f,
      156f
  hyaloid remnants, 152, 153f
  myelinated retinal nerve fibers, 152–153,
      153f
Pseudotumor cerebri, 57
Pulfrich's phenomenon, 66, 66f

Pupillary function testing
    in compressive optic neuropathy, 110*t*
    methods of, 28, 29*f*
    in optic neuritis, 66
    in papilledema, 49
Pupillography, 30

Radiation optic neuropathy (RON), 209–211,
    210*f*
Radiotherapy
    for chiasmal glioma, 115–116
    for craniopharyngioma, 118
    for meningiomas, 127, 127*f*
    for optic nerve sheath meningioma, 129
    for thyroid-associated orbitopathy, 140
RAPD. *See* Relative afferent pupillary defect
Recessive optic atrophy, 166–167
Relative afferent pupillary defect (RAPD)
    in compressive optic neuropathy, 106
    detection of, 28, 29*f*
    in pituitary adenomas, 119
    quantification of, 28, 30*f*
Retinal folds, circumferential, in fully-developed
    papilledema, 43, 47*f*
Retinal nerve fiber layer
    decreased thickness, in compressive optic
        neuropathy, 106, 107*f*
    elevation, in papilledema, 43, 44*f*–45*f*, 47*f*
    myelination, in pseudopapilledema, 152–153,
        153*f*
Retinal vasculitis, 218. *See also* Papillophlebitis
Retropulsion defect, in compressive optic
    neuropathy, 106
RON (radiation optic neuropathy), 209–211,
    210*f*
Russell's diencephalic syndrome, 114, 115

Sarcoidosis, with optic neuritis, 78–79, 80*f*
Sedimentation rate, in giant cell arteritis, 94
Seizures, in papilledema, 52
Sella, anatomy of, 102*f*–103*f*
Semustine (methyl-CCNU) neurotoxicity, 182
Serologic tests
    for arteritic anterior ischemic optic
        neuropathy, 94
    for neuroretinitis, 212
Sildenafil (Viagra)
    nonarteritic anterior ischemic optic
        neuropathy and, 92
    optic neuropathy and, 183
SMON (subacute myelo-optic neuropathy), 181
Snellen acuity, 26
Solvent toxicity, optic neuropathy from, 180
Sphenoid, lesser and greater wings,
    meningiomas of, 125
Spontaneous retinal venous pulsations, absence,
    in early papilledema, 43
Stellate maculopathy, 211
Stereopsis loss, in pituitary adenomas, 119
Styrene toxicity, optic neuropathy from, 180

Subacute myelo-optic neuropathy (SMON), 181
Subarachnoid hemorrhage, Terson syndrome
    from, 133, 133*f*
Superior segmental optic hypoplasia, 159, 159*f*
Supraclinoid cartoid artery aneurysm, 133
Surgery
    for chiasmal glioma, 114–115
    for craniopharyngioma, 117–118
    for decompression. *See* Decompression
    for intracranial aneurysms, 135–136, 136*f*
    for meningiomas, 127
    for papilledema, 60, 61*f*, 62*f*
Swinging-flashlight test
    description of, 28, 29*f*, 30*f*
    in papilledema, 66
Syphilis, optic perineuritis and, 78, 79*f*
Systemic disease, with optic neuritis, 78–79, 80*f*
Systemic lupus erythematosus, 96

TAB (temporal artery biopsy), for giant cell
    arteritis, 95
Tacrolimus (FK506) neurotoxicity, 181–182
Tadalafil (Cialis), nonarteritic anterior ischemic
    optic neuropathy and, 92, 183
TAO. *See* Thyroid-associated orbitopathy
Temporal artery biopsy (TAB), for giant cell
    arteritis, 95
Terson syndrome, 133, 133*f*
Testing, clinical
    assessment of findings, 31–37, 33*f*, 35*f*–38*f*
    for brightness comparison, 27–28
    for color vision, 27
    for contrast sensitivity, 28–29
    electrophysiologic, 30–31
    history taking and, 25–26
    imaging studies, 31, 32*f*
    ophthalmoscopy, 29–30
    for photostress recovery, 28
    pupillary, 28
    of visual acuity, 26
    of visual field, 26–27
"30-degree test," 31
Thyroid-associated orbitopathy (TAO)
    causes of, 136
    clinical features, 136–137, 138*f*–139*f*
    incidence, 136
    management, 137–138, 140, 138*f*–139*f*
Tilted optic discs, 161, 162*f*, 163*f*
Tobacco-induced toxic optic neuropathy, 182–183
Toluene toxicity, optic neuropathy from, 180
Toxic optic neuropathy, 177–185
    causality, criteria for, 178
    causes
        alcohol, 182–183
        carbon monoxide, 180
        ethylene glycol, 180
        medication-induced, 180–184, 181*f*
        methanol, 178–180, 179*f*
        solvents, 180
        tobacco, 182–183

clinical features, 177
clinical presentations, 178
differential diagnosis, 184
patient evaluation, 184
treatment, 184
Toxin, definition of, 178
Toxoplasmosis optic neuritis, macular star, 78, 80*f*
"Tram-track sign," 128
Transverse myelitis, with bilateral optic neuritis, 74
Traumatic optic neuropathy, 191–203
    from direct optic nerve injury, 193–195, 194*f*, 195*t*
    from optic nerve evulsion, 191–193, 192*f*, 193*f*
Tuberculum sellae, meningioma of, 124
Tubulin, 17

Uhthoff's symptom, in optic neuritis, 67
Ultrasonography
    of anterior optic nerve injury, 198
    supplemental, for CT and MRI studies, 31
Uremia, nonarteritic anterior ischemic optic neuropathy and, 93

Valsalva's maneuver, intracranial hypertension headache and, 52, 58
Vascular tone, 15
Vasospasm, of optic nerve vessels, 93
Venous sinus thrombosis, papilledema from, 53, 55*f*
VEP. *See* Visual evoked potential
VER. *See* Visual evoked response
Viagra. *See* Sildenafil
Vigabatrin-induced optic neuropathy, 182
Vincristine neurotoxicity, 182
Viral infections, causing optic neuritis, 76–77
Vision loss
    with associated symptoms, 26
    binocular, 25–26
    in carcinomatous optic neuropathy, 213–214
    in compressive optic neuropathy, 106
    from direct optic nerve injury, 193–194
    functional, diagnosis of, 34, 37*f*
    in nonarteritic anterior ischemic optic neuropathy, 87
    onset or tempo of, 26
    in optic nerve sheath meningioma, 127–128

in optic neuritis, 65–66, 66*f*
in papilledema, 47
in pituitary adenoma, 119–120
in radiation optic neuropathy, 209–210
subacute, causes of, 103, 105, 105*f*
in thyroid-associated orbitopathy, 136
in toxic optic neuropathy, 177
Visual acuity
    in compressive optic neuropathy, 110*t*
    in nonarteritic anterior ischemic optic neuropathy, 87
    in papilledema, 48
    in pituitary adenoma, 119
    testing methods, 26
    in toxic optic neuropathy, 177
Visual evoked potential (VEP)
    description of, 30
    diagnosis of functional visual loss, 34, 37*f*
Visual evoked response (VER)
    in indirect optic nerve injury, 197
    in optic neuritis, 67, 69, 69*f*
Visual field testing
    Amsler grid, 27
    bowl perimetry, 27
    of confrontation defects, 27
    defects
        arcuate and nasal "step," 6
        in chiasmal glioma, 114
        in compressive optic neuropathy, 110*t*
        in indirect optic nerve injury, 197
        in nonarteritic anterior ischemic optic neuropathy, 87, 87*f*
        in optic nerve disease, 26–27
        in optic neuritis, 67, 68*f*
        in papilledema, 48, 51*f*, 52*f*
        in tilted optic discs, 161, 163*f*
        in toxic optic neuropathy, 177
    methods, 26–27
Vitamin B$_{12}$ deficiency
    diagnosis, 185–186
    optic neuropathy and, 185, 185*f*, 186
    treatment, 186
Vomiting, in papilledema, 52

Wegener's granulomatosis, 96
Weight loss, compressive optic neuropathy and, 105
Wilbrand's knee, 12
Wolfram's syndrome (DIDMOAD), 167, 170*t*